OPHTHALMOLOGY
Oral and Practical

OPHTHALMOLOGY
Oral and Practical

As per the Competency Based Medical Education Curriculum (NMC)

Fifth Edition

Samar K Basak MD (AIIMS) DNB FRCS
Director and Founder Member
Disha Eye Hospitals
Kolkata, West Bengal, India
Email: basak_sk@hotmail.com

Soham Basak MS DNB FRCS
Consultant
Cataract, Cornea and External Disease
Disha Eye Hospitals
Kolkata, West Bengal, India
Email: sohambasak88@gmail.com

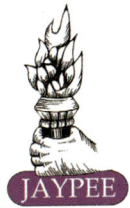

JAYPEE BROTHERS MEDICAL PUBLISHERS
The Health Sciences Publisher
New Delhi | London

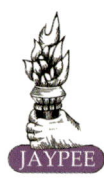 **Jaypee Brothers Medical Publishers (P) Ltd**

Headquarters
Jaypee Brothers Medical Publishers (P) Ltd
EMCA House
23/23-B, Ansari Road, Daryaganj
New Delhi - 110 002, India
Landline: +91-11-23272143, +91-11-23272703
+91-11-23282021, +91-11-23245672
Email: jaypee@jaypeebrothers.com

Corporate Office
Jaypee Brothers Medical Publishers (P) Ltd
4838/24, Ansari Road, Daryaganj
New Delhi 110 002, India
Phone: +91-11-43574357
Fax: +91-11-43574314
Email: jaypee@jaypeebrothers.com

Overseas Office
J.P. Medical Ltd
83 Victoria Street, London
SW1H 0HW (UK)
Phone: +44 20 3170 8910
Fax: +44 (0)20 3008 6180
Email: info@jpmedpub.com

Website: www.jaypeebrothers.com
Website: www.jaypeedigital.com

© 2022, Jaypee Brothers Medical Publishers (P) Ltd

The views and opinions expressed in this book are solely those of the original contributor(s)/author(s) and do not necessarily represent those of editor(s) and publisher of the book.

All rights reserved. No part of this publication may be reproduced, stored or transmitted in any form or by any means, electronic, mechanical, photocopying, recording or otherwise, without the prior permission in writing of the publishers.

All brand names and product names used in this book are trade names, service marks, trademarks or registered trademarks of their respective owners. The publisher is not associated with any product or vendor mentioned in this book.

Medical knowledge and practice change constantly. This book is designed to provide accurate, authoritative information about the subject matter in question. However, readers are advised to check the most current information available on procedures included and check information from the manufacturer of each product to be administered, to verify the recommended dose, formula, method and duration of administration, adverse effects and contraindications. It is the responsibility of the practitioner to take all appropriate safety precautions. Neither the publisher nor the author(s)/editor(s) assume any liability for any injury and/or damage to persons or property arising from or related to use of material in this book.

This book is sold on the understanding that the publisher is not engaged in providing professional medical services. If such advice or services are required, the services of a competent medical professional should be sought.

Every effort has been made where necessary to contact holders of copyright to obtain permission to reproduce copyright material. If any have been inadvertently overlooked, the publisher will be pleased to make the necessary arrangements at the first opportunity.

Inquiries for bulk sales may be solicited at: jaypee@jaypeebrothers.com

Ophthalmology: Oral and Practical

Fifth Edition: **2022**

ISBN 978-93-5465-661-3

Printed at: Samrat Offset Pvt. Ltd.

Dedicated to
*My beloved teacher
Late Professor DC Dutta
a successful author
who has taught me many things
except ophthalmology*

Preface

In the world of medicine, there is only one constant: change. Therefore, it has been essential to bring out the fifth edition of this book. Another constant, the appreciation and feedback from the undergraduate students, and the teachers from all over India, has encouraged me to improve and update the book. As a teacher, it has been a pleasure to see the readership of *Ophthalmology Oral and Practical* grow and now after 25 years, and with over 80,000 copies sold, the book is stepping into a new era!

Ophthalmology course and syllabus has changed considerably. Recently, the "Competency based undergraduate curriculum for the medical graduates 2018" has been published by the National Medical Commission (NMC). All items and integrations as advised in the curriculum are included in this book. Theories, common questions, viva voce, instruments, common eye surgeries have also been included.

The highlights of this edition are—plenty of new colored diagrams and photographs, latest medical and surgical management of important diseases, and updates on newer investigations. The bulleted format of the book, point-to-point answers—all will be helpful before examination.

Finally, this edition marks the handover of the book from Current Books International to Jaypee Brothers Medical Publishers. I take this opportunity to thank my old publisher for taking care of this book for so many years, and extend my thanks to my new publisher as well, who has published five of my ophthalmology books previously. I take this opportunity to acknowledge Gauder Ophthalmology Division, Germany, who has kindly granted us permission to use their instrument images.

A special thanks to Dr Soham Basak, a budding ophthalmologist, who has also helped me with his insights and suggestions. From now on, the responsibility lies with the younger generation to carry it forward. Lastly, as always, my sincere thanks to my wife Dr Bani and my daughter, Sohini.

I hope this edition with current syllabus will enhance your understanding of the subject in this new format. Readers are welcome to send in their constructive criticism.

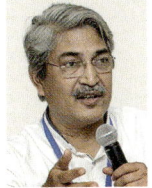
Samar K Basak

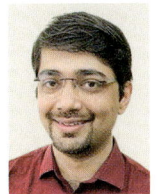
Soham Basak

Disha Eye Hospitals, Kolkata 700120, India

Date: April, 2022

Contents

1. **History Taking and Examination of an Eye Case** 1
   - Ocular Symptoms 2
   - Ocular Examination 6

2. **Practical: Clinical Cases** 21
   - List of Long and Short Cases 21
   - Immature Senile Cataract 21
   - Mature Senile Cataract 24
   - Hypermature Cataract 24
   - Aphakia 26
   - Pseudophakia 29
   - Posterior Capsular Opacification 31
   - Pterygium 33
   - Phlyctenular Conjunctivitis 35
   - Subconjunctival Hemorrhage 37
   - Corneal Ulcer 38
   - Leucoma 42
   - Adherent Leucoma 45
   - Anterior Staphyloma 46
   - Phthisis Bulbi 48
   - Chalazion 50
   - Stye (Hordeolum Externum) 52
   - Bitot's Spot and Conjunctival Xerosis 53
   - Acute Iridocyclitis (Red Eye) 55
   - Chronic Iridocyclitis 56
   - Chronic Dacryocystitis 60
   - Acute Dacryocystitis 61
   - Episcleritis 64
   - Trichiasis 65
   - Blepharitis 65

3. **Brief Theories and Viva** 68
   - Ocular Anatomy 68
   - Layers and Regions of Retina 72
   - Ocular Pharmacology 74
   - Antiglaucoma Medications 78
   - Physiology of Vision 79
   - Optics and Refraction of the Eye 80
   - Refractive Errors of the Eye 81

Contents

- Indications and Principles of Refractive Surgery 84
- Amblyopia 85
- Lid and Adnexal Conditions 86
- How to Give Lacrimal Sac Massage in Congenital Dacryocystitis 89
- Trichiatic Cilia (Eyelash) Removal by Epilation 90
- Orbital Cellulitis 90
- Proptosis and Orbital Tumors 92
- Intraocular Tumors 93
- Red Eye (Conjunctivitis) 94
- Trachoma 97
- Vernal Conjunctivitis 99
- Pterygium 100
- Symblepharon 100
- Technique of Removal of Foreign Body from Eye 101
- Correct Technique of Instillation of Eye Drops 102
- Cornea 103
- Causes of Corneal Blindness 105
- Indications and Types of Keratoplasty 107
- Sclera 110
- Iris and Anterior Chamber 113
- Glaucoma 117
- Investigations of a Patient with Uveitis 121
- Crystalline Lens and Cataract 123
- Etiopathogenesis, Stage of Maturation and Complications of Cataract 124
- Retina and Optic Nerve 128
- Indications of Laser Therapy in Retinal Diseases 129
- Diseases of Optic Nerve and Visual Pathways 133
- Miscellaneous 135
- Strabismus (Squint) and Indications for Referral 136
- Avoidable Blindness, NPCBVI and Vision 2020 139
- Evaluation, Initial Management and Referral in Patient with Ocular Injury ...142
- Ocular Manifestations and Associations of COVID-19 143
- Explain Effect of Pituitary Tumors on Visual Pathway 143
- Describe Anatomical Basis of Horner's Syndrome 144
- Explain the Anatomical Basis of Oculomotor, Trochlear and Abducent Nerve Palsies Along with Strabismus 144
- Describe and Demonstrate Parts and Layers of Eyeball 145
- Describe the Position, Nerve Supply and Actions of Intraocular Muscles 145
- Describe and Discuss Functional Anatomy of Eye, Physiology of Image Formation, Physiology of Vision Including Color Vision, Refractive Errors, Color Blindness, Physiology of Pupil and Light Reflex 145
- Describe and Discuss the Physiological Basis of Lesion in Visual Pathway 146
- Describe the Etiology, Genetics, Pathogenesis, Pathology, Presentation, Sequelae and Complications of Retinoblastoma 148
- Describe Drugs used in Ocular Disorders 149
- Visual Loss in the Elderly 149

4. Common Eye Instruments 151
- Eye Speculums 151
- Barraquer's Wire Speculum 152
- Artery Forceps (Hemostat) 152
- Fixation Forceps (Eyeball Fixation Forceps) 152
- Scalpel Handle (Bard Parker Handle) 153
- Blade Breaker 153
- Thermocautery (Heat Cautery) 154
- Corneal Spring Scissors (Universal) 154
- Iris Forceps 155
- De-Wecker's Iris Scissors 156
- Lens Expressor (Lens Hook) 156
- Iris Repositor 156
- Needle Holder (Barraquer's and Castroviejo's) 157
- Colibri Forceps 157
- St. Martin's Forceps 157
- Lim's Sclerocorneal Forceps 157
- Superior Rectus Holding Forceps 157
- Suture Tying Forceps 158
- Cystitome or Capsulotome 158
- Capsulorhexis Forceps (Utarata Forceps) 158
- Irrigating Vectis 159
- Vectis (Wire Vectis) 159
- Irrigation-Aspiration Cannula (Simcoe) 159
- McPherson's Forceps 160
- Vannas' Scissors 160
- IOL Dialer (Sinsky's Hook) 160
- Crescent Knife (Sclerocorneal Splitter) 161
- Angular Keratome 161
- Side-Port Blade 161
- Phaco Chopper 162
- Phaco Handpiece with Connecting Cord 162
- Epilation Forceps (Cilia Forceps) 162
- Strabismus Hook (Muscle or Squint Hook) 163
- Lid Retractor (Desmarre's) 163
- Chalazion Forceps (Clamp) 163
- Chalazion Scoop (Curette) 164
- Punctum Dilator (Nettleship's) 164
- Lacrimal Cannula 165
- Lacrimal Dissector with Scoop (Lang's) 165
- Rougine 165
- Muller's Retractor 166
- Cat's Paw Retractor 166
- Bone Punch 166
- Hammer, Chisel and Bone Gouge 166

- Evisceration Scoop or Spoon 167
- Enucleation Scissors and Spoon 167
- Lacrimal Probe (Bowman's) 168
- Lid Spatula (Plate) 168
- Entropion Forceps 169
- Entropion Clamp 169
- Caliper (Castroveijo's) 169
- Corneal Trephine (Castroveijo's) 170
- Pin-Hole 170
- Stenopaeic Slit 170
- Trial Frame and Ophthalmic Lenses 171
- Retinoscope 172
- Jackson's Cross Cylinder 174
- Maddox Rod 174
- Placido's Disc 175
- Methods of Sterilization of Instruments 175

5. **Few Common Eye Surgeries** 177
   - Cataract Surgery 177
   - Intraocular Lens 181
   - Dacryocystorhinostomy 183
   - Enucleation 183
   - Evisceration 184
   - Pterygium Operation 184
   - Chalazion Operation 185
   - Indications and Methods of Tarsorrhaphy 185
   - Incision and Drainage of Lacrimal Abscess 186
   - Incision and Drainage of Lid Abscess 186

Index *187*

Competency Table

Undergraduate Ophthalmology Curriculum—2018
With Code Number, Topics and Page Number

Code number	Topics	Assessment methods	Page
OP 1: Visual Acuity Assessment			
OP 1.1	Describe the physiology of vision	Written/Viva voce	79
OP 1.2	Define, classify, and describe the types and methods of correcting refractive errors	Written/Viva voce	80
OP 1.3	Demonstrate the steps in performing the visual acuity assessment for distance vision, near vision, color vision, the pin-hole test and the menace and blink reflexes	Skill assessment/Logbook	6, 8
OP 1.4	Enumerate the indications and describe the principles of refractive surgery	Written/Viva voce	84
OP 1.5	Define, enumerate the types and the mechanism by which strabismus leads to amblyopia	Written/Viva voce	85
OP 2: Lids and Adnexa, Orbit			
OP 2.1	Enumerate the causes, describe, and discuss the etiology, clinical presentations and diagnostic features of common conditions of the lid and adnexa including Hordeolum externum/internum, blepharitis, preseptal cellulitis, dacryocystitis, hemangioma, dermoid, ptosis, entropion, lid lag, lagophthalmos	Written/Viva voce	50, 53, 60, 86
OP 2.2	Demonstrate the symptoms and clinical signs of conditions enumerated in OP 2.1	Skill assessment	50, 53, 60, 86, 87
OP 2.3	Demonstrate under supervision clinical procedures performed in the lid including Bell's phenomenon, assessment of entropion/ectropion, perform the regurgitation test of lacrimal sac massage technique in congenital dacryocystitis, and trichiatic cilia removal by epilation	Skill assessment	12, 65, 89-90, 135
OP 2.4	Describe the etiology, clinical presentation. Discuss the complications and management of orbital cellulitis	Written/Viva voce	90
OP 2.5	Describe the clinical features on ocular examination and management of a patient with cavernous sinus thrombosis	Written/Viva voce	91
OP 2.6	Enumerate the causes and describe the differentiating features, and clinical features and management of proptosis	Written/Viva voce	92

Competency Table

Code number	Topics	Assessment methods	Page
OP 2.7	Classify the various types of orbital tumors. Differentiate the symptoms and signs of the presentation of various types of ocular tumors	Written/Viva voce	92, 93
OP 2.8	List the investigations helpful in diagnosis of orbital tumors. Enumerate the indications for appropriate referral	Written/Viva voce	92
OP 3: Conjunctiva			
OP 3.1	Elicit document and present an appropriate history in a patient presenting with a "red eye" including congestion, discharge, pain	Skill assessment	3, 5, 12, 38, 94
OP 3.2	Demonstrate document and present the correct method of examination of a "red eye" including vision assessment, corneal lustre, pupil abnormality, ciliary tenderness	Skill assessment	3, 37, 94
OP 3.3	Describe the etiology, pathophysiology, ocular features, differential diagnosis, complications. and management of various causes of conjunctivitis	Written/Viva voce	35, 94
OP 3.4	Describe the etiology, pathophysiology, ocular features, differential diagnosis, complications and management of trachoma	Written/Viva voce	97
OP 3.5	Describe the etiology, pathophysiology, ocular features, differential diagnosis, complications, and management of vernal catarrh	Written/Viva voce	99
OP 3.6	Describe the etiology, pathophysiology, ocular features, differential diagnosis, complications and management of pterygium	Written/Viva voce	33
OP 3.7	Describe the etiology, pathophysiology, ocular features, differential diagnosis, complications, and management of symblepharon	Written/Viva voce	100
OP 3.8	Demonstrate correct technique of removal of foreign body from the eye in a simulated environment	Skill assessment	101
OP 3.9	Demonstrate the correct technique of instillation of eye drops in a simulated environment	Skill assessment	102
OP 4: Cornea			
OP 4.1	Enumerate, describe, and discuss the types and causes of corneal ulceration	Written/Viva voce	103
OP 4.2	Enumerate and discuss the differential diagnosis of infective keratitis	Written/Viva voce	39–41
OP 4.3	Enumerate the causes of corneal edema	Written/Viva voce	103
OP 4.4	Enumerate the causes and discuss the management of dry eye	Written/Viva voce	53, 103–104
OP 4.5	Enumerate the causes of corneal blindness	Written/Viva voce	42, 105
OP 4.6	Enumerate the indications and the types of keratoplasty	Written/Viva voce	107
OP 4.7	Enumerate the indications and describe the methods of tarsorrhaphy	Written/Viva voce	185

Competency Table

Code number	Topics	Assessment methods	Page
OP 4.8	Demonstrate technique of removal of foreign body in the cornea in a simulated environment	Skill assessment	101
OP 4.9	Describe and discuss the importance and protocols involved in eye donation and eye banking	Written/Viva voce	107
OP 4.10	Counsel patients and family about eye donation in a simulated environment	Skill assessment	109
OP 5: Sclera			
OP 5.1	Define, enumerate, and describe the etiology, associated systemic conditions, clinical features complications indications for referral and management of episcleritis	Written/Viva voce	64, 110
OP 5.2	Define, enumerate, and describe the etiology, associated systemic conditions, clinical features, complications, indications for referral and management of scleritis	Written/Viva voce	111
OP 6: Iris and Anterior Chamber			
OP 6.1	Describe clinical signs of intraocular inflammation and enumerate the features that distinguish granulomatous from non-granulomatous inflammation. Identify acute iridocyclitis from chronic condition	Written/Viva voce	55–57, 96
OP 6.2	Identify and distinguish acute iridocyclitis from chronic iridocyclitis	Written/Viva voce	55–57, 96
OP 6.3	Enumerate systemic conditions that can present as iridocyclitis and describe their ocular manifestations	Written/Viva voce	114
OP 6.4	Describe and distinguish hyphema and hypopyon	Written/Viva voce	115
OP 6.5	Describe and discuss the angle of the anterior chamber and its clinical correlates	Written/Viva voce	15, 116
OP 6.6	Identify and demonstrate the clinical features and distinguish and diagnose common clinical conditions affecting the anterior chamber	Skill assessment	15
OP 6.7	Enumerate and discuss the etiology, the clinical distinguishing features of various glaucomas associated with shallow and deep anterior chamber. Choose appropriate investigations and treatment for patients with above conditions	Written/Viva voce	117
OP 6.8	Enumerate and choose the appropriate investigation for patients with conditions affecting the uvea	Written/Viva voce	121
OP 6.9	Choose the correct local and systemic therapy for conditions of the anterior chamber and enumerate their indications, adverse events, and interactions	Written/Viva voce	78
OP 6.10	Counsel patients with conditions of the iris and anterior chamber about their diagnosis, therapy, and prognosis in an empathetic manner in a simulated environment	Skill assessment	122
OP 7: Lens			
OP 7.1	Describe the surgical anatomy and the metabolism of the lens	Written/Viva voce	123, 124

Competency Table

Code number	Topics	Assessment methods	Page
OP 7.2	Describe and discuss the etiopathogenesis, stages of maturation and complications of cataract	Written/Viva voce	124
OP 7.3	Demonstrate the correct technique of ocular examination in a patient with a cataract	Written/Viva voce	21–24
OP 7.4	Enumerate the types of cataract surgery and describe the steps, intraoperative and postoperative complications of extracapsular cataract extraction surgery	Skill assessment	26, 29, 177–81
OP 7.5	To participate in the team for cataract surgery	Skill assessment/Logbook	126
OP 7.6	Administer informed consent and counsel patients for cataract surgery in a simulated environment	Skill assessment	126
OP 8: Retina and Optic Nerve			
OP 8.1	Discuss the etiology, pathology, clinical features and management of vascular occlusions of the retina	Written/Viva voce	128
OP 8.2	Enumerate the indications for laser therapy in the treatment of retinal diseases (including retinal detachment, retinal degenerations, diabetic retinopathy and hypertensive retinopathy)	Written/Viva voce	129
OP 8.3	Demonstrate the correct technique of a fundus examination and describe and distinguish the funduscopic features in a normal condition and in conditions causing an abnormal retinal examination	Skill assessment	19
OP 8.4	Enumerate and discuss treatment modalities in management of diseases of the retina	Written/Viva voce	130
OP 8.5	Describe and discuss the correlative anatomy, etiology, clinical manifestations, diagnostic tests, imaging, and management of diseases of the optic nerve and visual pathway	Written/Viva voce	133
OP 9: Miscellaneous			
OP 9.1	Demonstrate the correct technique to examine extraocular movements (uniocular and binocular)	Skill assessment	10
OP 9.2	Classify, enumerate the types, methods of diagnosis and indications for referral in a patient with heterotropia/strabismus	Skill assessment; Written/Viva voce	11, 136
OP 9.3	Describe the role of refractive error correction in a patient with headache and enumerate the indications for referral	Written/Viva voce	138
OP 9.4	Enumerate, describe, and discuss the causes of avoidable blindness and the National Programmes for Control of Blindness (including Vision 2020)	Written/Viva voce	139
OP 9.5	Describe the evaluation and enumerate the steps involved in the stabilization, initial management, and indication for referral in a patient with ocular injury	Written/Viva voce	37, 142

INTEGRATION

The undergraduate training curriculum is aligned and integrated horizontally and vertically to allow the students to understand the structural basis of ophthalmological problems, their management and correlation with function, rehabilitation, and quality of life.

Code number	Topics	Assessment methods	Page
	Integration		
Anatomy			
AN 30.5	Explain effect of pituitary tumors on visual pathway	Written	143
AN 31.3	Describe anatomical basis of Horner's syndrome	Written	144
AN 31.5	Explain the anatomical basis of oculomotor, trochlear and abducent nerve palsies along with strabismus	Written	144
AN 41.1	Describe and demonstrate parts and layers of eyeball	Written/Viva voce	68
AN 41.2	Describe the anatomical aspects of cataract, glaucoma and central retinal artery occlusion	Written	116, 123, 145
AN 41.3	Describe the position, nerve supply and actions of intraocular muscles	Written/Viva voce	71, 73
Physiology			
PY 10.17	Describe and discuss functional anatomy of eye, physiology of image formation, physiology of vision including color vision, refractive errors, color blindness, physiology of pupil and light reflex	Written/Viva voce	79, 80, 145
PY 10.18	Describe and discuss the physiological basis of lesion in visual pathway	Written/Viva voce	146
PY 10.19	Describe and discuss auditory and visual evoke potentials	Written/Viva voce	79
PY 10.20	Demonstrate testing of visual acuity, colour and field of vision in volunteer/simulated environment	Skill assessment/Viva voce	7–9
Pathology			
PA 36.1	Describe the etiology, genetics, pathogenesis, pathology, presentation, sequelae and complications of retinoblastoma	Written/Viva voce	148
Pharmacology			
PH 1.58	Describe drugs used in ocular disorders	Written/Viva voce	74
Internal Medicine			
IM 24.15	Describe and discuss the etiopathogenesis, clinical presentation, identification, functional changes, acute care, stabilization, management and rehabilitation of vision and visual loss in the elderly	Written/Viva voce	149

CHAPTER 1

History Taking and Examination of an Eye Case

Case No: Date:
Name of the Patient:
Age/Gender:
Occupation:
Address of the Patient:
History:
1. **Chief presenting complaints with its duration:**

   The common symptoms in ophthalmology are:
   - Painless progressive dimness of vision
   - Sudden loss of vision
   - Pain ⎫
   - Redness ⎬ may be together as acute pain, redness and watering
   - Watering ⎭
   - Discharge
   - Itching
   - Foreign body sensation
   - Photophobia and glare
   - Dimness of vision at night
   - Double vision or multiple vision
   - Distortion of vision
   - Floaters (like small flies)
   - Flash of light
   - Headache
   - Stickiness of the eyelids
   - Small swelling on the eyelids
   - Abnormal fleshy mass in the eye
   - Disfigurement of the eyeball
   - White opacity over the black of the eye
   - Smallness of the eyeball
   - Abnormal deviation of the eyeball
   - Field defect and/or black shadow (scotoma)
   - Trauma

2. **History of presenting complaints:** To be written in chronological orders.
3. **Past history:**
   - Acute pain, redness and watering in the same or the other eye.
   - Ocular trauma (any type)
   - Wearing of spectacles and its power
   - Acute infectious fever with rash
   - Similar problem in the other eye
4. **Medical history:**
   - Diabetes, hypertension, cardiac problem with medicines
   - Bronchial asthma, COPD, tuberculosis
   - Rheumatoid arthritis or other collagen diseases
   - Enlarged prostate with medicines, etc.
   - Thyroid disorder
5. **Treatment history:** Prior or current ocular medication
6. **Surgical history:**
   - Any surgery in the same, or the other eye with date/year
   - Any known operative complication
7. **Personal and allergy history:**
   - Tobacco and/or alcohol
   - Using computer or digital devices for long hours
   - Systemic allergy or atopy
   - *Drug allergy*: For any systemic or topical medication
8. **Family history:** If any, e.g., high refractive error, glaucoma, cornea or retinal diseases. Family history of any systemic illness.
9. **Others if any:**

Physical examination: Built, pallor, jaundice, abnormal head posture, mental status, hearing problem, facial asymmetry or any obvious abnormality, etc.

General examination: Pulse; respiration rate; blood pressure; CVS; lungs; CNS; GIT; skin

Chapter 1: History Taking and Examination of an Eye Case

Examination of the Eye
Summary:
Provisional Diagnosis

OCULAR EXAMINATION		
Right eye		**Left eye**

	1. Visual acuity
	2. Ocular movements
	3. Eye lids
	4. Conjunctiva
	5. Sclera
	6. Cornea
	7. Anterior chamber (A/C)
	8. Iris
	9. *Pupil:* Size, shape, appearance
	10. *Light reflex:* Direct and consensual
	11. Lens
	12. Lacrimal apparatus
	13. Intraocular pressure
	13. Fundus
	14. Brow position and facial asymmetry
	15. Others, if obvious:
	   • Visual axes (Hirschberg's test)
	   • Palpation
	   • Pre-auricular and sub-mandibular lymph nodes
	   • Any swelling related to the eye
	   • Transillumination (only if there is a large mass)
	   • Also note for facial appearance and head posture	

Summary:		
Provisional diagnosis:		
Investigations:		
Management plan:		

In undergraduate examination, examiner may ask to examine one eye only. In that case write your findings for that eye only. For the other eye, just have a look with the torch light, and keep the findings in your mind. This is for better correlation with your diagnosis and management while answering.

OCULAR SYMPTOMS

Painless Progressive Loss of Vision

The common causes are:
1. Senile cataract
2. Primary open angle glaucoma
3. Age-related macular degeneration (AMD)
4. Diabetic retinopathy
5. Presbyopia
6. Degenerative myopia
7. Retinitis pigmentosa
8. Papilledema

Differential diagnosis:
1. **Senile cataract:** Aged patient; greyish-white or white reflex at the pupillary area; iris shadow—present in immature type; normal IOP; and poor or absent fundal glow.
2. **Primary open angle glaucoma:** Aged patient; high IOP; typical glaucomatous field defects and cupping of the optic disc.
3. **Age-related macular degeneration (AMD):** Aged patients; progressive central loss of vision; anterior segment and IOP are essentially normal; retinal pigment

epithelium (RPE) atrophy; detachment of RPE with sub-retinal neovascular membranes (SRNVMs) formation; macular OCT and fundus fluorescein angiography (FFA) is diagnostic.
4. **Diabetic retinopathy:** Young adult or aged patient; history of long-standing diabetes, often uncontrolled; anterior segment normal; typical fundus picture—dot and blot hemorrhage, hard exudates; diabetic macular edema, neovascularization; FFA is diagnostic.
5. **Presbyopia:** Aging process; gradual D/V in near only; no lens opacity; normal IOP; no cupping of the disc and near vision is regained by simple 'plus-power' glasses.
6. **Degenerative myopia:** Younger subject; increasingly high 'minus-power' glasses; normal IOP; typical myopic degenerative changes in the fundus.
7. **Retinitis pigmentosa:** Middle-aged patient; positive family history; night blindness; tubular field defect; normal IOP; typical fundus findings—bone-corpuscle pigments/bony spicule pigmentation, arteriolar attenuation and waxy pallor of the disc.
8. **Papilledema:** Any age; bilateral onset; associated headache and vomiting; normal reacting pupil; normal IOP; bilateral optic disc swelling and may be with superficial hemorrhage, soft exudates and macular star; CT scan or MRI may detect intracranial SOL.

Sudden Loss of Vision

Unilateral Causes

Painless:
- Optic neuritis or retrobulbar neuritis (sometimes with mild pain on looking up due to involvement of superior rectus muscle sheath)
- Vitreous hemorrhage, e.g., in Eales' diseases, hypertension, diabetes, trauma, retinal tear, posterior vitreous detachment (PVD), etc.
- Central serous retinopathy (CSR)
- Central or branch retinal venous occlusion (CRVO/BRVO)
- Central retinal artery obstruction (CRAO)
- Retinal detachment

With moderate to severe pain:
- Acute iritis or keratitis/corneal ulcer
- Acute attack of angle closure glaucoma
- Orbital apex syndrome

Bilateral causes:
- **Methyl alcohol poisoning:** After consuming spurious liquor or hooch poisoning and usually painless
- **Chemical or thermal burn:** With pain and photophobia
- **Epidemic dropsy glaucoma:** Usually painless
- **Photokeratitis:** With pain and severe photophobia
- **Bilateral optic neuritis:** Associated with paraplegia (Devic's disease)

Acute Pain in the Eye *(OP 3.1)*

Ocular structures like the cornea, sclera and iris are very richly innervated, and hence, very delicate and sensitive.

Pain sensation from these structures is carried through the nasociliary nerve (a branch of ophthalmic division of the 5th cranial nerve).
- Foreign body on ocular surface
- Corneal abrasion or erosion
- Keratitis/corneal ulcer
- Acute iridocyclitis
- Scleritis
- Acute attack of angle-closure glaucoma
- Endophthalmitis/panophthalmitis
- Lens-induced glaucoma
- Ocular injuries—blunt, open globe, or chemical injuries

These are the also the causes for "redness of eye with pain".

Red Eye *(OP 3.1 and 3.2)*

The classical causes are:
- Acute conjunctivitis
- Acute iridocyclitis
- Angle closure glaucoma
- Subconjunctival hemorrhage
- Episcleritis/scleritis
- Inflamed pinguecula

Watering from the Eye *(OP 3.1)*

May be: (A) Lacrimation or (B) Epiphora

A. **Lacrimation:** Excessive secretion of tears.
   Causes:
   - Emotional (as in weeping or laughing).
   - Irritation of the eye due to dust, fumes, chemicals, foreign body, inflammation, etc.
   - In yawning, sneezing, coughing or vomiting.
   - Exposure to bright light.
   - Irritation of nasal mucosa.

B. **Epiphora:** Secretion of tears is normal but there is obstruction in normal drainage into the nose.
   Causes:
   - Congenital absence or occlusion of the puncta
   - Punctal stenosis—drug induced, e.g., latanoprost, netersudil, etc.
   - Ectropion of lower eyelid
   - Canalicular block by foreign body (like, by eyelash) or atresia
   - Nasolacrimal duct block as in chronic dacryocystitis or congenital
   - Nasal polyp, tumors in the inferior meatus of nose
   - Lacrimal pump failure as in Bell's palsy

Causes of watering in children:
- Conjunctivitis including ophthalmia neonatorum.
- Congenital dacryocystitis.
- Buphthalmos or congenital glaucoma.

Ophthalmia neonatorum: Any discharge from the eyes of an infant before 4 weeks of life.

Causes are:
- **Gonococcal conjunctivitis:** Previously, it was synonymous with ophthalmia neonatorum. It is rare nowadays because of good antenatal care, but most serious.
- **Inclusion conjunctivitis:** By *Chlamydia oculogenitalis* (commonest)
- **Chemical conjunctivitis:** Antibiotic drops, Detol, Savlon or soap.
- **Other bacterial conjunctivitis:** *Streptococci, Staphylococci,* etc.

Discharge *(OP 3.1)*

- ❖ **Watery:** Viral infection, toxic irritation
- ❖ **Mucoid:** In allergic conjunctivitis, mucocele of lacrimal sac
- ❖ **Serous (slight yellow tint):** Viral or allergic conjunctivitis
- ❖ **Ropy (stringy) discharge:** Typically, vernal conjunctivitis
- ❖ **Mucopurulent:** Acute mucopurulent conjunctivitis, corneal ulcer
- ❖ **Purulent:** Gonococcal conjunctivitis, any severe infection
- ❖ **Serosanguineous:** Hemorrhagic or membranous conjunctivitis
- ❖ **Sanguineous:** Bloody tears (vicarious menstruation)

Itching of Eyes (Itchy Eyes)

- ❖ Typically, allergic conjunctivitis (seasonal or perineal)
- ❖ Atopic individual along with rhinitis
- ❖ Dry eye syndrome
- ❖ Meibomian gland dysfunction
- ❖ Blepharitis (mainly due to *Demodex folliculorum*)
- ❖ Computer vision syndrome
- ❖ Contact lens solution
- ❖ Allergy to specific eye drop or its preservative, or ointment

Foreign Body Sensation

- ❖ Foreign body on the ocular surface (cornea, tarsal conjunctiva, etc.)
- ❖ Trichiasis/entropion
- ❖ Corneal abrasion/recurrent erosion
- ❖ Dry eye syndrome
- ❖ Conjunctivitis
- ❖ Blepharitis

Glare

Excessive awareness of light, causing visual discomfort or disability but without any significant pain.

Causes

- ❖ Immature cataract
- ❖ Albinism
- ❖ Altered pupillary size/shape
- ❖ Aniridia
- ❖ Post-LASIK eyes, in multifocal IOL eyes (during night driving), etc.
- ❖ Corneal opacity on the visual axis

Photophobia and Blepharospasm

Photophobia: Abnormal ocular discomfort, pain or intolerance—induced by normal light or dim light.

Causes

- Pharmacological dilation of the pupil
- Keratitis or corneal ulcer
- Corneal abrasion or erosions
- Acute attack of angle closure glaucoma
- Corneal edema due to any other cause
- Acute iridocyclitis
- Congenital glaucoma
- Migraine

Blepharospasm: Involuntary, sustained and forcible closure of eyelids.

Causes

- May occur spontaneously—**essential blepharospasm**
- Precipitated by sensory stimuli—**reflex blepharospasm,** e.g., in:
  - Keratitis or corneal ulcer
  - Corneal abrasion
  - Foreign body on the cornea
  - Dust, fumes or chemical irritants

Blepharospasm and photophobia are not synonymous, though all the causes of photophobia may also produce blepharospasm.

True reflex blepharospasm is not abolished in the dark; but is abolished by topical anesthesia as it involves the 5th nerve, not the optic nerve.

But true photophobia is abolished in the dark.

Colored Halos

Patient notices rainbow-colored halos around light (bulb).

Causes

- Angle closure glaucoma (*see* page 119).
- Immature cataract.
- Mucopurulent conjunctivitis (due to mucus flecks).
- Corneal edema due to other cause

Rainbow halos are due to diffraction of light rays by the refracting media of the eyeball.

One can do *"Fincham's stenopaeic slit test"* to differentiate between a rainbow halo of angle closure glaucoma with that of immature cataract.

Nyctalopia (Night Blindness)

Means night blindness, i.e., difficulty in vision at night.

Causes

- Vitamin A deficiency
- Retinitis pigmentosa (other rod dystrophies)
- High myopia
- Open angle glaucoma
- Nuclear cataract
- Oguchi's disease (usually found in Japan)

Among these, vitamin A deficiency and retinitis pigmentosa are most important. Family history is usually positive in retinitis pigmentosa. In vitamin A deficiency other signs like conjunctival xerosis, Bitot's spots or corneal xerosis may be present.

Treatment

- **In vitamin A deficiency:** Vitamin A supplementation (*see* page 105).
- **In retinitis pigmentosa:** No treatment is available, only genetic counseling may help.

Hemeralopia

Means day blindness, i.e., inability to see as clearly in bright light as in dim light.

Causes

- Central cataract, posterior subcapsular/polar cataract
- Cone dystrophy
- Achromatopsia
- Antiepileptic drug-like, trimethadone

Treatment

- May benefit from sunglasses
- Dilated examination to find out the cause
- Treat underlying disorders

Diplopia

Diplopia means double vision. Polyopia means multiple vision.

It must be ascertained whether the diplopia is binocular or uniocular.

Causes of binocular diplopia are (diplopia will disappear after closure of one eye):
- Paralytic squint.
- Anisometropia—as in aphakia with conventional glasses, another eye being normal.
- Displacement of the eyeball (as in uniocular proptosis by space-occupying lesions of the orbit).
- Mechanical restriction of movements of the eyeball (as in large pterygium, symblepharon, blow-out fracture of orbit, etc.)
- Dislocated IOL.
- Faulty spectacles power

Causes of uniocular diplopia are (diplopia will persist even after closure of one eye):
- Immature cataract—in some eyes—polyopia
- Iridodialysis
- Large peripheral iridectomy
- Polycoria
- Subluxation of the lens.
- Decentration of an IOL beyond pupillary margin.
- Keratoconus: Polyopia; multiple smaller images like Japanese kite.

Treatment (binocular diplopia):
- Temporary patching of the worse eye.
- Investigations to find out the cause.
- Treatment of the cause.

Distortion of Vision

Distorted image, also known as metamorphopsia.

Causes
- **Macular pathologies:** Central serous retinopathy, macular edema, AMD, CNVMs due to other causes.
- Corneal irregularities
- High astigmatism

Floaters (Black Spots) in Front of Eyes

Causes
- *Muscae volitantes* (commonest)
- Posterior vitreous detachment
- Retinal tears/holes
- Intermediate or posterior uveitis
- Fresh small vitreous hemorrhage
- Migraine—it is transient

Flashes of Light
Causes
- Retinal break (tear/hole)
- Retinal detachment
- Posterior vitreous detachment
- Migraine
- Oculodigital stimulation

White Pupillary Reflex in Children (Amaurotic Cat's Eye Reflex)

The common causes are:
1. Congenital cataract
2. Retinoblastoma
3. Toxocara endophthalmitis
4. Persistent hyperplastic primary vitreous (PHPV)
5. Retinopathy of prematurity
6. Coat's disease
7. Choroidal coloboma
8. Retinal dysplasia

OCULAR EXAMINATION

Visual Acuity Testing *(OP 1.3)*

Definition: It is the ability or power of the eye by which objects are distinguished one from the other. It also measures the smallest retinal image, formed at the foveal region which can be appreciated regarding shape and size (central vision).

Visual acuity is tested for distant and near objects, called as distant vision and near vision. Each eye is to be tested separately without spectacles (*unaided*), with spectacles (*aided*) and with pin-hole if the visual acuity is less than 6/6. Pin-hole visual acuity is tested for distant vision only.

Principle of normal visual acuity: It means when two distinct points can only be recognizable as separate when they subtend an angle of 1 minute of an arc at the nodal point of the eye. *Nodal point* is an imaginary optical center (or point) which lies just in front of the posterior pole of the crystalline lens in the schematic eyes.

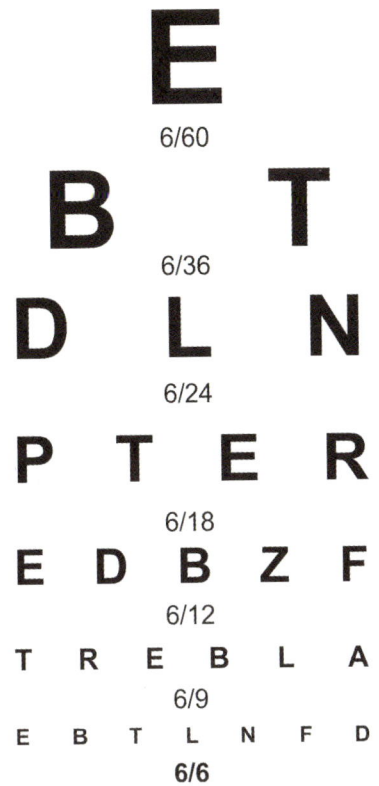

Fig. 1.1: Snellen's distant vision chart.

accommodation does not come to play. Visual acuity is written as numerator/denominator.

Numerator is the distance of the patient from the chart and usually it is 6 meters or 20 feet. *Denominator* is the distance at which a normal person or the distance at which patient should be able to read.

As for example, 6/36 means that the patient reads from a distance of 6 meters what a normal person can read from a distance of 36 meters, or the patient reads from a distance of 6 meters what the patient should read from 36 meters. The normal distant visual acuity is recorded as 6/6 or 20/20.

Procedures of Recording Distant Vision

- ❖ The patient is asked to sit or stand at 6 meters distance (i.e., 20 feet). He is asked to close his left eye with the cup of the palm, little bit obliquely to cross the opposite forehead. He is asked to read with his *right eye first* from the top line to downward. The last line that he reads, is recorded as the visual acuity of the right eye, e.g., top letter is 6/60, 2nd line is 6/36, 3rd line is 6/24 and so on. If he can read some letters (not all letters) of a line, in that case visual acuity is recorded as part (e.g., 6/9p or 6/12p, etc.).
- ❖ If the patient cannot read the first line (i.e., his visual acuity is less than 6/60), then he is brought nearer to the chart at a distance of 5 meters, 4 meters, 3 meters, and so on, till he is able to read the top letter of the chart. The vision is then recorded as 5/60, 4/60, 3/60 respectively and so on.
- ❖ If the patient cannot read the top letter at 1 meter distance, he is then asked to count the examiner's finger against an illuminated background. The rough distance at which he can count finger is recorded, e.g., visual acuity FC at 1/2 meter (FC = Finger counting).
- ❖ If vision is still less, the examiner will move his hand infront of the patient's eye. If he can appreciate the movements of the hand, then vision is recorded as HM or hand movement (from that distance or close to face, etc.).

Distant Vision

In case of Snellen's chart (**Fig. 1.1**), each letter is perfectly placed in a square which is divided into 25 small squares. Each single letter subtends an angle of 5 minute and each component part of the letter subtends an angle of 1 minute at the nodal point of the eye, from a given distance in meters.

Snellen's Distant Vision Chart

Various charts are available in different languages, for illiterate (E chart or Landolt's broken ring) and for children (toys or picture chart).

The Snellen's chart should be read at a distance of 6-meters or 20 feet. If the room is 3 meters, with the help of a plane mirror and reverse chart, this 6-meter distance is achieved. In newer digital charts, the size of the letters can be calibrated for the testing distance.

Rays coming from 6 meters or more are parallel for all practical purposes, hence

If the patient cannot perceive hand movements—*he is then taken to a dark room (ideally)* and asked to close one eye firmly with the palm and look straight or look at his thumb of the other hand, held in front of the eye to be tested and advised not to move that eye. The pencil light is thrown on the open eye from all direction, i.e., up, down, nasal and temporal. If the patient can recognize the light and indicate its direction correctly, his vision acuity is PL and PR present.

PL means: Perception of light
PR means: Projection of rays.
This vision is recorded as PL + PR ✴ in the right eye or left eye.

- If the patient is not able to perceive light from a particular quadrant, then a negative sign is put against that quadrant, e.g.,

VA = PL + PR ✴, i.e. patient is having inaccurate PR.

> **Note**
> When light is thrown from one quadrant—the retina of the opposite quadrant is stimulated. "PL present" indicates that optic nerve is healthy with normal functioning nerve fiber layer of retina. PL is absent in optic atrophy.

"PR accurate" indicates the normal function of peripheral four quadrants of the retina. PR may be defective in detachment of retina, big patch of chorioretinal atrophy, advanced open angle glaucoma, etc.

- If the patient can see the glow of light only, but cannot indicate the side of the projected rays, his VA is recorded as 'only PL' with 'inaccurate' PR.
- Last of all, if the patient cannot see or perceive the glow of the torch light—his vision is recorded as VA = 'No PL (NPL)'. (ideally, the illumination in the Snellen's chart is 100 foot candles, but it should not be less than 20 foot candles.)

The other eye, i.e., left eye is to be tested in a similar manner. Lastly, one should record the distant visual acuity with both eyes open, i.e., binocular distant visual acuity.

Near Vision

It is always tested and corrected after correcting the distant vision. Different charts are used to record near vision;

- **Jager's chart:** J_1, J_2, J_3, J_4, etc.
- **Printer's types of N (point) series:** N_6, N_8, N_{10}, N_{12}, etc.
- **Snellen's near chart:** It is 1/17th times photographic reduction of the original Snellen's chart for distance.

Procedure: The patient is asked to sit in a brilliantly illuminated place. Near vision chart is held at a distance of 25–33 cm depending upon the patient's nature of near work. The patient is asked to read the chart from bigger print size to smaller prints. The line that he reads up to, is recorded, e.g., N_{12}, N_8, N_6, etc. Each eye should be tested separately first, and then binocularly, normal near acuity is N_6 (6 point) in printer's type.

Pin-hole Vision Testing *(OP 1.3)*

Method: Patient complaining of dimness of vision, is asked to look at the Snellen's chart. Then a pin-hole **(Fig. 1.2)** is placed in front of his eye, the other eye is being closed. He is asked whether his vision is better or worse, or unchanged.

Pin-hole: It is a black disc with a small central hole, attached to a small handle.

Principle of pin-hole: When it is held in front of eye, only a small pencil of rays get through, which passes through the axis of dioptric system of the eye, and is therefore, unaffected by it.

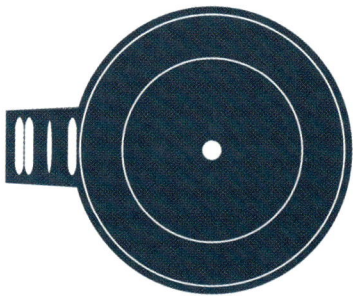

Fig. 1.2: Pin-hole.

Chapter 1: History Taking and Examination of an Eye Case

It follows that if the hole is small enough, all refraction would be eliminated, and a clear image thus be formed in the same manner as seen in a pin-hole camera.

Uses

- To differentiate dimness of vision is due to refractive error or due to organic diseases of the media; or due to macular or neuro-ophthalmologic disease.
  - In case of refractive error or in minor opacity in the media; there will be a substantial improvement of vision.
  - In case of macular or neurological disease, and major opacity in the media—there will be no improvement, rather some worsening may occur.
- During prescription of the glasses in refractive error, achieved by proper lenses or not.
- During follow-up after cataract surgery or keratoplasty, the potential visual acuity can be judged.

Color Vision Testing (OP 1.3 and PY 10.20)

Pseudoisochromatic (Ishihara's) test (Figs. 1.3A to C) is used for routine screening in most ophthalmologist's office. Here, a series of plates containing panels that are filled by colored dots in which bold numerical or different lines (for illiterates) are represented in dots of various tinted sets. This gives a fair assessment, especially for red-green (R-G) blindness.

Farnsworth-Munsell 100 hue test: It is scientifically most accurate and of academic interest.

Edridge-Green lantern test: It is modified by various filters (e.g., to simulate mist, rain, fog, etc.). Mainly important for engine drivers.

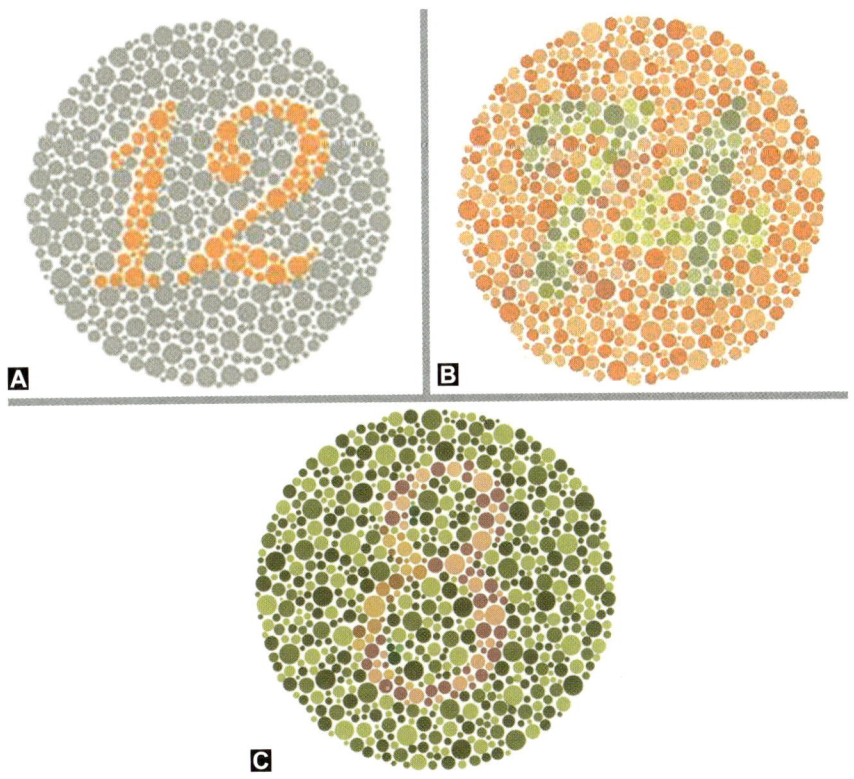

Figs. 1.3A to C: Ishihara's charts—for normal color vision and color blind people: (A) Normal and color blind should read the number 12; (B) Normal should read 74, but red-green (R-G) blind people will read the number as 21; (C) Normal should see the number 8, but R-G blind people will read the number as 3.

Holmgren's wools test: Color matches are done with different shades of colored wool.

Nagel's anamaloscope: It is used to measure the qualitative and quantitative anomalies of color perception.

Visual Field Testing by Confrontation Method *(OP 9.1)*

The visual fields of both eyes overlap. Therefore, each eye is to be tested independently.

The patient is asked to cover right eye with right palm (vice versa when testing the opposite eye). With the examiner seats directly across from the patient, the patient should direct their gaze to the opposite eye of the examiner. The testing is performed using moving targets (disk mounted on a stick or examiner's fingers).

A moving target should start outside the usual 180° visual field, then move slowly towards a more central position until the patient confirms visualization of the target. All four quadrants (upper and lower, temporal and nasal) should be tested for both eyes separately.

The Menace Reflex (*Blink Reflex to Visual Threat*) *(OP 1.3)*

It is the reflex blinking of the eyelids in order to protect the eyes from potential damage, in response to the rapid approach of an object. It is elicited by advancing a closed fist quickly toward the eye and observing a blink, turning of head and neck away from optical stimulus, or all of these.

The menace reflex tests the visual processing at the bedside, in patients who cannot participate in normal visual field testing.

Ocular Movements *(OP 9.1)*

Any deviation of the eye, uniocular and binocular, is to be noted.

Uniocular movements are called—**duction** and consist of adduction, abduction, supraduction (elevation), infraduction (depression), incycloduction (intorsion) and excycloduction (extorsion).

The sign used for ocular movements is "Union Jack' position, i.e., in 6 cardinal positions of gaze.

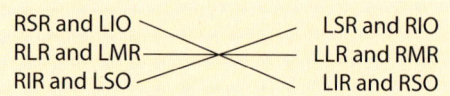

(RMR: right medial rectus; RLR: right lateral rectus; RSO: right superior oblique; RSR: right superior rectus; RIR: right inferior rectus; RIO: right inferior oblique; LMR: left medial rectus; LLR: left lateral rectus; LSR: left superior rectus; LIR: left inferior rectus; LSO: left superior oblique; LIO: left inferior oblique)

Any under-action or over-action is noted with '–' (minus) or '+' (plus) sign. Normally, a person is orthophoric. Any abnormality in the ocular movements is to be noted.

Binocular Movements (Version)

* Dextroversion (right gaze), levoversion (left gaze), supraversion (up gaze), and infraversion (down gaze). These are secondary positions of gaze.
* Dextroelevation (gaze up and right), dextrodepression (gaze down and right), levoelevation (gaze up and left) and levodepression (gaze down and left). These oblique movements are tertiary positions of gaze.
* Dextrocycloversion (rotation of upper limbus of both eyes to the right) and levocycloversion (rotation to the left).
* **Convergence** is also to be checked.

Examination of the Ocular Adnexa and Anterior Segment of the Eye *(OP 9.1)*

Examination Methods

Examination of the anterior segment of the eye (up to the lens-iris diaphragm) can be done by three methods:
1. Diffuse illumination with a good torch light
2. Focal/oblique illumination using a pencil torch and *corneal loupe* (uniocular or binocular)
3. Focal/oblique illumination with the help of a *slit lamp microscope*.

Methods of Examination by Torch and Uniocular Loupe

Patient is placed in a dark room, with a pencil torch light focussed about 2 feet away from the patient's side. The surgeon holds the loupe by thumb and index finger while lifting the upper lid by middle finger, and two other fingers rest on eyebrow. Surgeon moves very close to the loupe to see the enlarged image of the cornea, iris or lens in details. It is useful to search for *superficial punctate keratitis (SPK), keratic precipitates (KPs), minute foreign body, caterpillar hairs,* etc.

Uniocular Loupe (Dioptric Power = +40.0 D)

Advantages
- 10 times magnified image
- Small and handy instrument

Disadvantages
- Both hands are engaged during examination
- Inconvenience due to closeness to the patient
- No depth perception

Binocular Loupe (Dioptric Power = +7.5 or +10.0 D)

It is kept fixed before the surgeon's eyes by an elastic band or a belt attached to the forehead.

Advantages
- Both hands are free during examination
- Depth of lesion is better judged
- Convenient, as surgeon is away from the patient

Disadvantages
- Low magnification (three or four times)
- Interpupillary distance may be difficult to adjust

Examination with a Slit Lamp Biomicroscope (Fig. 1.4)

It is the best method as bright illumination, slit section and various grades of magnification are used. A slit lamp has three parts:
1. Illumination system
2. Viewing system, and
3. Mechanical devices to adjust the slit lamp

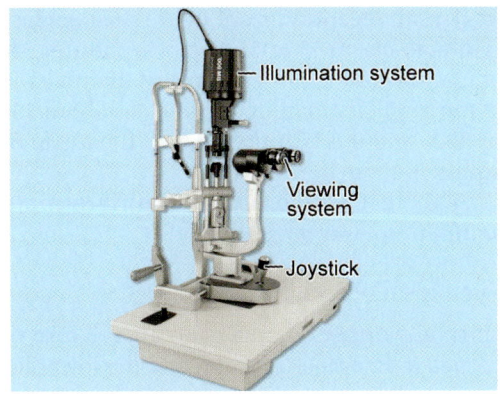

Fig. 1.4: Slit-lamp biomicroscope.

Depth perception is accurate as it is binocular. In fact, one can cut a cross section (optical section) of the eyeball layer by layer for detailed examination at various magnifications.

Uses
- Detailed microscopic examination of anterior segment and anterior 1/3 of vitreous.
- For fundus examination by high powered convex lenses (+90 D, +78 D or +60 D lens) or Hruby (pronounce as Ruby) lens (55.0 D)
- For examination of the *anterior chamber angle* by gonioscope.
- To measure IOP by Goldmann's applanation tonometer.
- For fluorescein staining, along with cobalt blue filter.
- For anterior segment photography.
- As a delivery system for different LASERs e.g., argon, YAG or diode laser

Visual Axes *(OP 9.2)*

Normally, visual axes of both eyes are parallel (orthophoria). This is normal ocular muscle balance. Any deviation of visual axes can be assessed by corneal reflection test or **Hirschberg's test.**

A fixing pencil torch light is held at a distance of 30 cm in front of the patient's eyes and the distance of corneal light reflex (first Purkinje's image) is estimated from the pupillary center.

1 mm decentration of light reflex corresponds to about 7° or 15Δ (prism diopter) of ocular deviation. For example, if the reflex is at the pupillary margin, the angle is about 15° or 30Δ, and if it is at the limbus, the angle of squint is about 45°.

This test is also useful to differentiate squint from pseudo-squint.

Eye Lids *(OP 2.3)*

Normally upper lid covers about 1-2 mm of cornea at 12 o'clock position and the lower lid just touches the limbus at 6 o'clock position. Eyelids are examined for congenital or acquired lesion.

Lid Margin

- Thickened—multiple chalazion, blepharitis
- Inverted (entropion) or everted (ectropion)
- Any ulcer or scales (blepharitis)
- Meibomian duct openings (meibomitis)

Eyelashes

- **Misdirected** and touching the globe (trichiasis)
- **Loss or scantiness of eyelashes** (*Madarosis*): in blepharitis, leprosy
- **Matting of the eyelashes:** Due to mucopurulent discharge
- **Gray eyelashes:** *Poliosis*—in extreme old age, VKH syndrome

Lid Proper

- **Thickened:** Multiple chalazion, blepharitis
- **Edema:** Blepharitis, Stye (Hordeolum externum), allergic conjunctivitis, insect bite, corneal ulcer, lid abscess, trauma, cellulitis, etc.
- **Localized mass:** Chalazion, Stye, cyst, growth

Palpebral aperture: 8-9 mm vertically and 20-25 mm horizontally.

- **Narrow:** Phthisis bulbi, ptosis, lid edema, Horner's syndrome, enophthalmos, microphthalmos
- **Wide:** Lid retraction (thyroid exophthalmos), protopsis, other eye in unilateral ptosis.

Any other specific lid sign: Lid lag, lagophthalmos, black eye, coloboma or pigmentation to be noted.

Conjunctiva *(OP 3.1)*

Conjunctiva is the mucous membrane covering the sclera and the back of the eyelids. It is examined for congestion, inflammatory or allergic reactions, degenerative lesions and foreign bodies.

Bulbar conjunctiva, palpebral conjunctiva (lower and upper), limbal conjunctiva and fornix—all are to be examined.

- *Examination of the lower palpebral conjunctiva, lower fornix and lower part of bulbar conjunctiva* can be easily done by pulling down the lower lid by the thumb or index finger, while the patient is asked to look upwards.
- *Examination of upper palpebral conjunctiva* is done by everting the upper lid.
- *Examination of upper fornix* requires double eversion, with the help of a lid retractor.
- *Examination of bulbar conjunctiva and limbal conjunctiva* are done by separating both lids while the patient is asked to move his eyeball in different directions.

Bulbar Conjunctiva

Note for:
- Lustre
- **Congestion:** Both conjunctival and ciliary congestion
- Discharge
- Edema or chemosis
- Subconjunctival hemorrhage
- Pterygium
- Pinguecula
- Bitot's spot
- Symblepharon, and
- Cyst, nodule, naevus or growth.

Palpebral Conjunctiva

Note for:
- Papillae
- Follicles
- Concretions
- Scarring (as in trachoma)

- Foreign body
- Any tumor mass
- Arrangement of blood vessels

Limbal Conjunctiva

Note for:
- Circumcorneal (ciliary) congestion (CCC)
- Phlycten
- Nodules
- Follicles
- Scar or filtering bleb of previous surgery

Differences between Conjunctival and Ciliary Congestion

Conjunctival congestion	Ciliary congestion
1. Bright red in color	1. Pinkish or dusky red in color
2. Mostly near the fornix	2. Around the limbus (circum-corneal)
3. Branched dichotomously	3. Radially arranged
4. Branches of posterior conjunctival vessels	4. Branches of anterior ciliary vessels
5. Easily blanched by pressure or phenylephrine (10%) drop	5. No such blanching
6. Vessels fill up from the fornix	6. Vessels fill up from the limbus
7. Indicates superficial involvement, e.g., conjunctivitis, simple hyperemia.	7. Indicates deeper tissue involvement, e.g., iritis, keratitis or scleritis.

Cornea (OP 4)

It is avascular, transparent structure forming the anterior 1/6th of the eyeball. It is examined for its size, shape, surface, curvature, transparency, opacity, staining, vascularization, sensation and KPs.

Size

Horizontally 12 mm, vertically 10–11 mm.
- **Size increased:** Megalocornea, buphthalmos
- **Size decreased:** Microcornea, microphthalmos

Shape

Normally, it is like a part of a sphere.
It may be flat, conical or globular.
- **Flat:** Cornea plana, phthisis bulbi, corneal scar
- **Conical:** Keratoconus, pellucid marginal degeneration
- **Globular:** Keratoglobus, buphthalmos

Surface

Normally, it is smooth and regularly curved. Surface and curvature are tested with:
- Slit lamp microscope
- Keratometer
- Photokeratoscope, corneal topography or tomography and anterior segment OCT.
- Window reflex
- Placido's disc
  There will be distortion of the images of window reflex or placido disc in case of keratoconus, corneal edema, corneal ulcer, opacity, etc.

Corneal Staining

Not necessary in all cases.
- **Flourescein staining:** For denuded epithelium (corneal abrasion, erosions, keratitis or ulcers), filaments.
- **Rose Bengal staining:** For devitalized cells. Useful in xerosis of the conjunctiva and cornea (dry eye), dendritic keratitis.
- **Alcian blue:** It stains the mucus selectively.
- **Lissamine green:** To stain xerotic area of conjunctiva and cornea in dry eye.

Transparency

The cornea is optically transparent. This transparency is due to certain anatomical and physiological factors. They are:
- Avascularity of the cornea.
- Demyelinated nerve supply.
- Regular arrangement of the stromal collagen fibrils
- Active endothelial Na-K ATPase pump mechanism.
- Optimum intraocular pressure.
  Any interference with these factors affects the corneal transparency. Thus, the cornea becomes hazy in corneal edema, ulcers, scars, xerosis, vascularization, mucopolysaccharidosis (MPS), acute attack of angle-closure glaucoma, absolute glaucoma, etc.

Opacity

For development of a corneal opacity at least the Bowman's membrane must be damaged.

Grades of Opacity

- **Nebula:** Only Bowman's membrane is involved. Faint opacity which allows iris details to be seen clearly.
- **Macula:** Bowman's membrane and part of the anterior stroma are involved. Moderately dense opacity where iris details are seen but with loss of details.
- **Leucoma:** Full thickness cornea is involved. Dense opacity and underlying anterior chamber details are not seen.
- **Adherent leucoma:** A full thickness corneal opacity with iris inclusion. It indicates perforation of a corneal ulcer or a penetrating injury in the past.

In case of corneal opacity look for:

- Its density (grade)
- Situation and extent in relation to the pupillary axis and limbus
- Any pigmentation
- Any vascularization—superficial or deep
- Iris adherence is present or not
- Its sensation

Causes of corneal opacity:

- Healed infection (keratitis or corneal ulcer)
- Degeneration
- Dystrophy
- Trauma—surgical or non-surgical
- Congenital (sclerocornea, MPS).

Corneal Sensation

Method of examination: Patient is asked to look straight with both eyes wide open. A wisp of cotton is brought close to the patient's eye from the temporal side (to avoid optical blinking reflex) and the lower part of the cornea is touched with it. The blinking reflex of the lids is observed. Avoid any accidental touch to the eyelashes (a false blinking will result). It can be measured by Asthesiometer.

Cornea is supplied *by ophthalmic division of 5th cranial nerve* and it has no kinesthetic sensation.

Causes of Loss of Corneal Sensation

- Herpetic keratitis
- Acute attack of angle-closure glaucoma
- Keratomalacia
- Leprosy
- 5th nerve damage
- After corneal surgery (e.g., keratoplasty, LASIK)
- Neuroparalytic keratitis
- Long-standing corneal edema.

Vascularization

Note:
- Is it localized or circumferential?
- Its site and extent.
- Is it superficial or deep?

Causes of Corneal Vascularization

- Corneal ulcers
- Trachoma
- Interstitial keratitis
- Leprosy
- Contact lens wear
- After penetrating keratoplasty.

Differences between Superficial and Deep Vascularization

Superficial vascularization	Deep vascularization
1. Can be traced over the limbus into the conjunctiva	1. Seems to come from an abrupt end at the limbus
2. Bright red and well defined	2. Greyish red (red blush); ill defined
3. Branches in an arborescent fashion and runs dichotomously	3. Branches at acute angles and runs in a radial fashion
4. May raise the epithelium over them and corneal surface is uneven	4. Deep inside the stroma and corneal surface remains smooth

Keratic precipitates (KPs): These are deposits of inflammatory cells on the lower part of corneal endothelium and best seen by slit lamp examination. They may be:
- Fine
- Medium
- Mutton fat

- ❖ Pigmented
- ❖ They may be fresh or old.
- This is due to inflammation of the anterior uveal tract (anterior uveitis or iridocyclitis).

Keratitis or corneal ulcer: Details of ulcer, e.g., size, shape, extent, margin, floor, central or peripheral, etc., are to be noted. Also note the staining pattern with fluorescein dye if necessary.

Sclera *(OP 5)*

It is dense tough fibrous envelope that covers 5/6th of the eyeball. Normally, the sclera is whitish in adult, and bluish in newborn and is covered by the conjunctiva.

Note for:
- ❖ **Nodule:** Episcleritis, scleritis
- ❖ **Congestion:** Dusky ciliary congestion in scleritis
- ❖ **Ectasia:** Ciliary or equatorial staphyloma
- ❖ **Thinning:** Scleritis, post-surgical
- ❖ **Thickening:** Long-standing scleritis
- ❖ **Blue sclera:** Buphthalmos, *osteogenesis imperfecta*, healed scleritis.

Anterior Chamber *(OP 6.6; 6.7)*

It is the space between the cornea and the iris. It contains aqueous humor. It is approximately 2.5 mm in depth at its center.

Depth

(i) Normal, (ii) Shallow or flat, (iii) Deep and (iv) Irregular.

Causes of Shallow of Flat Anterior Chamber

- ❖ Hypermetropia
- ❖ Hypermature cataract (Morgagnian type)
- ❖ Intumescent cataract
- ❖ Angle closure glaucoma
- ❖ Choroidal detachment
- ❖ Pupillary block
- ❖ Cornea plana
- ❖ Wound leak after intraocular surgery
- ❖ Perforating injury or perforating corneal ulcer.

Causes of Deep Anterior Chamber

- ❖ Myopia
- ❖ Aphakia, pseudophakia
- ❖ Keratoconus, keratoglobus
- ❖ Buphthalmos
- ❖ Posterior dislocation of the lens.

Causes of Irregular Anterior Chamber

- ❖ Subluxation of the lens
- ❖ Iris bombe (funnel shaped A/C)
- ❖ Adherent leucoma
- ❖ Iris cyst
- ❖ Angle recession.

Abnormal Contents of the Anterior Chamber

- ❖ Blood *(hyphema)*, e.g., traumatic, post-operative, herpetic iridocyclitis, spontaneous, iris neovascularization.
- ❖ Pus *(hypopyon)*, e.g., in corneal ulcer, acute iridocyclitis, endophthalmitis or panophthalmitis.
- ❖ Malignant cells *(pseudohypopyon)*, e.g., in retinoblastoma.
- ❖ Emulsified silicone oil after vitreoretinal surgery *(inverse hypopyon)*.
- ❖ Lens or cortical matter (after ECCE or after penetrating injury).
- ❖ Albuminous material (aqueous flare) as in iridocyclitis.
- ❖ IOL (anterior chamber IOL or iris-claw IOL).
- ❖ Vitreous (after ICCE or after accidental rupture of posterior capsule in ECCE).

Angle of the anterior chamber is examined by *gonioscope*. Normally, it is not possible to see angle structure due to high corneal refractive power and iris-corneal interface which causes total internal reflection of the rays.

Iris *(OP 6)*

It is a brown or black diaphragm hanging in front of the lens and is perforated centrally which is known as pupil.

Color

Difference in color of the iris between two eyes is called heterochromia.

Causes of Heterochromia

- ❖ Congenital
- ❖ Horner's syndrome

- Iris atrophy
- Heterochromic cyclitis of Fuchs
- Pigmented tumor of the iris
- Siderosis bulbi, etc.

Pattern

'Muddy iris' in iridocyclitis where the pattern is lost. Here, the iris becomes edematous, swollen, water-logged and shows impaired mobility.

Iridodonesis

Tremulousness of the iris (due to loss of support of the lens). This is elicited by asking the patient to move the eyeball in different directions.

Causes of Iridodonesis

Aphakia, dislocation or subluxation of the lens, some cases of pseudophakia and buphthalmos.

Synechiae

Abnormal adhesions of the iris are called synechiae. Adhesion of iris with the cornea is called *anterior synechia*; and adhesion of iris with the anterior lens capsule, IOL or vitreous face is called *posterior synechia*.

Causes of Anterior Synechia

- Perforated corneal ulcer
- Penetrating injury, post-surgical wound leak
- Angle closure glaucoma
- Iris bombe (iridocyclitis)
- Neovascular glaucoma
- Iridocorneal endothelial (ICE) syndrome
 In case of small central perforation of cornea, one may not find anterior synechia, instead, anterior polar cataract is found.
Causes of posterior synechia: Iridocyclitis.

Neovascularization

Called "*Rubeosis iridis*", found in diabetes, central retinal venous thrombosis, heterochromic cyclitis of Fuchs', etc.

Any Gap in the Iris

Congenital gap (coloboma of iris found at the inferonasal region) or marks of iridectomy (peripheral or complete) is to be noted.

Peripheral iridectomy (PI) is done in cataract surgery (11 and/or 1 o'clock position), in angle-closure glaucoma, trabeculectomy, penetrating keratoplasty operation, etc. Inferior PI is done in vitreoretinal surgery and endothelial keratoplasty. YAG laser PI is done at any place as prophylaxis of angle-closure glaucoma.
Complete iridectomy (large defect) may be found in aphakic patient (if there is any vitreous loss during ICCE, in small pupil situation, cataract surgery in pseudoexfoliation or in presence of extensive posterior synechiae).

Pupil

It is a circular aperture at the center of the iris. It regulates the amount of light entering the eye; and helps in maintaining the depth of focus. Pupil is examined for its position, size, shape, reactions, and color of its reflex (appearance).

Position

The pupil is situated just inferior and nasal to the center of the iris. It may be eccentric, known as corectopia, as seen in congenital corectopia, iridocorneal endothelial (ICE) syndrome, after penetrating injury or after vitreous loss in cataract surgery (updrawn pupil).

Size

Normally, it varies between 2 to 4 mm. It may be smaller (miosis) or larger (mydriasis).

Causes of Miosis (Pupil Size <2 mm)

- Extreme of ages
- In bright light
- Opium addict
- Morphine intoxication
- Pontine hemorrhage
- Acute iritis
- During sleep
- Use of miotics (*e.g.*, pilocarpine).

Causes of Mydriasis (Pupil Size 6 mm or More)

- In dark
- Optic atrophy
- Acute attack in angle-closure glaucoma

- Absolute glaucoma
- Comatose patient
- Head injury
- 3rd nerve palsy
- Use of any mydriatics (e.g., atropine, homatropine, phenylephrine, etc.).

Shape

Normally it is perfectly circular. It may be:
- **Irregular:** Iritis, post-traumatic
- **D-shaped:** Iridodialysis
- **Boat or Hammock-shaped:** Optic capture of PC IOL, vitreous loss in cataract surgery
- **Pear-shaped:** Incarceration of iris with corneal wound.
- **Festooned:** Iridocyclitis.
- **Mid-dilated and oval:** Acute attack in angle-closure glaucoma
- **Inverted pear-shaped and inferonasal:** Coloboma of the iris.
- **Key-hole appearance:** After optical iridectomy or sphincterotomy

Light Reactions

The pupil constricts briskly on exposure to bright light and dilates in the dark. The afferent pathway is via the optic nerve and the efferent, via the third cranial nerve.

Light reactions are: Direct and consensual.

Direct Light Reaction

The patient is asked to cover one eye with his own palm, and the beam of pencil light is thrown on the pupil of uncovered eye from one side, noting the nature of pupillary contraction. Normally, the reaction is brisk and sustained.

Consensual Light Reaction

Pupil of the ipsilateral eye contracts when the light beam is thrown on the contralateral eye.

Ill-sustained pupillary reaction is a sign of early optic neuritis.

In optic atrophy: Direct light reaction is absent but consensual reaction is present.

In **relative afferent pupillary defect (RAPD)** or Marcus-Gunn pupil, both pupils dilate when the light is moved (*swinging flash light test*) from the unaffected eye to the affected eye. RAPD is mostly seen in unilateral optic neuritis.

Color (Appearance) of the Pupillary Area

Normally, it is black in young individual. It may be grayish haze in old age even in absence of cataract. This is due to increased light scattering.
- **Jet black pupillary reflex:** Aphakia
- **White or brown pupillary reflex:** Cataract
- **Glassy pupillary reflex:** Pseudophakia
- **Amaurotic cat's eye reflex** (white pupillary reflex) in children

Crystalline Lens

The crystalline lens is a transparent biconvex structure with a nucleus, cortex and the capsule. It is supported by suspensory ligaments, called zonules, attached to the ciliary processes and the valleys between them.

Color of the Lens

Normally, it is transparent.
- **Grayish white:** Immature cortical cataract.
- **White or pearly white:** Mature cataract.
- **Milky white:** Hypermature cataract.
- **Shrunken and white with calcified spots on the anterior capsule:** Hypermature sclerotic cataract.
- **Amber:** Early nuclear cataract.
- **Brown:** *Cataracta brunescens* (nuclear cataract).
- **Black:** *Cataracta nigra* (advanced nuclear cataract).

Position

Normally, it is in the pupillary area. Note any subluxation or dislocation is present or not. *Phacodonesis or tremulousness* is seen in lens subluxation. Opacity or any subluxation is better judged with dilated pupil.

Aphakia means absence of crystalline lens from its normal anatomical position (i.e., from the pupillary area).

Ectopia lentis is the congenital malposition of the lens, due to faulty development of the lens zonules, as seen in Marfan's syndrome,

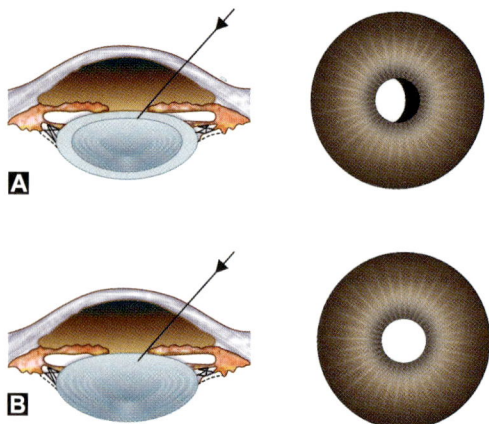

Figs. 1.5A and B: Iris shadow. (A) Present—immature cataract; (B) Absent—mature or hypermature cataract.

homocystinuria, Weil Marchesani's syndrome, etc.

Pseudophakia means the presence of an intraocular lens (IOL) in the eye after cataract operation with IOL implantation.

Iris Shadow (Figs. 1.5A and B) (Also Figs. 2.1A and 2.2A)

It is a concave shadow of the pupillary margin of the iris, cast upon the lens when light is thrown obliquely. This shadow is formed on the same side as the direction of incident light.

It signifies that some clear cortical fibers are still present beneath the lens capsule (i.e., between the iris margin and the actual opacity of the lens). It is present in immature cataract.

But it is absent in mature or hypermature cataract. In case of mature cataract all the substance of lens become opaque, so iris margin lies almost in contact with the opaque lens surface—so no iris shadow will form if light is thrown obliquely.

Pigmentation Over the Anterior Lens Surface

- **Congenital iris pigments:** Epicapsular stars
- A sign of posterior synechiae in old irido-cyclitis
- In traumatic cataract (Vossius's ring)

Purkinje's Images

Note the 3rd and 4th Purkinje's images in a dark room. 3rd image is formed by the anterior convex surface of the lens. It moves in the same direction and is erect. 4th image is formed by the posterior concave lens surface. It is inverted and moves in the opposite direction. In *aphakia*: Both the 3rd and 4th images are absent.

In mature or hypermature cataract: 3rd image is present but the 4th image is absent.

In immature cataract: 3rd image is present, but 4th image may be absent or distorted.

The structures beyond the lens—like the vitreous, retina and optic nerve are not possible to examine with a torch and loupe and beyond the scope of undergraduate examination.

Lacrimal Apparatus

Lacrimal Puncta

They are situated on the medial side of the lid margins on the papilla. They are always in contact with the eyeball.

Note:
- They are open or stenosed
- Any eversion or non-contact
- Any inflammation

Lacrimal Sac

1. **Skin over the sac area:** Swollen, inflamed, any excoriation of skin, fistula or scar mark.
2. **Regurgitation test of lacrimal sac *(OP 9.1)* regurgitation on pressure over the lacrimal sac (ROPLAS):** Anterior lacrimal crest is identified by tracing the inferior orbital margin medially and superiorly. The index finger is then directed behind the crest and used to apply pressure on the sac area in an upward and medial direction so as to express the lacrimal sac contents into the conjunctiva.

Any reflux of fluid or purulent material from the puncta is noted.
  - Regurgitation of mucoid material (mucocele), pus (Pyocele) through the puncta.

- *Swelling is present but no regurgitation via puncta:* Encysted mucocele.
- *Sometimes regurgitate may go into the nasopharynx,* i.e., there is block in common canaliculus.

3. **Signs of acute inflammation (i.e., swelling, redness, raised temperature and tenderness):** Acute dacryocystitis.

Nasal cavity is better to be examined grossly for DNS, polyps, hypertrophied inferior turbinate, etc., as in chronic dacryocystitis.

Digital Tonometry (Finger Tension)

Technique

Rough assessment of intraocular pressure (IOP) by eliciting the fluctuation of the eyeball.

The patient is asked to look downwards at his feet.

Examiner places both index fingers side by side above the upper border of the tarsal plate on the upper lid, resting the other fingers lightly on the forehead.

One index finger is stationary and the other one presses the globe, thereby conveying the amount of fluctuation to the stationary finger. Fluctuation is well appreciated by regular practice. The intraocular tension is graded as normal, high or low.

The eyeball is harder in all primary and secondary glaucomas. It is *stony hard* (the fluctuation is absent) in absolute glaucoma.

The eyeball is soft in chronic uveitis, recent penetrating injury, wound leak and choroidal detachment. In phthisis bulbi, it is soft as water bag.

Other means of recording IOP:
- **Goldmann applanation tonometer:** Greatest accuracy of IOP is determined by this method by applanating the central portion of the cornea. This instrument is an optional attachment to the slit lamp. It can also be done by a portable hand-held applanation tonometer (Perkins tonometer).
- **Non-contact or air-puff** tonometry
- **Schiotz tonometer:** By indentation of the cornea with this instrument, IOP can be recorded from a chart after getting the scale reading.

Normal IOP is about 14–21 mm of Hg

Facial Asymmetry

In a normal ophthalmic case, there is a symmetry between two halves of the face.

In some congenital diseases (like craniosynostosis, hemifacial atrophy, or orbitopalpebral cyst), or orbital diseases (like malignant nasopharyngeal tumor or sphenoidal-ridge meningioma)—there may be asymmetry between two sides of the face.

Head Posture

Normally, the head posture is straight while fixing an object at any given distance.

Most of the time, the abnormal head posture is purposive and compensatory. It is found in:
- **Nystagmus, especially in spasmus nutans:** Here, the patient tries to find out a neutral or null point where the nystagmus is minimum.
- **Paralytic squint:** Here, the patient tries to neutralize diplopia by 'chin elevation or depression', 'turning the face right or left' or by 'tilting the head' towards right or left shoulder. It may be alone or in combination. This is to neutralize the angle of deviation of squint or to separate the image maximally, so as to avoid binocular diplopia.

Abnormal head posture is not seen in concomitant squint.

Examination of the Fundus
(OP 8.3 and 9.1)

- **Examination with a retinoscopic plane mirror at 1 meter distance:** To know the fundal glow and refractive status of the patient's eye.
- **Examination by an ophthalmoscope or a plane mirror at 22 cm distance (distant**

direct ophthalmoscopy): Opacities in the anterior segment or a bullous retinal detachment can be readily visualized.
- **Direct ophthalmoscopy:** The details of central retina are examined under higher magnification (15 times). Uniocular, direct and erect image.
- **Indirect ophthalmoscopy:** With this, up to the peripheral portion of retina is visualized. Magnification is 3–5 times. But the image is real and inverted. Depth of lesion is judged accurately as it is binocular.
- **Slit lamp and with special lenses:**
  - +90 D lens, + 78 D lens or + 60 D lens.
  - Hruby lens
  - Fundus contact lens
  - 3-mirror contact lens

Method of Direct Ophthalmoscopy (OP 8.3)

- Ophthalmoscope is held close to the observer's eye and approximately 15 cm from the patient's eye.
- It is held in the right hand to examine patient's right eye and in the left hand to examine patient's left eye.
- Observer uses their right eye to examine patient's right eye and left eye for patient's left eye.
- Patient should fix on a distant target with the eye as steady as possible.
- Observer has to adjust ophthalmoscope power setting to accommodate for the patient's refractive error and/or their own.
- If both patient and observer are emmetropic, the lens is set at zero. A red reflex will be seen and is considered normal.
- Moving the ophthalmoscope as close to the patient's eye as possible and using the plus or minus lens, the observer will be able to see central retina in detail up to the equator.

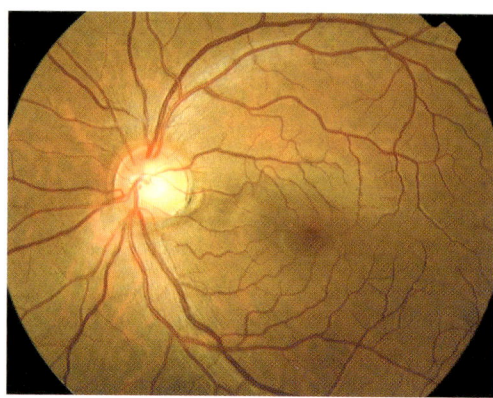

Fig. 1.6: Normal fundus.

Fundus Examination in Abnormal Retinal Conditions (Fig. 1.6)

- **Fundal glow:** Good, poor or hazy, or absent.
- **Optic disc:** Margin, color, size, shape, cup:disc (C:D) ratio, neuroretinal rim, venous pulsation, any abnormal vessels, hemorrhages, or any lesions.
- **Retinal blood vessels:** Vascular reflexes, artery: vein (A:V) ratio, A-V crossing, any abnormal or new vessels.
- **Macula and foveal reflex:** Any abnormality, i.e., cyst, hole, hemorrhage, edema, scar, etc.
- **General fundus:** Any abnormality, e.g., exudates (soft/hard), hemorrhage, pigmentation, scar, new vessels, detached area, coloboma, folds, etc.
- **Peripheral fundus (best seen by an indirect ophthalmoscope):** For retinal break (hole/tear) degenerative area, pigmentation, exudation, localized detachment, etc.
- **Choroidal blood vessels:** Normally not visible, but in case of choroidal sclerosis they are visible as ribbons.

CHAPTER 2

Practical: Clinical Cases

SELF-ASSESSMENT QUESTIONNAIRE

These are representative samples—discussed as long case format. But they are interchangeable as long and short cases.

Long case involves structured case writing—like, any branch of clinical medicine, to be approached, examined (in detail), and documented properly up to provisional diagnosis, investigations and management plan.

For short cases: Chief complaints, positive and relevant negative findings to be written point-wise to establish a provisional diagnosis.

* **In practical**
  * *Long cases:* 2 cases = 20 × 2 = 40
  * *Short cases:* 4 cases = 5 × 4 = 20
  * *Spotter:* 10 = 10 × 1 = 10
* **Viva** = 10 + 10 = 20: One internal and one external in each group
* **Record** = 10
* **Total** = 100

Clinical cases and skill assessment procedures—have been prescribed for the undergraduate students, and published curriculum by the Indian Medical Council in 2018. All have been incorporated under the ocular examination of different cases with code.

LIST OF LONG AND SHORT CASES

* Immature cataract
* Mature/hypermature cataract
* Pseudophakia
* Aphakia
* Subconjunctival hemorrhage
* Phlyctenular conjunctivitis
* Bitot's spot
* Pinguecula
* Pterygium
* Phlyctenular conjunctivitis
* Symblepharon
* Corneal ulcer
* Leucoma
* Adherent leucoma
* Anterior uveitis
* Chalazion
* Blepharitis
* Chronic dacryocystitis
* Anterior staphyloma
* Phthisis bulbi

IMMATURE SENILE CATARACT (ISC) *(OP 7.3 AND OP 9.1)*

A. **Patient's particulars:**
B. **Chief complaints with duration:** Painless, progressive loss of vision in RE/LE for 6–12 months.
C. **History of present illness:** Elaborate the patient's complain. History of colored halos, polyopia, glare at night especially during driving, etc. Negative history—like, blunt trauma, use of systemic or topical steroids, etc.
D. **Medical history:** Diabetes, hypertension, cardiac problems on anticoagulants (blood thinners), COPD; history of COVID-19 recently (self or among family members).
   For male patient, enquire about BHP on alpha-1 antagonist (Tamsulosin), etc.
E. **Surgical history:** History of any surgery in the same eye or other eye

F. **Personal and allergy history:** Allergy to any eye drops, or systemic drug, alcoholism, smoking, etc.
G. **General examination:** Overall built, obesity, pallor, deep socket.
  Look carefully for any lung and heart problem, check BP, pulse and *oxygen saturation* (PO_2), if possible.
H. **Ocular examination:**
- **Vision:**
  - *Uncorrected vision:* Finger counting—3 mt to 6/12
  - *Vision with glasses:* May improve
  - *Vision with pinhole, if possible:* Usually 6/6 or 6/9
- **Ocular movement:** Full
- **Eyelids:** Normal
- **Conjunctiva:** Normal; pinguecula or early pterygium may be present
- **Cornea:** Arcus senilis may be present. Corneal clear.
- **Anterior chamber:** Normal depth, clear
- **Iris:** Brown or dark brown, normal pattern, no iridodonesis
- **Pupil:** Circular, 3–4 mm.
  - *Direct and consensual light reflex:* Present (brisk).
  - *Pupillary area:* Grayish white appearance
  - *Iris shadow:* Present **(Fig. 2.1A)**
    [Pupil may be dilated for examination. Pupillary reaction may be absent in that case.]
- **Lens:** Grayish white, often radial spoke-like: **(Fig. 2.1B).**
- **Purkinje's images** (better in a dark room):
  - 3rd image—present.
  - 4th image—may be visible and distorted in early IMSC.
- **Lacrimal sac:** No regurgitation on pressure over the sac region
- **Digital (finger) tension (IOP):** Normal.
- **Any other:** No abnormal head posture or no obvious defect
I. **Summary:**
J. **Provisional diagnosis:** Immature senile cataract of RE/LE

Self-assessment Questionnaire *(OP 7.2)*

1. **Define cataract:** (means – 'waterfall'). Any opacity in the lens or its capsule, causing visual impairment is called cataract.
2. **Prevalence of cataract blindness in India:** 66.2% among all blindness—National RAAB (Rapid Assessment of Avoidable Blindness) Survey, 2015–2019
3. **Causes of diplopia or polyopia:** (*see* page 5).
4. **Causes of colored halos:** (*see* page 5 and 19).
5. **Causes of painless progressive loss of vision:** (*see* page 2).
6. **Differential diagnosis:** Age-related macular degeneration (AMD); refractive error; diabetic retinopathy
7. **Points favor of diagnosis:**
   - Colored halos, glare at night, polyopia in early stage followed by painless progressive diminution of vision as symptoms.

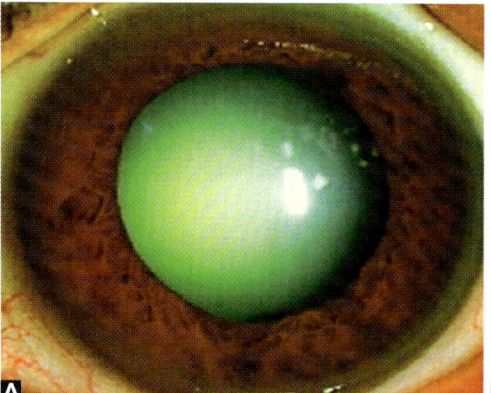 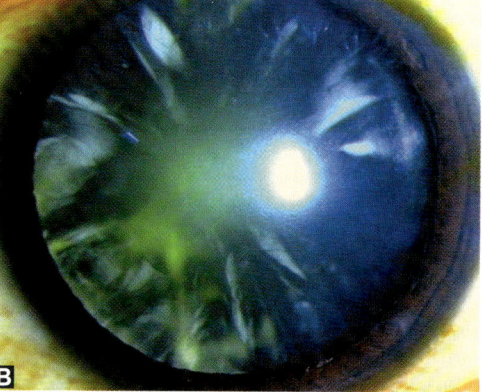

Figs. 2.1A and B: (A) Iris shadow present; (B) Immature senile cataract.

- On examination—reduced spectacles—corrected vision, grayish white opacity of lens with iris shadow and presence of 4th Purkinje's image
8. **Stages of maturation of cataract:** *See* page 124
9. **Management of immature senile cataract:**
   - Dark room examination and refraction.
   - If the vision improves satisfactorily with glasses—prescribe glasses and ask the patient to come for follow up at a regular interval of 3–6 months.
   - If the vision does not improve satisfactorily—advise for cataract surgery.
10. *Timing of surgery:* In spite of spectacles correction when the vision is reduced to such an extent that the patient cannot carry out his day-to-day work efficiently.
11. **Reasons for cataract operation:**
    - For regaining visual loss caused by cataract.
    - To correct the early visual symptoms, and also to correct preoperative high plus or minus power
    - To avoid difficult surgery as in mature stage when the cataract is hard
    - To prevent future complications of hypermature stage, e.g., lens-induced glaucoma, iridocyclitis, and subluxation or dislocation of lens.
12. **Investigations before cataract operation:**
    Details ocular examination:
    - Slit lamp evaluation of the cornea for specular reflection to see endothelial cell status.
    - Dilatation of the pupil to know:
      - Extent of dilatation
      - Presence of synechia
      - Grade of cataract
      - Any subluxation or zonular weakness
      - Presence of pseudo-exfoliation
      - Vitreous and fundus details.
    - Applanation, non-contact or Schiotz tonometry to know exact IOP.
    - *Syringing:* To know the patency of nasolacrimal passage
    - Specular microscopy to study corneal endothelial cell count and morphology.
    - Macular optical coherent tomography (OCT)
    - USG B-scan (if fundus details—not clearly visible)
    - Biometry—to calculate IOL power
    - Conjunctival swab for culture and sensitivity (not a routine).

    Systemic
    - *Blood sugar (PP), HbA1C:* In presence of high blood sugar, there is higher chance of delayed wound healing, wound infection and endophthalmitis. Suboptimal visual outcome in presence of pre-existing diabetic retinopathy. Even, cataract surgery may also aggravate it.
    - *Blood pressure:* more chance of intra-operative bleeding including suprachoroidal hemorrhage, sometimes, cardiovascular accident.
    - *ECG,* and cardiological check-up if necessary
    - *Dental check-up:* To avoid patient with dental/gum infection
    - *Physician's check-up*, if necessary
13. **Important medicine-intake history before surgery:**
    - *Antidiabetic medicines*
    - *Blood thinners:* Like, aspirin; clopidogrel, or similar, etc. It is to be stopped 5 days before cataract surgery, as there is chance of intraoperative bleeding.
    - *Alpha-1 adrenergic blockers:* Tamsulosin, which is used for BHP in male and sometime, for urinary incontinence in female. Poor pupillary dilatation and *intraoperative floppy iris syndrome (IFIS)* are the problems during cataract surgery. IFIS is characterized by progressive miosis, billowing of flaccid iris which tends to prolapse through the wounds during surgery, especially in phaco. Pupil-expand devices (ring or hooks) are used commonly in these cases.
14. **Surgical management in immature cataract:** Phacoemulsification with foldable posterior chamber intraocular lens implantation (phaco with foldable PCIOL), alternately, manual small incision cataract surgery (SICS) with PMMA PCIOL

Or, conventional extracapsular cataract extraction (ECCE) with PCIOL with 4–5 stitches.
15. **Cataract surgery details with complications:** *See* Page: 177–181

MATURE SENILE CATARACT (MSC) (OP 7.3)

A. **Patient's particulars:**
B. **Chief complaints with duration:**
- Gradual, painless, complete loss of vision in RE/LE for few weeks to months
- White opacity—noticed for few days/weeks

C. **History of present illness:** Elaborate the patient's complain. History of gradual, painless loss of vision in RE/LE for few months. Recently, complete loss of vision for few weeks or so. White opacity noticed by patient, or relatives for few days/weeks. The loss of vision is not sudden onset. No history of blunt trauma; or use of systemic or topical steroids, etc.

D. **Medical history:** Diabetes, hypertension, cardiac problems on anticoagulants (blood thinners), COPD, for male patient, enquire about BHP on alpha-1 antagonist (Tamsulosin), etc.

E. **Surgical history:** History of any surgery in the same eye or other eye
F. **Personal and allergy history:** Allergy to any eye drops, or systemic drug, alcohol intake, smoking, etc.
G. **General examination:** Overall built, obesity, pallor, deep socket.
H. Look carefully for any lung and heart problem, check BP, pulse and oxygen saturation (PO_2), if possible.
I. **Ocular examination:**
- **Vision:**
  - *Uncorrected vision:* Only perception of light (PL). Projection of rays (PR)—accurate all quadrants
  - *Vision with glasses and pin-hole:* No improvement
- **Ocular movement:** Full
- **Eyelids:** Normal
- **Conjunctiva:** Normal; pinguecula or early pterygium may present
- **Cornea:** Arcus senilis may be present. Corneal clear.
- **Anterior chamber:** Normal depth, clear
- **Iris:** Brown or dark brown, normal pattern, no iridodonesis
- **Pupil:** Circular, 3–4 mm.
  - *Direct and consensual light reflex:* Present (brisk).
  - *Pupillary area:* Milky white appearance
  - *Iris shadow:* Absent (**Fig. 2.2A**)
  - *Pupil may be dilated for examination. Pupillary reaction is absent in that case.*
- **Lens:** White *or* milky white (**Fig. 2.2B**)
- **Purkinje's images** (better in a dark room):
  - 3rd image—present.
  - 4th image—absent
- **Lacrimal sac:** No regurgitation on pressure over the sac region
- **Digital (finger) tension (IOP):** Normal
- **Any other:** No abnormal head posture or no obvious defect

J. **Summary:**
K. **Provisional diagnosis:** Mature senile cataract of RE/LE

HYPERMATURE CATARACT (HMSC) (OP 7.3)

Almost same as mature senile cataract—*except:*
- **In chief complaints:** Duration of complete loss of vision—more
- **On examination:**
  Color of lens: Pearly white ('mother of pearl' appearance) in Morgagnian cataract. Brown-colored lens nucleus may sink at the bottom of the capsular bag (**Fig. 2.3A**). Calcified white spots on the anterior capsule in sclerotic cataract (**Fig. 2.3B**).

Self-assessment Questionnaire

1. **Differential diagnosis:** Immature cataract
2. **Define mature cataract:** When the entire lens cortex becomes opaque and white, it is called mature cataract. Crystalline lens swells up due to imbibition of water.
   Points favor of mature cataract:
   - *Visual acuity:* Reduced to PL only with accurate PR

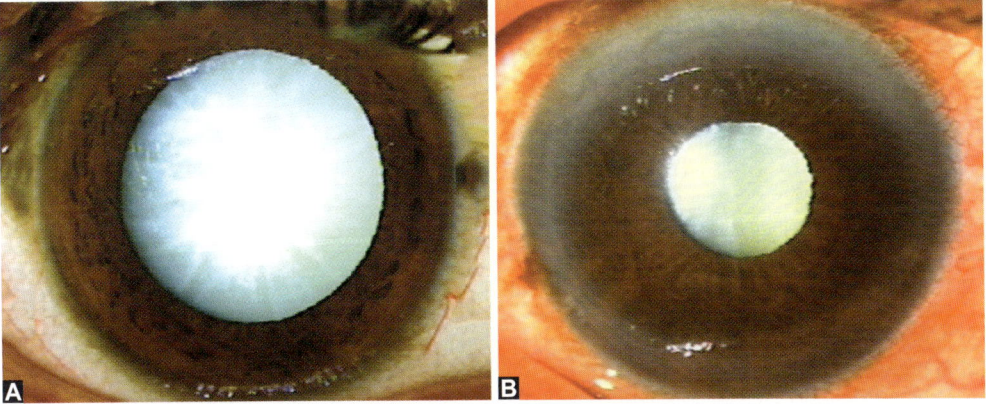

Figs. 2.2A and B: Iris shadow absent; (B) Mature cataract.

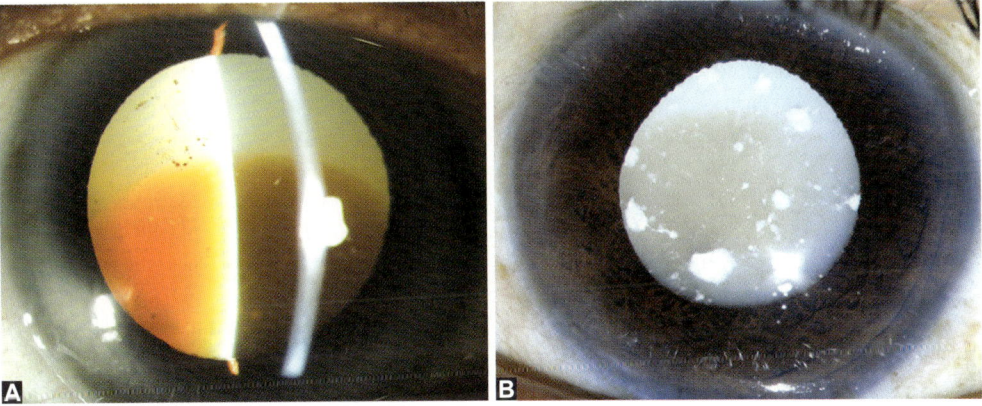

Figs. 2.3A and B: (A) Hypermature Morgagnian cataract; (B) Hypermature sclerotic cataract.

- Absence of iris shadow
- Color of lens—white or milky white
- Absence of 4th Purkinje's image

3. **Management of mature cataract:** Extracapsular cataract extraction with posterior chamber IOL implantation (ECCE with PCIOL) under peribulbar block or topical anesthesia.
   Phacoemulsification with foldable PCIOL is mostly preferred method. Alternately, manual SICS with single-piece PCIOL. Very rarely, conventional ECCE with PCIOL with sutures.

4. **Timing of surgery:** As soon as possible after both ocular and systemic investigations.
   If not operated early, the possible complications are: Hypermature cataract, phacolytic glaucoma in morgagnian type, zonular dehiscence with subluxation, dislocation of lens and eventually, patient may present with blind eye with inaccurate PR or with no PL.
   Also, cataract surgery becomes more difficult as the nucleus becomes harder and zonules are weaker with time.

5. **Investigations in this case:** Same as in immature cataract. Additionally, USG B-scan is a must to rule out any posterior segment pathology.

6. **Possible problems encountered during cataract surgery in mature cataracts:** As the lens nucleus is bigger and harder with some degree of zonular weakness—there is more chance of:
   - Corneal endothelial cell damage
   - Posterior capsular rent with vitreous loss

TABLE 2.1: Differences between immature and mature cataract.

	Immature cataract	Mature cataract
A. Symptoms:	• Partial loss of vision • Diplopia/polyopia • Rainbow halos	• Total loss of vision. • White opacity noticed by patients or relatives
B. Sign: 1. Visual acuity 2. Color of the lens 3. Iris shadow 4. Purkinjie's images 5. Fundal glow 6. Retinoscopy 7. Spectacles correction	• Vision reduced to varying degree • Gray/grayish white • Present • 3rd image is seen, 4th image may be distorted • Present • Possible • May improve vision	• Vision reduced to HM or PL • White/pearly white • Absent • Only 3rd image is seen, 4th image is absent • Absent • Not possible • Does not improve vision

TABLE 2.2: Differences between cortical and nuclear cataract.

Cortical cataract	Nuclear cataract
1. Usually starts at late 50s	1. Tends to occur earlier than cortical variety
2. Starts with uniocular diplopia or polyopia and colored halos	2. No such symptoms
3. Gives rise to index hypermetropia	3. Gives rise to index myopia. Neutralizes the 'plus power' of presbyopia ('Second sight')
4. Appears grayish to white to milky white with maturity of the cataract	4. Appears yellow, brown or black with progression of cataract
5. Progress is gradual and ultimately progress into hypermature stage with liquefaction of cortex	5. Progress is very slow and the entire lens functions as a nucleus, but hypermaturity does not occur
6. More chance of lens-induced secondary glaucoma	6. Little chance of lens-induced secondary glaucoma

  ➢ Zonular dehiscence
  ➢ Nucleus drop into the vitreous cavity
  ➢ Wound-related problems (e.g., wound burn in case of phacoemulsification)
7. **Differences between immature and mature cataract** (Table 2.1)
8. **Differences between cortical and nuclear cataract** (Table 2.2)
9. **Current grading system of cataract:** See page 125

APHAKIA *(OP 7.4)*

A. **Chief complaints with duration:** Gross dimness of vision without glasses after cataract extraction for (certain duration).

B. **History of present illness:** Elaborate the patient's complain. History of loss of vision without glasses in RE/LE for few years or months after cataract surgery. He also gives the distortion of objects after wearing thick-lens spectacles.

C. **Medical history:** Diabetes, hypertension, cardiac problems on anticoagulants (blood thinners), COPD, etc.

D. **Surgical history:** History of cataract surgery in the same eye. There may be history of some complications during or after the cataract surgery.

E. **Personal and allergy history:** Allergy to any eye drops, or systemic drug, alcohol intake, smoking, etc.

F. **General examination:** Overall built, obesity, pallor, etc.

G. Look carefully for any lung and heart problem, check BP, pulse and oxygen saturation (PO_2), if possible.

H. **Ocular examination:**
- ❖ **Distant vision:**
  - ➢ Unaided—finger counting—1 mt.
  - ➢ With glasses (thick plus power lens):
- ❖ **Near vision:** Unable to see near objects without glasses.
- ❖ **Conjunctiva:** Scar mark may be present.
- ❖ **Cornea:** Limbal scar with suture marks 120–180° in the upper half may be present.
- ❖ **Anterior chamber:** Deep.
- ❖ **Iris:** (a) Iridodonesis or tremulousness of the iris, (b) Peripheral buttonhole iridectomy mark(s) at 11 o'clock and/or 1 o'clock position **(Fig. 2.4).**
- ❖ **Pupil:** Jet-black appearance—3 mm size; direct and consensual light reflexes: present and brisk.
- ❖ **Lens:** Absence of 3rd and 4th Purkinje's images.
- ❖ **Lacrimal sac:** Normal.
- ❖ **Digital (finger) tension:** Normal.

I. **Provisional diagnosis:** Aphakia—RE/LE

Self-assessment Questionnaire

1. **Define aphakia:**
   - ➢ *Anatomically,* aphakia means absence of crystalline lens from the eyeball.
   - ➢ *But optically,* aphakia means absence of crystalline lens from its normal position (i.e., from the pupillary area).
2. **Causes of aphakia:**
   - ➢ Congenital primary aphakia (very rare).
   - ➢ Operative—cataract operation, needling operation and couching (an ancient form of cataract surgery, where cataractous lens was forcibly pushed backward into the vitreous cavity).
   - ➢ Traumatic/spontaneous dislocation of the lens into the vitreous.
3. **Differences from posterior dislocation of lens (traumatic or spontaneous):**
   - ➢ History of blunt injury to the eye
   - ➢ No history of surgery
   - ➢ No limbal scar mark
   - ➢ No iridectomy mark
   - ➢ Vision is poor even with glasses because of other complications.
   - ➢ Usually, there is no astigmatism
   - ➢ Associated uveitis or secondary glaucoma
4. **Mechanism and causes of iridodonesis:** Normally, iris rests upon the anterior surface of the lens, but in aphakia there is loss of support.
   The causes are:
   - ➢ Aphakia
   - ➢ Subluxation of the lens
   - ➢ Dislocation of the lens
   - ➢ Shrunken sclerotic hypermature cataract
   - ➢ Buphthalmos
   - ➢ Sometimes, in pseudophakia.
5. **Phakia and pseudophakia (definition):**
   - ➢ *Phakia* means eyeball with natural crystalline lens. Normal person is phakic and the eye is called *phakic eye.*
   - ➢ *Pseudophakia* means eyeball with an artificial lens, i.e., with an IOL. The eye is called *pseudophakic eye.*
6. **Normal dioptric power of eye:**
   Total = + 58 D to + 60 D.
   Lens = + 15 D to + 18 D and cornea = 43 D to + 45 D.
7. **What are the optical defects in aphakia?**
   - ➢ High hypermetropia.
   - ➢ Astigmatism *"against the rule"*, since cornea is flatter in vertical meridian than the horizontal. This due to fibrosis or contraction of limbal scar.
   - ➢ Loss of accommodation.
8. **Treatment of aphakia:**
   - ➢ Spectacles correction
   - ➢ Contact lens

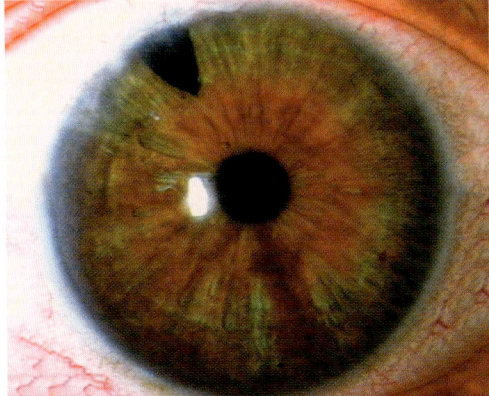

Fig. 2.4: Aphakia.

- Secondary intraocular lens (IOL) implantation:
  - Anterior chamber IOL (AC IOL)
  - Posterior chamber scleral fixation IOL (SF IOL), also called glued IOL
  - Iris retro-fixated posterior chamber IOL
  - Sulcus-supported posterior chamber IOL, if posterior capsue is intact.
9. **Prescription of aphakic glasses:** If the patient is emmetropic preoperatively—the spectacles power will be approximately for:
   - Distant vision = + 10.0 D Sph with + 2.00 D Cyl × 180°
   - Near vision = + 13.0 D Sph with + 2.00 D Cyl × 180°

   Two glasses are given separately for distant and near vision. Bifocal glasses are usually not prescribed, because the patient cannot tolerate the high plus-power bifocal glasses due to more spherical and prismatic aberrations.

   + 3.00 D Sph is added to near vision as there is loss of accommodation due to absence of lens in aphakia and the comfortable reading distance is 33 cm (i.e., 100/33 = + 3.0 D).

   Glasses are prescribed usually 4 to 6 weeks after the surgery as by this time proper healing of the wound is completed.

   Aphakia glasses are presently required in operated bilateral congenital cataract before 2 years of age. Here, the spectacle power is approx +14 to +18 D Sph determined after refraction.

10. **Disadvantages of aphakic glasses:**
    - An image magnification of about 25–30%.
    - Spherical aberration producing "pincushion effect".
    - Lack of physical coordination in finer movements.
    - Roving ring scotoma or 'Jack-in-the-box' phenomenon due to high prismatic aberration.
    - Reduced peripheral field and poor eccentric visual acuity.
    - *In monocular cases*—there will be high aniseikonia (difference in retinal image sizes between two eyes) resulting in diplopia.
    - High degree of chromatic aberration.
    - Physical inconvenience and cosmetic deficiency due to thick and heavy aphakic spectacle lenses.

11. **Advantages and disadvantages of contact lens in aphakia:**

    Advantages:
    - Image magnification is about 7–8% and can be well tolerated.
    - All the aberrations are less, so there is increase in visual field and improvement of hand-eye coordination and spatial sensation.
    - In monocular cases, diplopia is almost absent.
    - Cosmetically, it is well accepted.
    - Valuable in unilateral operated congenital cataract before in children

    Disadvantages:
    - Lack of dexterity in old patients.
    - Foreign body sensation.
    - Lens spoilage (due to loss, breakage, dislodgement)—leading to high recurrent expenditure.
    - Corneal problems, like erosions, ulceration, vascularization, edema, etc., may be troublesome in future.

12. **Advantages and disadvantages of IOL implantation (pseudophakia):**

    Advantages:
    - Image magnification is virtually nil.
    - No spherical or prismatic aberration.
    - No aniseikonia—so rapid return of binocularity.
    - Normal peripheral visual field and eccentric vision.
    - Freedom from handling the optical devices (e.g., contact lens or heavy spectacles).
    - Good hand-eye coordination and spatial sensation.
    - Cosmetically, best accepted by the patient.

Disadvantages:
- Risks and complications are more in inexperienced hands, e.g., corneal decompensation, lens displacement, iridocyclitis, posterior capsular rent with vitreous loss, PCO (after cataract) formation, etc.
- Needs special trained surgeons, operative microscope and other microsurgical instruments.
- Initially, it appears costly.

13. **Intraocular lens details:** *See* page 181.

PSEUDOPHAKIA *(OP 7.3)*

A. **Patient's particulars:**
B. **Chief complaints with duration:**
- History of cataract microsurgery operation in R/E or L/E on ....
- Associated dimness of vision for near and/or distant without glasses

C. **History of present illness:** Patient complains of difficulty in near vision without glasses. Patient also gives the history of irritation and watering of the operated eye for few days/months. No other significant history.

D. **Past history:** Nothing significant

E. **Medical history:** Diabetes, hypertension, cardiac problems on anticoagulants (blood thinners), COPD, etc.

F. **Surgical history:** History of cataract surgery with IOL implantation in the same eye .... weeks/months/years back. There were no complications during or immediately after the cataract surgery.

G. **Personal and allergy history:** Allergy to any eye drops, or systemic drug, alcohol intake, smoking, etc.

H. **General examination:** Overall built, obesity, pallor, etc.

Check BP, pulse and oxygen saturation (PO_2), if possible. Look carefully for any lung and cardiac problem.

I. **Ocular examination:**
- **Vision:** (a) Uncorrected: ... (b) with glasses: ... and (c) Pin-hole vision: ....
- **Eye lids:** Normal
- **Conjunctiva:** Scar mark may be present at superior or temporal bulbar conjunctiva. In early postoperative period, there may be patchy area of subconjunctival hemorrhage.
- **Cornea:** Minimal scarring 2 mm inside from limbus in manual SICS or phacoemulsification. Limbal scar with interrupted suture marks from 2–10 o'clock position at the upper part. Also 1–2 small side port marks.
- **Sclera:** A frown-shaped incision mark (5.5–6.5 mm in length) is seen superiorly.
- **Anterior chamber:** Normal or slightly deeper.
- **Iris:** Brown, patchy areas of iris atrophy, peripheral iridectomy mark may be present. Iridodonesis may be present.
- **Pupil:** Shiny glassy reflex of intraocular lens is observed in the pupillary area. Direct and consensual reaction present **(Fig. 2.5A)**.
- **Lens:** Reflex (seen as 3rd Purkinje's image) from intraocular lens present **(Fig. 2.5B)**. There may be posterior capsular opacification (PCO) which is appreciated through dilated pupil.
- **Ocular movements:** Normal
- **Lacrimal sac:** Normal.
- **Digital tension:** Normal.

J. **Provisional diagnosis:** Pseudophakia in RE/LE.

Self-assessment Questionnaires

1. **Differential diagnosis:** Aphakia
2. **Define pseudophakia:** Pseudophakia means eyeball with an artificial lens, i.e., intraocular lens (IOL). The eye is called *pseudophakic eye*.
3. **Points favor of pseudophakia:**
   - History of cataract surgery with IOL implantation
   - Incision mark at superior or temporal cornea just inside limbus. In manual SICS, a curved (frown) incision about 2 mm away from limbus in the superior area.
   - Shiny glassy reflex of intraocular lens in the pupillary area.

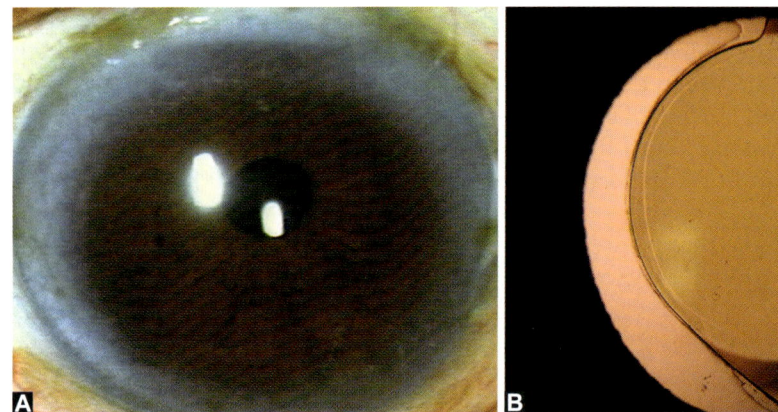

Figs. 2.5A and B: (A) Pseudophakia; (B) Pseudophakia (after dilation).

4. **Probable type of cataract surgery done in this case:** Probably manual SICS or probably phacoemulsification. Before answering check for:
   - Definite history given by the patient
   - Incision length
   - *Site of incision:* In manual SICS, mostly superior. But in phaco, it may be temporal or superior
5. **Type of IOL implanted in this case:** Posterior chamber IOL. In manual SICS, it is mostly PMMA IOL and in phaco, it is usually a foldable IOL (hydrophobic or hydrophilic)
6. **Differentiate between pseudophakia and aphakia (Table 2.3):**
7. **Advantage of pseudophakia over aphakia:** See page 28
8. **Parts of intraocular lens:** (See page 182).
9. **Types of IOL:** (See page 181).
10. **IOL power calculation:** There are many ways to decide on IOL power:
    - *Using standard IOL power (+19D):* No longer acceptable.
    - *Based on 'basic refraction':* Formula for posterior chamber IOL is: $P = +19D + (R \times 1.25)$ (P = IOL power and R = Basic refraction of '+' or '−' power lens).
    - Using SRK formula (SRK = Sanders, Retzlaff and Kraff): $P = A - 2.5 \times AL - 0.9 \times K$ (where P = IOL power, L = axial length, K = average keratometry in diopter and A = specific constant which varies with the type of IOL and written in IOL box).

TABLE 2.3: Differentiate between pseudophakia and aphakia.

	Pseudophakia	Aphakia
Surgical history from the patient	Cataract surgery with IOL implantation	Without IOL. may had some complication
Incision scar mark	Smaller scar mark in manual SICS, smallest in phaco	Larger incision mark at the limbus
Anterior chamber depth	Slightly deeper than normal	Deep
Iris	No or mild iridodonesis	Obvious iridodonesis
Iridectomy	Absent in most cases	Always present
Pupillary area	Black. Shiny glassy reflex of IOL visible	Jet black pupil
Purkinje's image	3rd image brightly visible	3rd and 4th images—absent

- Axial length (AL) is calculated by USG A-scan, K is calculated by keratometry. Both are manual methods.
- Currently, IOL power calculation is mostly automatic and done with sophisticated machine, called *"Optical Biometry"* (e.g., IOL master, Lenstar, etc.). Here, axial lenghth, keratometry, anterior chamber depth, white to white diameter—all automatically measured and IOL power is calculated according to the choice of specific IOL.

- SRK II or SRK T formula is mostly used for emmetropic eyes
- Barrett universal II formula also gives predictive IOL power
- For long (myopic) eyes—SRK II and Holladay-1 formulas are more accurate
- For very short (hypermetropic) eyes—Hoffer-Q and Holladay-2 formulas are used.
- All formulas are incorporated in current *"Optical biometers"* available in the market.

11. **Relative contraindications of IOL implantation:**
    - Congenital cataract if operated under 2 years of age
    - Rubella cataract
    - Recurrent severe iridocyclitis
    - Microphthalmos
    - Sometimes, in bilateral subluxated/dislocated lens.

12. **Ideal intraocular lens implantation:** Posterior chamber IOL with 'in-the-bag' placement is the "ideal IOL implantation". Because:
    - It is the safest of all IOL implantations.
    - Most physiological as natural crystalline lens.
    - Perfect centering is possible.
    - Pupil remains central, perfectly circular and mobile.
    - Safer for the corneal endothelium, iris and ciliary body.
    - Least chance of iritis, glaucoma and lens displacement.

POSTERIOR CAPSULAR OPACIFICATION (PCO) *(OP 7.4)*

A. **Patient's particulars:**

B. **Chief complaints:** Dimness of vision after cataract surgery—few months/years

C. **History of present illness:** Patient was operated for cataract in R/E or L/E about ..... months/years back. After spectacles correction, patient regained good vision which he enjoyed for sometimes. But now he is complaining of gradual loss of vision both for distant and near, even with corrected glasses. No history of acute pain, redness or watering from the same eye.

D. **Ocular examination:**
  - **Vision:** Uncorrected and with glasses—vision with pin-hole.
  - **Lids:** Normal.
  - **Conjunctiva:** Normal.
  - **Cornea:**
    - A linear scar mark at upper limbus from 3–9 o'clock position, or
    - Minimal scarring 2 mm inside from limbus in manual SICS or phacoemulsification.
    - 1–2 small side port marks at the limbus
    - A point scar may be seen in the cornea on its temporal side (in case of needling for congenital cataract).
  - **Anterior chamber:** Slightly deeper in pseudophakia, or deep in aphakia
  - **Iris:** Iridectomy mark may be present at 11 o'clock and/or at 1 o'clock position. Iridodonesis may be present.
  - **Pupil (after dilatation):**
    - A whitish dense membrane-like structure is seen in the pupillary area in aphakia, or behind the IOL in pseudophakia
    - Pupil—normal; may be irregular and with posterior synechiae
  - **Lens:** Absence of 3rd and 4th Purkinje's images.
  - **Digital tension:** Normal.

E. **Provisional diagnosis:** Posterior capsular opacification (PCO).

Self-assessment Questionnaires

1. **Define PCO:** It is the whitish opacity that follows extracapsular cataract extraction (ECCE) or discission (needling) in congenital cataract. It is also known as secondary cataract. Previously, it was called as "After-cataract".
   Posterior capsular opacification or PCO is a new terminology for after-cataract as the term 'after-cataract' is confusing, especially to the layman.
2. **Mechanism of formation of PCO:**
   - Even after good cortical cleaning, the cuboidal cells lining the periphery

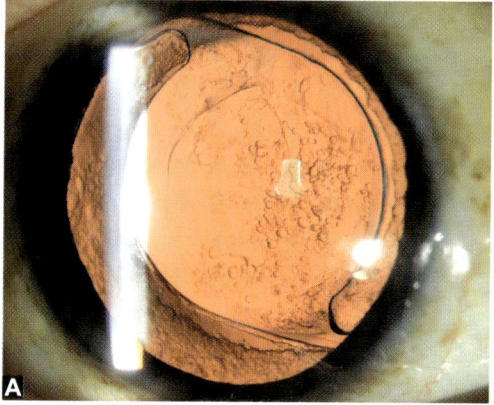
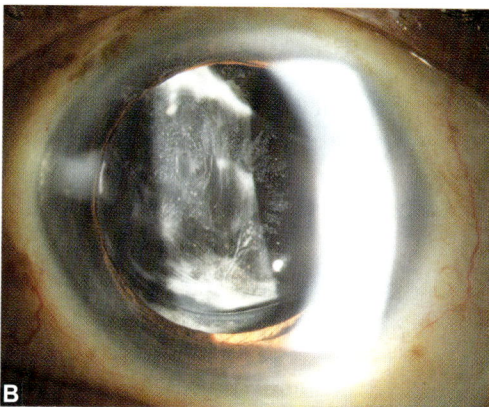

Figs. 2.6A and B: (A) PCO with Elschnig's pearl; (B) PCO: Fibrous type.

of the anterior capsule and equator, continue to grow to form new lens fibers. These lens fibers under the abnormal conditions are abortive and opaque.
- This gets partially absorbed by the action of the aqueous, but often gets entrapped by adhesion of the remnants of anterior capsule to the posterior capsule.
- Along with it, inflammatory materials (form iridocyclitis) or fibrin (from hyphema)—may also contribute to the formation of PCO.

3. **Types of PCO:**
   - *Elschnig pearls:* Sometimes, the sub-capsular cuboidal cells instead of forming lens fibre, develop into large balloon-like cells which fill the pupillary aperture. This balloon lens cell looks like pearl and is known as Elschnig's pearl **(Fig. 2.6A)**.
   - *Fibrous PCO:* When the PCO originates from abnormal lens fibers and it appears as whitish thin sheet **(Fig. 2.6B)**.

4. **Define Soemmerring's ring:** It is a ring behind the iris formed by the lens fibers enclosed between the two layers of the lens capsule. It is found in some cases of PCO, with incomplete cleaning of peripheral cortical. It may be visible after full dilatation of the pupil.

5. **PCO rate:** Incidence varies between 1% to 100%.
   - In pediatric cataract, the incidence is almost 100% even after best surgery and best IOL. That is why a posterior capsular opening (posterior capsulorhexis—PCCC) is done along with in-the-bag IOL implantation.
   - PCO rate is also higher—with younger age, with PMMA IOL, round-edge optic, and also with hydrophilic IOL.
   - PCO rate is lower—in elderly patients, mature/hypermature cataracts, with hydrophobic and silicon IOLs, and also with square-edge design IOLs.
   - *Capsulorrhexis size should be optimum (5.0–5.5 mm) so that the rhexis margin should cover nicely the IOL-optic all 360° in case of in-the-bag implantation.*

6. **Treatment of PCO:**
   - *Nd-YAG (Neodymium Yttrium Aluminum Garnet)* laser capsulotomy—useful in ECCE with IOL and subsequent formation of PCO. This laser acts by photodisruption of tissues.
   Advantages: It is non-invasive OPD procedure without any chance of infection. It is also very safe and painless.
   - *Discission or needling:* If the PCO is thicker membrane—the opening can be done with the help of a Bowman's needle or Zeigler's knife.
   - Alternately, very thick PCO can be removed by a vitreous cutter.

Repeated needling or YAG capsulotomy disturbs the anterior face of the vitreous and subsequently the vitreous gets organized at places which may lead to retinal detachment in future.

PTERYGIUM (OP 3.6)

A. **Patient particulars:**
B. **Chief complaints:**
- Slowly progressive fleshly mass on inner side of the white of R/E or L/E for 1 year or more
- Persistent redness on inner side of eye for same duration

C. **History of present illness:** The patient was apparently all right few months to years back. The appearance of fleshy mass with redness is gradual, painless and slowly progressive. The look of the eye is cosmetically unacceptable to the patient. No improvement with application of different eye drops. There is no history of diplopia.

D. **Medical history:**

E. **Surgical history:** May be present (if it is present, note the date and type of surgery).

F. **Personal history:** Patient spends several hours in sunlight for some outdoor activities.

G. **Family history:** Nothing significant.

H. **Systemic examination:**

I. **Ocular examination:**
- **Visual acuity:** Uncorrected:.....; with glasses: ......; with pin-hole:........
- **Ocular movements:** Normal; or may be restricted in recurrent type.
- **Eye lids:** Normal.
- **Conjunctiva and cornea:**
  - A wing-shaped triangular vascularized fleshly mass arising from nasal side of the conjunctiva (rarely temporal) and encroaching towards the cornea about ... mm inside the limbus.
  - The upper and lower borders of the mass appear folded
  - A faint white semilunar opacity in the cornea just in front of the apex of the mass.
  - Rest of the cornea is normal.
    [Always draw a line diagram of the mass in reference to limbus and pupil.]
- **Sclera:** Normal
- **Anterior chamber:** Normal
- **Iris and pupil:** Normal
- **Lens:** Normal. There may be associated cataract.
- **Lacrimal sac:** Normal
- **Digital tension:** Normal

J. **Provisional diagnosis:** Pterygium (may be progressive or atrophic).

May be recurrent pterygium (if there is history of operation of pterygium in the same eye).

Self-assessment Questionnaires

1. **Differential diagnosis:** Pseudopterygium
2. **Define pterygium (literal meaning—wing):** It is a degenerative condition of the sub-conjunctival tissues which proliferate as a triangular vascularized fleshy tissue-mass to invade the cornea involving the Bowman's membrane the whole thing being covered by the conjunctival epithelium.
3. **Points favor for pterygium:**
   - Painless, triangular fleshy mass from conjunctiva encroaching over the cornea
   - The apex of this triangular mass is on the cornea
   - Vascularized and pink-red in color
   - Situated in the nasal side of interpalpebral area
4. **Points in favor of "progressive" type:**
   - History of gradual increase in size
   - Thick and fleshy appearance
   - vascularized and reddish in color
   - A faint semilunar opacity (cap) is present in front of apex or head
5. **Types of pterygium:**
   True:
   - *Progressive:* It is thick, fleshy with prominent vascularity, and gradually increasing in size and encroaching towards the central part of the cornea. Cap is present **(Fig. 2.7A)**.
   - *Atrophic or stationary:* It is thin, attenuated with poor vascularity. No progression is seen. Cap is absent **(Fig. 2.7B)**.

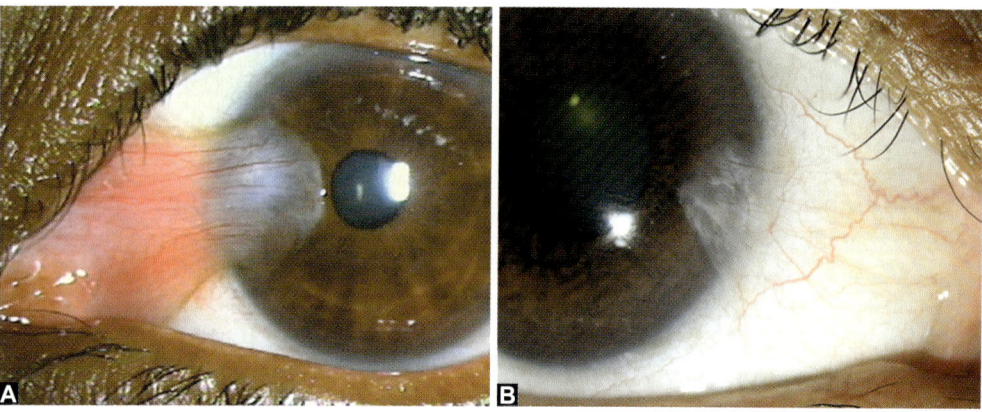

Figs. 2.7A and B: (A) Progressive pterygium; (B) Atrophic pterygium.

Pseudo (false)
6. **Differences between true and pseudo-pterygium (Table 2.4)**
7. **Grade of pterygium (Table 2.5):**
8. **Etiology:** Not precisely, known but few factors are responsible.
    ➢ *Ultraviolet irradiation:* Pterygium is more common among farmers and outdoor workers.
    ➢ Hot, sandy and dusty weather.
    ➢ More in tropical countries, where UV radiation is maximum.
    ➢ Pinguecula may be a precursor.
9. **Parts of a pterygium (Fig. 2.8):**
    ➢ *Apex or head:* Apex of the triangular mass.
    ➢ *Neck:* Constricted portion at the limbus.
    ➢ *Body:* Remaining bulky part beneath the conjunctiva.

TABLE 2.4: Differences between true and pseudo-pterygium.

True pterygium	*Pseudo-pterygium*
1. Found in elderly persons	1. Found at any age
2. Usually, bilateral	2. Usually, unilateral
3. Degenerative process	3. Inflammatory process
4. Always in the interpalpebral area and more on nasal side	4. At any meridian
5. Progressive; sometimes stationary	5. Always stationary
6. Previous history of pain, redness absent	6. Previous history of pain, redness present
7. Probe cannot be passed under the neck of the true pterygium	7. Probe can be passed underneath the neck of the pseudo-pterygium

TABLE 2.5: Grade of pterygium.

Grade	Extent	Problems
Grade I	<2 mm onto the cornea	• Usually, asymptomatic • Occasionally red • Cosmetic blemish
Grade II	2–4 mm onto the cornea	• Usually, red and flesh • Distort corneal topography • Induces "against the rule" astigmatism
Grade III	>4 mm onto the cornea	• Involves visual axis • More visual loss • Can extend up to medial canthus with limitation of movement

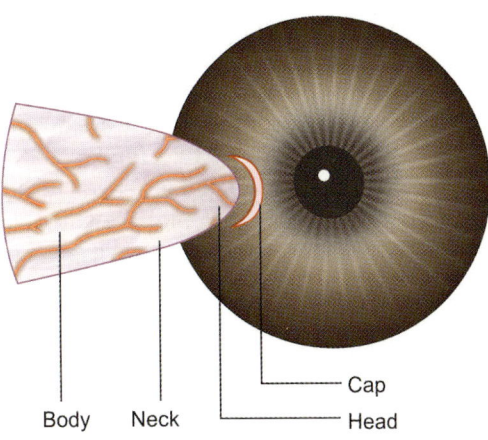

Fig. 2.8: Parts of a pterygium.

- *Cap:* A semilunar white opacity may present just in front of the apex or head.

10. **Visual problems with pterygium:**
    - *Dimness of vision:*
        - This is due to induced astigmatism due to corneal flattening in the axis of pterygium
        - Obstruction of visual axis when the pterygium covers the pupil.
    - *Diplopia:* This is rare and due to limitation of ocular movement.

11. **Management:**
    - *Atrophic pterygium or if it is just at the limbus* is best left alone with periodic follow-up of the patient.
    - *Progressive pterygium: Treatment of choice* is pterygium excision, and the bare sclera is covered with conjunctival autograft.
    - Bare sclera may be covered by human amniotic membrane.
    - Bare sclera may be treated with mitomycin C (0.02%) during the surgery.
    - *Recurrence after pterygium surgery is common (2–50%).*
    - *In Recurrent pterygium* (and also to prevent recurrence):
        - The bare sclera is covered *with conjunctival limbal autograft.*
        - After excision of pterygium, the bare scleral area is treated with—mitomycin-C (0.02%)—locally during operation or as drop postoperatively.
    - Lamellar keratoplasty of the affected area of the cornea.

- *If the pterygium involves the pupillary area:* Resection of pterygium with anterior lamellar keratoplasty may be required along with conjunctival autograft.

PHLYCTENULAR CONJUNCTIVITIS (OP 3.3)

A. **Patient particulars:**
B. **Chief complaints:**
   ❖ Redness with formation of nodule(s) or bleb(s) on the white of R/E or L/E for ….
   ❖ Watering and irritation for same duration.
   ❖ Pain and photophobia may be present (if the cornea is also involved).
C. **History of present illness:**
D. **Past history:** Similar problem may be present.
E. **Personal history:** Rhinitis, chronic tonsillitis, adenoids, tuberculosis, sore throat, otitis media, etc.
F. **General examination:** Upper respiratory tract and chest. Examine for lymph nodes of the neck.
G. **Ocular examination:**
   ❖ **Visual acuity:** Normal
   ❖ **Lids:** Normal; matting of the eyelashes may be present.
   ❖ **Conjunctiva:**
      - One or multiple small, round and raised nodule(s), (… mm in diameter), gray or pinkish-white in color on bulbar conjunctiva at or near the limbus.
      - Localized bulbar congestion surrounding the bleb.
      - The bleb may be ulcerated.
      - Discharge and whole conjunctiva may be congested.
   ❖ **Cornea:**
      - Usually, normal.
      - Similar nodule may be on the cornea, adjacent to the limbus.
      - Ciliary congestion may be seen on adjacent conjunctiva.
   ❖ *Sclera, anterior chamber, iris and pupil, lens, digital tension and lacrimal sac*—all normal.

H. Provisional diagnosis: Phlyctenular conjunctivitis, or phlyctenular kerato-conjunctivitis (if the cornea is involved simultaneously).

Self-assessment Questionnaires

1. **Define phlycten (*means—bleb*):** It is an allergic condition of the conjunctiva caused by endogenous bacterial toxins, characterized by bleb formation. Histologically, it is composed of a compact mass of mononuclear lymphocytes and polymorphs.
2. **Casual factors:** Endogenous bacterial toxins
   - Tuberculosis or
   - Nonspecific lymphadenitis
   - Chronic tonsillitis or adenoids *(Streptococcal or Staphylococcal)*
   - Chronic suppurative otitis media
3. **Types of clinical presentation:**
   - When conjunctiva alone is involved—*phlyctenular conjunctivitis* (**Fig. 2.9A**).
   - When at the limbus, and both the conjunctiva and cornea are involved—*phlyctenular keratoconjunctivitis* (**Fig. 2.9B**).
   - When cornea only is involved—*phlyctenular keratitis*.
4. **Treatment:**
   - *Local:*
     - Steroid (like, dexamethasone, fluorometholone or Loteprednol) drops—4 to 6 times daily.
     - If it is secondarily infected—first treat conjunctivitis with topical antibiotic (ciprofloxacin or gatifloxacin) drops. Then treat with local steroids.
     - *When cornea is involved:* Cycloplegics, like homatropine eye drop—3 times daily is to be added.
   - *General:* Improvement of general health by vitamins, minerals, nutritious diet, etc.
   - *Treatment of the causal factor:* If any, e.g.,
     - Treatment of tuberculosis.
     - Treatment of upper respiratory tract infection.
     - Treatment of adenoids or tonsillitis, etc.
5. **Investigations:** It is only indicated if the phlycten is multiple or recurrent in nature. They are:
   - Blood for TLC, DLC, ESR and Hb.
   - Mantoux test.
   - X-ray chest (PA).
   - ENT consultation to exclude chronic tonsillitis or adenoids.
6. **Complications of phlycten:**
   - Ulcerations,
   - Corneal involvement (keratitis),
   - Phlyctenular pannus,
   - Fascicular ulcer, and rarely, ring ulcer.
7. **Differential diagnosis of nodules at the limbus:**
   - *Phlyctenular conjunctivitis:* Young patients, at or away from the limbus, at any clock-hour, small bleb-like lesion with surrounding vessels, may be with poor nutrition with tubercular diathesis or chronic adenoids.

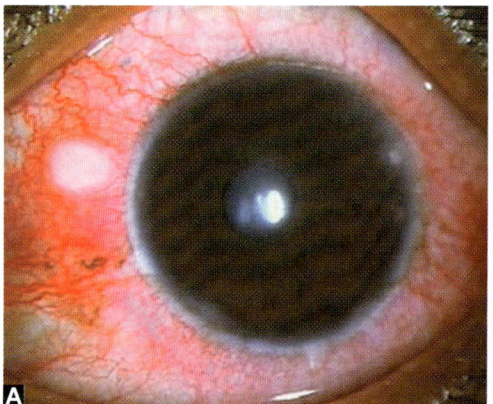 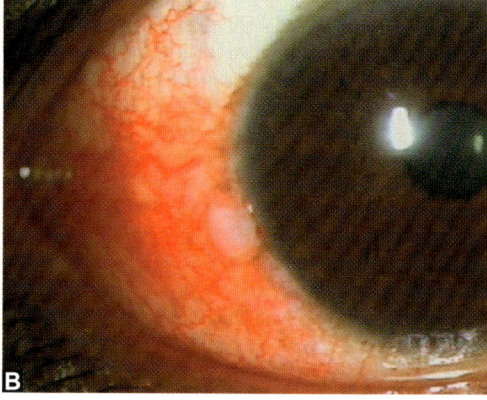

Figs. 2.9A and B: (A) Phlyctenular conjunctivitis; (B) Limbal phlycten.

- *Inflamed pinguecula:* Elderly subject; away from the limbus at nasal side in horizontal plane; triangular with apex towards medial canthus; bilateral similar lesion; well defined and moves with the conjunctiva.
- *Nodular episcleritis or scleritis:* Aged patient; away from the limbus at any place; usually unilateral; painful and tender; larger and not well defined; it does not move with the conjunctiva.
- *Limbal dermoid:* Usually in children; present since birth; mostly inferotemporal in location; commonly involves the cornea; epidermis like structures and hair may be present.
- *Vernal keratoconjunctivitis (limbal form)*
- *Ocular surface squamous neoplasia (OSSN)*
- *Ciliary staphyloma*
- *Cystic changes of pterygium*
- *Pyogenic granuloma after pterygium excision*
- *Post-trabeculectomy cystic bleb*

SUBCONJUNCTIVAL HEMORRHAGE (OP 3.2 AND 9.5)

A. **Chief complaints:**
- Bright red coloration of the white of right or left eye since ….
- History of blunt injury with ball, stone, fist, etc., in the same eye for same duration or history of straining factors.

B. **Medical history:** Bleeding disorder, e.g., purpura

C. **Personal history:** Chronic severe cough (whooping cough or chronic bronchitis), hypertension, vomiting, lifting heavy weight, etc.

D. **General examination:**
  Pulse: BP: Chest:

E. **Ocular examination:**
- **Visual acuity:** Usually normal.
- **Movements:** Normal.
- **Lids:** Black coloration or ecchymosis may be present.
- **Conjunctiva:**
  - Bright red coloration, which is flat homogenous and with sharply defined margin without any branching (**Fig. 2.10**).
  - There may be associated conjunctival chemosis.
  - Posterior limit of the hemorrhage is visible in blunt injury.
- **Cornea:** Normal.
- **Anterior chamber:** Normal.
- **Iris and pupil:** Normal.
- **Lens:** Normal.
- **Digital tension:** Normal.
- **Lacrimal sac:** Normal.

F. **Provisional diagnosis:** Subconjunctival hemorrhage RE or LE.

Self-assessment Questionnaire

1. **Causes of subconjunctival hemorrhage:**
   - *Traumatic:*
     - Due to direct injury to the eyeball and consequently rupture of minute conjunctival blood vessels.
     - Head injury or orbital bony injury. (In head injury—subconjunctival hemorrhage appears late, and posterior limit of the hemorrhage is not visible).
   - *Infective:* Conjunctivitis, *bacterial*, especially due to *Pneumococcus* or *viral* (*hemorrhagic conjunctivitis* due to picoRNA virus), etc.
   - *Mechanical:* Due to venous congestion and subsequent rupture of small vessels,

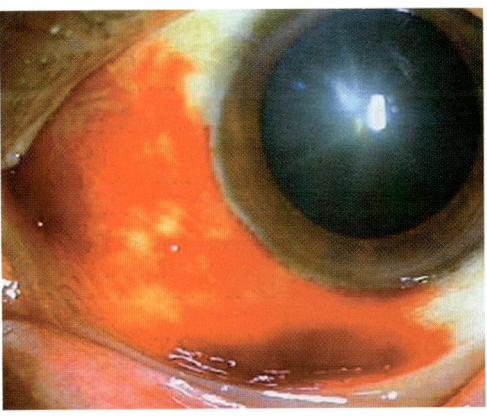

Fig. 2.10: Subconjunctival hemorrhage.

e.g., whooping cough, bronchitis, compression of the neck or chest, etc.
- *Arteriosclerosis and hypertension.*
- *Valsalva maneuver—heavy lifting, straining during constipation.*
- *Blood dyscrasias:* Leukemia, purpura, hemophilia, etc.
- Vicarious menstruation (leading to periodic bloody tears).
- *Idiopathic.*

2. **Site for subconjunctival hemorrhage:** Bulbar conjunctiva is the frequent site for hemorrhage as blood is easily accumulated in the loose subconjunctival tissue.

3. **Fate of subconjunctival hemorrhage:** At first, it is bright red in color. This is because of oxyhemoglobin as it is in constant contact with atmospheric oxygen. Subsequently, it changes to orange-yellow or blackish red, then yellow discoloration, this is due to breakdown of oxyhemoglobin. Ultimately, it gets absorbed within 2–4 weeks depending upon the amount of hemorrhage.

4. **Treatment:**
   - No treatment is necessary in most of the cases, as it is absorbed spontaneously within 2 to 4 weeks. Only assurance to the patient is important.
   - Initially cold compress is helpful as it constricts the blood vessels.
   - Tablet vitamin C (500 mg) may be given orally.
   - In severe cases, if the extravasated blood causes prolapse of the conjunctiva through interpalpebral fissure, subconjunctival space may be punctured to drain the blood.
   - Last but not the least, in selected cases, treatment of the cause, e.g., hypertension, chronic bronchitis, whooping cough, vomiting, etc.

5. **Enumerate the effects of blunt trauma on the eye:** (See page 142).

CORNEAL ULCER (OP 3.1)

A. **Patient particulars:**
Occupation: Farmer/factory worker/laborer

B. **Chief complaints:**
- Acute pain, redness and watering of RE or LE eye for .... days
- Dimness of vision in the same eye for ...

C. **History of present illness:** The patient was apparently alright about 2 weeks back. He gives the history of foreign body or trauma in the same eye. After that he develops acute pain redness and watering from the same eye which are increasing.

He also gives the history of dimness of vision which is increasing. He noticed white spot in the same eye which is also increasing. Patient consulted local doctor who gave some drops and ointment without much help.

There is no history of any recent surgery in that eye.

D. **Past history:** Patient may have similar history in the same eye or other eye, treated medically.

E. **Personal history:** Nothing significant

F. **Medical history:** Patient may be diabetic. No other systemic problem.

G. **Drug history:** There may be history of using topical steroids which was bought by the patient from pharmacy.

H. **Other history:** History of contact lens use.

I. **Systemic examination:** BP, pulse, chest, cardiac status, etc., all within normal limit

J. **Ocular examination:**
- **Vision:** Diminished, may be reduced to PL and PR. Look for accurate PR.
- **Ocular movements:** Full
- **Eye lids:**
  - Red and edematous.
  - Matting of the eyelashes.
  - Blepharospasm.
- **Conjunctiva:**
  - Mucopurulent, serous or purulent discharge.
  - Both conjunctival and circumcorneal ciliary congestion.
  - Chemosis may be present.
- **Cornea:**
  - Hazy, lustreless cornea.
  - Shallow, irregular ulcerated (whitish) area with surrounding infiltration.

[*Note and draw a schematic diagram*: Indicating the site (marginal, central or paracentral), size in mm (small, subtotal or total), shape (oval, round, geographical or ring-shaped) and vascularization].
  ➢ Note for satellite lesions.
  ➢ Or any endothelial plaque.
- **Corneal sensation:** Normal, diminished or absent.
- **Sclera:** Normal.
- **Anterior chamber:** Normal, or hypopyon. Note the height of hypopyon (in mm), its upper border—flat or convex, and whether it is fixed or mobile.
- **Iris:** Associated iritis may be present. May have posterior synechia formation.
- **Pupil:** Normal or dilated due to prior use of cycloplegic drop.
- **Lens:** Normal.
- **Digital tension:** Normal, high (secondary glaucoma due to hypopyon) or low (in case of perforation).
- **Lacrimal Sac:** Normal or may be associated chronic dacryocystitis.

K. **Provisional diagnosis:** Corneal ulcer or corneal ulcer with hypopyon of RE or LE.

Self-assessment Questionnaire *(OP 4.1)*

1. **What is corneal ulcer?** It is defined as a loss of corneal epithelium with underlying stromal infiltration and suppuration associated with signs of inflammation with or without hypopyon **(Fig. 2.11A)**.
2. **Types of corneal ulcer (Keratitis):**
    A. Infective corneal ulcer:
      ♦ Bacterial
      ♦ Fungal
      ♦ Viral
      ♦ Protozoal
    B. Non-infective corneal ulcer:
      ♦ Central:
        ○ Neurotrophic
        ○ Atheromatous
        ○ Following exposure
        ○ Keratomalacia
      ♦ Peripheral:
        ○ Marginal keratitis
        ○ Mooren's ulcer
        ○ Phlyctenular keratitis
        ○ Associated with collagen diseases, e.g., rheumatoid arthritis
3. **Predisposing factors for corneal ulcer:** Intact corneal epithelium cannot be penetrated by any organism except *N. gonorrhoeae* and *C. diphtheriae*. With other organisms, corneal ulcer is invariably associated with one or more of the following *predisposing factors*:
    ➢ Trauma to the corneal epithelium.
    ➢ Underlying corneal diseases, e.g., bullous keratopathy, keratomalacia, punctate keratitis.
    ➢ Neurotrophic or exposure keratopathy.
    ➢ Dry eyes.
    ➢ Dacryocystitis or blepharitis.
    ➢ Use of topical steroids.
    ➢ Vegetable foreign body *in fungal keratitis*.
    ➢ Contact lens wearer or pond bath—for *acanthamoeba*.
    ➢ Nutritional deficiency.
    ➢ Immunocompromised subject.
4. **Stages of corneal ulcer:** Uncomplicated localized corneal ulcer is having four stages:
    Stage 1: Stage of infiltration
    Stage 2: Stage of progression
    Stage 3: Stage of regression
    Stage 4: Stage of cicatrization
5. **What is hypopyon?** In any corneal ulcer, there is an associated iritis due to toxin being absorbed into the anterior chamber. This reaction is so toxic that leukocytosis takes place and PMNs pour out of the blood vessels into the aqueous and gravitate at the bottom of the anterior chamber. This is hypopyon and this pus remains sterile so long as the Descemet's membrane is intact except in fungal ulcer with hypopyon which may contain hyphae (fungal elements).
6. **Hypopyon corneal ulcer:** It is a typical bacterial ulcer which has a tendency to creep over the cornea in a serpiginous fashion and associated with hypopyon and violent iridocyclitis (also known as *ulcus serpens*).

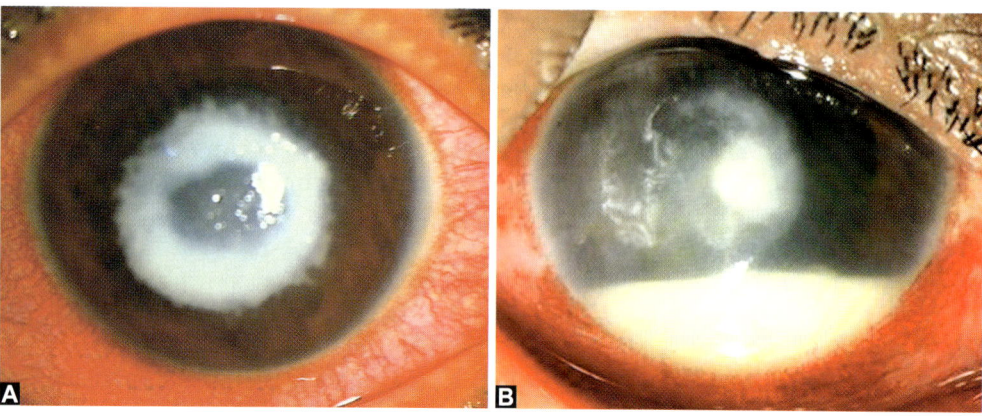

Figs. 2.11A and B: (A) Corneal ulcer; (B) Corneal ulcer with hypopyon.

It is caused by *Pneumococcus* and has a great tendency for early perforation.

It must be noted that any corneal ulcer (either bacterial or fungal) may be associated with hypopyon, and these are called 'corneal ulcer with hypopyon' **(Fig. 2.11B)**.

7. **Terminology of corneal ulcer:**
   - *Localized/focal:* Small to medium ulcer with strong tissue resistance.
   - *Perforating:* When ulcer penetrates through the corneal substance causing perforation.
   - *Sloughing:* When ulcer spreads so much that total or subtotal cornea sloughs off.
   - *Descemetocele (keratocele):* Herniation of the elastic Descemet's membrane through the ulcer as a transparent vesicle.
   - *Corneal abscess:* It is a localized collection of pus in the substance of cornea. Here, the corneal epithelium is usually intact.

8. **Fate of a corneal ulcer:**
   - Corneal ulcer usually heals with the formation of corneal scar. Depending upon the density it may be *nebula, macula* or *leucoma*.
   - It may perforate:
     - Smaller perforation → Iris prolapse → Adherent leucoma.
     - Larger perforation → Phthisis bulbi.
     - Larger perforation → Pseudocornea formation → Anterior staphyloma.
   - Infection may spread further into the deeper tissue → Panophthalmitis.
   - Very rarely, in case of small ulcers, it heals completely without leaving any scar formation.

9. **Relative advantages of perforation:** (See page 46).

10. **Complications of perforated corneal ulcer:** They vary according to the location and size of the perforation:
    - Adherent leucoma or anterior synechiae.
    - Due to leakage of aqueous, lens come forward with or without subluxation.
    - Anterior polar cataract when the perforation is at the center
    - Large perforation may lead to phthisis bulbi.
    - Large perforation, then pseudocornea formation which organizes, leading to anterior staphyloma.
    - Infection may spread further into the deeper tissue leading to panophthalmitis.
    - Choroidal detachment or may be frank expulsive hemorrhage due to sudden lowering of intraocular pressure.

11. **Clinical features of different types of infective corneal ulcer:**
    A. Bacterial (Fig. 2.12):
       - Mucopurulent or purulent discharge.
       - Wet look of the ulcer.
       - Surrounding area is edematous.
       - May be with mobile hypopyon and iritis.

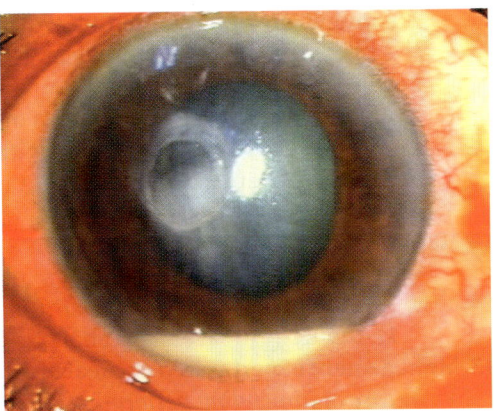

Fig. 2.12: Bacterial corneal ulcer.

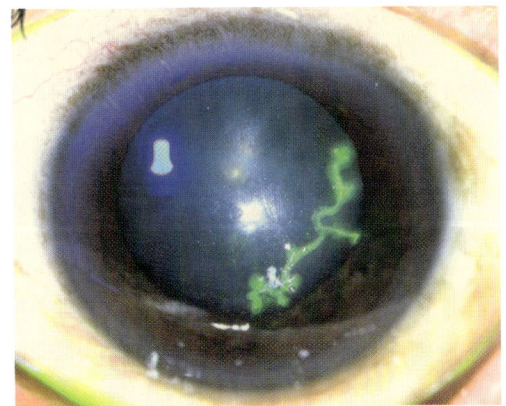

Fig. 2.14: Herpetic keratitis.

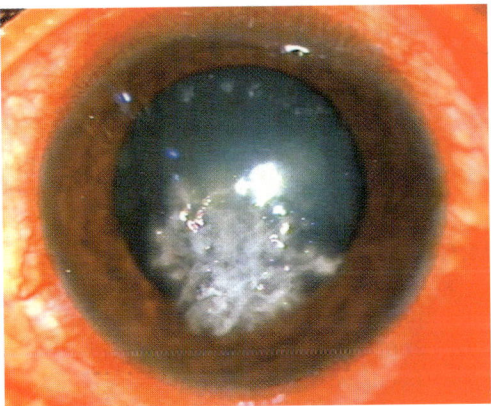

Fig. 2.13: Fungal corneal ulcer.

- Symptoms are proportionate with the signs.
- Corneal sensation is not affected.
- Rapid progression of the ulcer.

B. **Fungal (Fig. 2.13):**
- History of trauma with vegetable matters.
- Dry look of the ulcer.
- Raised from the surface.
- Infiltrates have feathery margins.
- Satellite lesions.
- Fixed (non-mobile) hypopyon with convex border.
- Endothelial plaque.
- Symptoms are less severe than the signs.
- Slow progression of the ulcer.

C. **Viral (Fig. 2.14):**
- Serous discharge.
- Usually superficial ulcer with less infiltration.
- Hypopyon is usually absent.
- Corneal sensation is diminished/absent.
- A positive Rose Bengal and fluorescein staining.
- Symptoms are more severe than the signs.
- Slow progression of the ulcer.

D. **Acanthamoebal (Fig. 2.15):**
- History of contact lens or bathing in swimming pool or pond.
- Pain is severe due to radial keratoneuritis.
- Lesion is raised above the surface.
- Ring-shaped lesion.
- Chronic indolent ulcer.

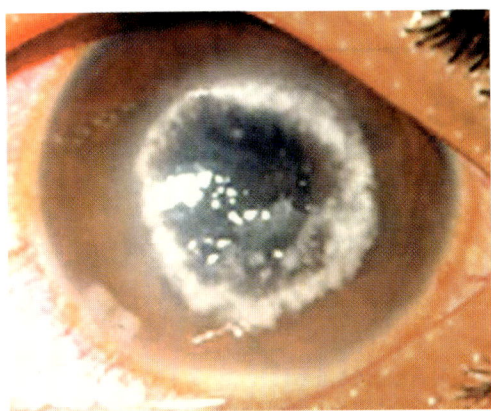

Fig. 2.15: Acanthamoebal keratitis.

- Not responding to conventional antimicrobial treatment.

12. **Treatment of corneal ulcer:**
    A. **Identification of organism:**
       - *Scraping and smear preparation:*
         - Gram stain
         - KOH mount preparation for fungal identification
         - Giemsa stain
       - *Culture:*
         - Bacterial (blood agar/chocolate agar/glucose broth)
         - Fungal (Saboraud's dextrose agar or potato dextrose agar)
    B. **Aggressive treatment with topical antibiotics/antifungals—according to smear report:**
       - Topical commercial broad-spectrum preparations, e.g., hourly moxifloxacin, gatifloxacin, ciprofloxacin, tobramycin, etc.
       - Topical fortified (concentrated) preparations, e.g., *cefazoline, tobramycin, vancomycin, or amikacin, etc.*—1 hourly
       - Sub-conjunctival injection of antibiotic and atropine.
       - Systemic antibiotic: Only required if there is:
         - Marginal corneal ulcer.
         - Perforating corneal ulcer.
         - Large sloughed-out corneal ulcer.
         - If the sclera is involved.
       - *For suspected fungal ulcer treatment with antifungal drugs*: Topical natamycin (5%), amphotericin B (0.15%) or voriconazole hourly, and systemic fluconazole, ketoconazole, or itraconazole.
    C. **Atropine sulphate (1%) eye drops:** 3 times daily to prevent ciliary spasm and control of iritis. It also prevents synechia formation and breaks away any existing synechia.
    D. **Analgesics with antacids.**
    E. **Oral and topical antiglaucoma preparation to control IOP.**
    F. **Treatment is to be continued according to sensitivity reports** till the ulcer gets healed.
    G. **If not responding to medical treatment:** Repeated debridement with repeat culture and sensitivity report is necessary.
    H. **Still if it does not respond:**
       - Temporary tarsorrhaphy
       - *And finally, therapeutic penetrating keratoplasty* to save the eyeball.

13. **Management of perforated corneal ulcer:**
    ▸ *In case of impending perforation:* Keep the IOP at lower level; and temporary tarsorrhaphy.
    ▸ *In frank perforation:*
       - If it is <2 mm—cyanoacrylate glue (tissue adhesive) with bandage contact lens (TA BCL)
       - If it is >2 mm—therapeutic penetrating keratoplasty. Alternately, Tenon's patch graft or amniotic membrane graft

14. **Causes of non-healing corneal ulcer:**
    ▸ *General cause:* Diabetes, malnutrition, patients on systemic steroids or immunosuppressants
    ▸ *Local causes:*
       - Wrong diagnosis or treatment without microbiology work up
       - Multidrug resistant organisms
       - Secondary glaucoma
       - Retained foreign body embedded within ulcer
       - Associated chronic dacryocystitis
       - Trichiatic eyelashes or entropion
       - Lagophthalmos
       - Dry eye, etc.

LEUCOMA (OP 4.5)

A. **Patient's particulars:**
   Occupation: Agriculture worker/factory worker/building labor

B. **Chief complaints:** White opacity and dimness of vision in RE or LE eye for ...

C. **History of present illness:** Patient was otherwise normal about few months or years back. He had history of acute pain, redness and watering of same eye and treated. White opacity developed after the treatment with dimness of vision. The symptoms remain stationary and not increasing.

D. **Past history:**
- A definite history of corneal ulcer in the same eye, or
- History of injury (mechanical, thermal or chemical)

E. **Medical history:** Otherwise not significant. Enquire about diabetic status.

F. **Personal history:** Nothing significant.

G. **Family history:** Nothing significant.

H. **Systemic investigations:** All vitals are normal

I. **Ocular examination:**
- **Vision:** Diminished, may be reduced to PL and PR. PR may be inaccurate. PH vision: may improve or remain same.
- **Eye lids:** Normal.
- **Ocular movements:** Full; there may be divergent squint of the involved eye
- **Conjunctiva:** Normal. In peripheral ulcer—there may be pannus formation
- **Cornea:**
  - *Type of opacity:* Nebula, macula or leucoma, or mixed **(Figs. 2.16A and B).**
  - *Site of opacity:* In relation to pupillary area and limbus.
  - *Size of opacity:* Approximate size in mm.
  - *Shape of opacity:* Linear, circular, oval or irregular.
  - *Vascularization:* Present or not; its extent (quadrant-wise) and type—superficial or deep, if it is present.
  - *Iris adherence:* Present or not; if present, note the extent of adherence and the shape of the pupil.
  - Any pigmentation
  - *Corneal sensation:* Present/reduced/absent.
    [Draw a schematic diagram indicating the site, size, shape and vascularization, etc. of the opacity.]
- **Sclera:** Normal.
- **Anterior chamber:** Normal or may be shallow.
- **Iris:** Normal or posterior synechia
- **Pupil:** Normal and reaction to light present.
- **Lens:** Normal or complicated cataract formation
- **Digital tension:** Normal.
- **Lacrimal sac:** Regurgitation present or not.
  (If the opacity is dense, i.e., *leucomatous and large, the deeper structures would not be visible through the cornea. Mention it.)*

J. **Provisional diagnosis:** Leucomatous corneal opacity RE or LE; or macular corneal opacity; or total (vascularized) leucomatous corneal opacity, etc.

Self-assessment Questionnaire

1. **Cause of corneal opacity in this particular case:** Probably healed corneal ulcer with scar formation

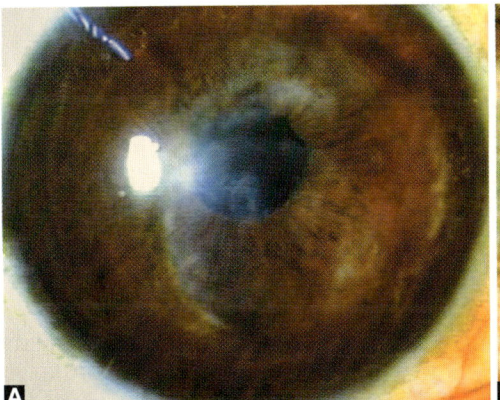 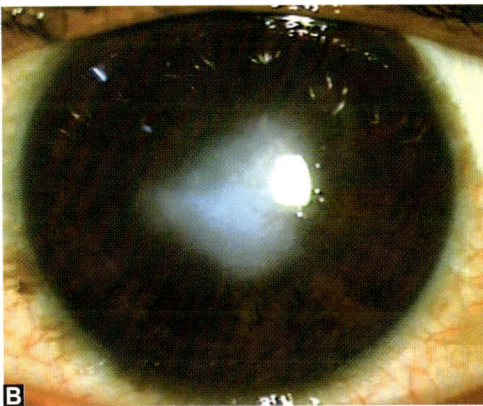

Figs. 2.16A and B: (A) Macular corneal opacity; (B) Leucomatous corneal opacity.

2. **What are the other causes of corneal opacity?**
   - *Congenital:* Central corneal opacity as in Peter's anomaly.
   - *Traumatic:* Blunt trauma, foreign body or penetrating injury.
   - *Chemical burn:* Acid or alkali burn
   - *Metabolic:* Mucopolysacharridosis (MPS)
   - *Hereditary:* Corneal dystrophy.
   - *Degenerative:* Band shaped keratopathy.
   - *Nutritional:* Vitamin A deficiency leading to keratomalacia.
   - *Surgical:* After any corneal surgery (e.g., pterygium).
3. **Differential diagnosis in this case:** Adherent leucoma; corneal degeneration; corneal dystrophy
4. **In case of corneal ulcer, the other fates beside a corneal opacity:**
   - Ulcer may penetrate into deeper tissue → Descemetocele → Perforation and phthisis bulbi.
   - Iridocyclitis → Hypopyon → Secondary glaucoma.
   - Ulcer may spread further → Sloughs out → Pseudocornea formation by fibrinous exudates → Secondary glaucoma → Anterior staphyloma.
   - Ulcer may spread deeper → Panophthalmitis.
5. **Define different types (grades) of corneal opacity:**
   - *Nebula:* It is the finest corneal opacity which is barely detectable with a torch light. It is due to damage of Bowman's layer only.
   - *Macula:* It is little more dense opacity, and the underlying structures are hazily visible through the opacity. It is due to damage of the Bowman's membrane and anterior corneal stroma.
   - *Leucoma:* It is the densest opacity, and the underlying structures are not visible through the opacity. It is due to damage of full thickness cornea.
   [A *nebular opacity in the pupillary region may be more harmful than a small clear cut leucoma. Because nebula causes irregular astigmatism which can only be treated with a contact lens whereas a small leucoma cuts only a few rays going inside the eye.*]
6. **Differences between superficial and deep vascularization (Table 2.6):**

TABLE 2.6: Differences between superficial and deep vascularization.

Superficial vascularization	Deep vascularization
1. Can be traced over the limbus into the conjunctiva	1. Seems to come from an abrupt end at the limbus
2. Bright red and well defined	2. Greyish red (red blush); ill defined
3. Branches in an arborescent fashion and runs dichotomously	3. Branches at acute angles and runs in a radial fashion
4. May raise the epithelium over them and corneal surface is uneven	4. Deep inside the stroma and corneal surface remains smooth

7. **Investigations in this case:**
   - *Ocular:* Good photographic documentation; anterior segment OCT to know the depth of scar; syringing for NLD patency; USG B-scan to evaluate posterior segment.
   - *Systemic:* BP; blood sugar; ECG; serology; physician's clearance for surgery, etc.
8. **Treatment of a corneal opacity:**
   Nebula: A contact lens is best to overcome irregular astigmatism.
   Macula or leucoma:
   - *Peripheral:* No treatment is necessary except refraction for optical reason
   - *If paracentral:* Atropine eye drop—once daily and refraction for better vision. But for cosmetic reason (also for central opacity with no PL or inaccurate PR):
     - Tattooing: Means coloring the cornea with chemical agents. Chemicals must be freshly prepared.
       - For brown coloration (against the iris): 4% gold chloride + 2% hydrazine hydrate (a reducing agent).

○ For black coloration (pupillary area): 2% platinum chloride + 2% hydrazine hydrate.
♦ Cosmetic soft contact lens.
➢ *Central opacity with good visual potential:*
♦ Ideally, full thickness or penetrating keratoplasty (PK) is considered for optical purpose.
♦ Optical iridectomy may be considered where the facilities of PK are not available.
♦ Anterior Lamellar keratoplasty (partial thickness) or deep anterior lamellar keratoplasty (DALK) may also be considered for superficial scars with good endothelial layer.
9. **Prognosis of PK in corneal opacity:**
➢ *If it is central and without vascularization:* Prognosis is good
➢ *If it is vascularized:* Prognosis is poor
10. **If left untreated, what changes that can occur in leucoma:**
➢ Pigmentation with Hudson-Stahli line
➢ More vascularization
➢ Hyaline degeneration
➢ Secondary calcific degeneration

ADHERENT LEUCOMA (OP 4.5)

A. The history and **presenting features** of an adherent leucoma are similar to those of a leucoma. But the ocular examination will differ as:

B. Ocular examination:
❖ **Vision:** May be only PL with accurate or inaccurate PR.
❖ **Lids, conjunctiva and sclera:** Normal.
❖ **Cornea:** Same as leucoma, a brown pigmentation (Hudson-Stahli's line) is usually present and deep vascularization is often present. Reduced corneal sensation on the opacity **(Fig. 2.17)**.
❖ **Anterior chamber:** Variable depth; shallower at the periphery; in the area of adherence—anterior chamber depth is virtually nil. Otherwise, AC is clear.
❖ **Iris:** Part of the iris, adherent with the corneal scar, is not visible, other part may be visible with atrophic patches.

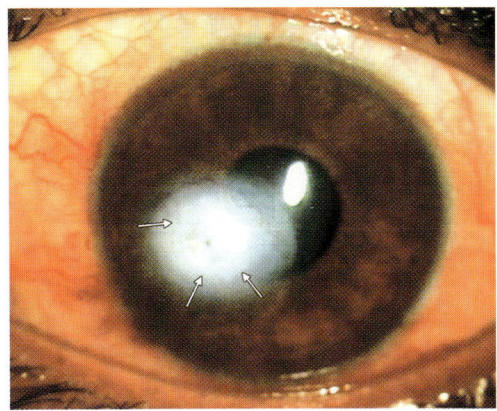

Fig. 2.17: Adherent leucoma.

❖ **Pupil:** Distortion is definitely present. It is dragged towards the adherent site. In central adherent leucoma pupil is not visible. Reactions may be difficult to assess.
❖ **Lens:** May be cataractous; may not be visible in central lesion.
❖ **Digital (finger) tension:** May be normal or higher.
❖ **Lacrimal sac:** Should be carefully examined.

[Like leucoma, it is better to draw a schematic diagram indicating the opacity, adherent area, pupillary distortion if visible, and extent of vascularization].

C. Provisional diagnosis: Adherent leucoma; vascularized central adherent leucoma, etc.

Self-assessment Questions

1. **Differential diagnosis:** Leucoma; partial anterior staphyloma or anterior synechia with opacity.
2. **Points in favor of adherent leucoma:**
   ➢ History of corneal ulcer in the past with perforation
   ➢ Profound loss of vision
   ➢ Dense white opacity in the cornea with iris inclusion within scar
   ➢ Areas of brown pigmentation within the opacity
   ➢ Variable anterior chamber depth— shallower at the periphery to nil at the area of adherence.

3. **Adherent leucoma versus anterior synechia:**
   - *Adherent leucoma* means iris tissue is incorporated with the corneal scar without any ectasia. This bond is firm, and difficult to separate iris tissue from the scarred cornea.
   - *Anterior synechia* is just a touch of iris with the back surface of the cornea. Initially, this is just an anatomical touch, but later on, the adhesion organizes. This bond can be separated with the help of an iris repositor.
4. **Mechanism of adherent leucoma:** When a corneal ulcer perforates (or any small perforation due to any other cause); the iris becomes gummed down to the opening with iris prolapse. With ulcer healing, this iris adhesion organizes, and then incorporated with the corneal scar—leading to the formation of an *adherent leucoma*.
5. **Causes of adherent leucoma:**
   - Perforated corneal ulcer.
   - Perforation of cornea by a penetrating injury.
   - Surgical wound.
   [Adherent leucoma does not usually occur when the perforation occurs just at the center of the cornea, because of absence of iris in pupillary region. But an anterior polar cataract may develop.]
6. **Relative advantages of perforation in corneal ulcer:**
   - Pain is relieved due to immediate lowering of intraocular pressure.
   - Better nutrition and more antibody (or antibiotics) will reach the cornea by diffusion of fluid and through the iris blood vessels.
   - Rapid healing of corneal ulcer.
7. **Investigations:** Same as leucoma. Gonioscopy and ultrasonic biomicroscopy (UBM) may be required in selective cases.
8. **Treatment:** Same as leucoma *except*:
   - Prognosis is poor in case of adherent leucoma.
   - *Treatment of secondary glaucoma* may be necessary prior to penetrating keratoplasty, either medically or by surgical means (trabeculectomy).
   - A *synechiotomy (synichiolysis)* is required to free the adhered iris during keratoplasty.
   - Simultaneous lens opacity, may be an indication of cataract surgery with IOL implantation along with it, called *triple procedure* (PK, cataract operation and IOL implantation).
   - Both in leucoma or adherent leucoma, *deep vascularization is an important prognostic factor for penetrating keratoplasty*. If it is present more than 2 quadrants, the chance of graft rejection is more than avascular opacity, due to more immunological tissue reaction.
   - *If the patient is one eyed and cornea is partially clear*—'optical iridectomy' is the choice to give ambulatory vision.
   - *In no PL eyes—tattooing:* Unlike, leucoma, in a case of adherent leucoma, before tattooing, it is better to do synechiotomy first, otherwise severe iridocyclitis may occur.
9. **Important complications of adherent leucoma:**
   - Secondary glaucoma due to shallow anterior chamber and secondary angle-closure and subsequent optic atrophy.
   - Deep vascularization of the opacity.
   - Visual disturbances if it is central.
   - Atheromatous ulcer in long standing cases

ANTERIOR STAPHYLOMA *(OP 4.5)*

A. **Patient's particulars:**
Occupation: Agriculture worker or may be a child.

B. **Chief complaints:**
- Disfigurement with bulging of the right or left eye for ....
- Complete loss of vision in same eye for same duration.

C. **History of present illness:** Patient was alright before ... months/years. Suddenly he had an attack of acute pain, redness and watering. He was treated for a long time with medicines for corneal ulcer. Consequently, he develops disfigurement of the eyeball with forward bulging. He has also total loss of vision in same eye for same duration. Patient also gives the history of intermittent pain redness and watering in the same eye.

He also complains about cosmetic blemish of that eye.

D. **Medical history:** Nothing significant.

E. **Past history:**
- History of corneal ulcer.
- History of systemic illness in a child (keratomalacia).
- History of coma for a prolonged period (exposure keratitis).

F. **Systemic examination:** Nutrition status; pulse; BP; all vitals

G. **Ocular examination:**
- **Vision:** Usually no PL, or PL present with inaccurate PR.
- **Ocular movement:** Full, there may be exophoria.
- **Lids:** Normal, may be mild lid retraction.
- **Conjunctiva:** Normal. Or mild congestion.
- **Cornea:**
  - A forward protrusion of pigmented scarred cornea, which has lobulated appearance with grayish-black color with bluish hue.
  - Thin fibrous band at some places with incarceration of altered iris tissues.
  - No definite cornea can be identified.
  - It may extent into surrounding part of the sclera.
  - If it is partial, part of the cornea is visible.
- **Anterior chamber, iris, pupil and lens:** Could not be visible *[in partial anterior staphyloma—they are partly visible.]*
- **Digital tension:** On higher side.
- **Lacrimal sac:** Normal.

H. **Provisional diagnosis:** Total/partial anterior staphyloma.

Self-assessment Questionnaire

1. **Staphyloma:**
   Definition and types: (*Means*—a bunch of grapes)
   It is an ectasia or bulging of the outer coat of the eyeball, lined by uveal tissue.
   Types:
   - *Anterior staphyloma:* It is an ectasia of the scarred cornea with incarceration of iris tissue. It may be total or partial **(Figs. 2.18A and B)**. Here, the bands of scar tissue on the staphyloma vary in breadth and thickness, producing a lobulated structure which is often blackened by uveal pigment (giving an appearance of a bunch of grapes).
   - *Posterior staphyloma:* Seen in case of degenerative or pathological myopia at the posterior pole of the eyeball.
   - *Equatorial staphyloma:* At the equator.

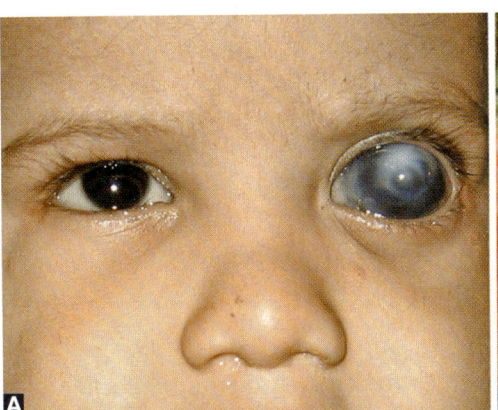 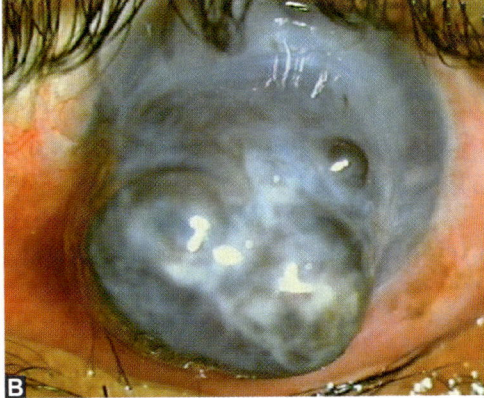

Figs. 2.18A and B: (A) Total anterior staphyloma; (B) Partial anterior staphyloma.

- *Ciliary staphyloma:* Near the ciliary body region.
- *Intercalary staphyloma:* In between ciliary body and the limbus. Last three types may be seen in resolved scleritis or trauma.

2. **Differential diagnosis in this case:** Adherent leucoma
3. **Probable mechanism of anterior staphyloma formation:** In case of sloughed out corneal ulcer, the exposed iris becomes inflamed with exudation. The exudate which covers the prolapse, becomes organized and form a thin layer of connective tissue, over which conjunctival or corneal epithelium rapidly grows. This is called *pseudocornea*. Simultaneously, there is rise in intraocular pressure due to closed angle.

   This *pseudocornea* is thin, and too weak to withstand high intraocular pressure. Naturally, it bulges forward, and known as anterior staphyloma.

   Thereafter, more irregular scarring giving rise to lobular appearance.
4. **Complications of anterior staphyloma:**
   - Secondary glaucoma due to complete abolition of the anterior chamber with its angle.
   - Absolute glaucoma (i.e., painful blind eye).
   - In recent cases—there may be chance of infection leading to panophthalmitis.
5. **Preoperative investigation:** As in leucoma. Enucleation surgery should be performed preferably under GA, as it is psychologically traumatic.
6. **Treatment option for anterior staphyloma:**
   - *In partial anterior staphyloma:* Trabeculectomy with iridectomy may be done to treat secondary glaucoma. Then, a corneal patch graft can be tried in case of PL positive eye.
   - *In total anterior staphyloma:* Enucleation with orbital implant is the choice. It is the followed by artificial prosthetic eye.
   - *Indication:*
     - With absolute glaucoma (painful blind eye)
     - For cosmetic reason.

     [Evisceration is not advised as there may be chance of *sympathetic ophthalmia of the opposite eye later on.*]
   - *Alternate option:* Staphylectomy and keratoplasty followed by cosmetic contact lens may be tried.

PHTHISIS BULBI (OP 4.5)

A. **Chief complaints:**
   - Smallness and cosmetic disfigurement of the eye for ....
   - Loss of vision in the same eye for ....

B. **History of present illness:** Patient was apparently all right few moths/year back. He complains of disfigurement and smallness of the eye with complete loss of vision after an episode of acute red eye for which he was treated for few weeks/months. He also complains of periodic watering and mild pain. There is no other history.

C. **Past history:**
   - Acute pain, redness, watering and loss of vision of the same eye few months/years back.
   - Open globe injury or history of surgery of the same eye.

   In either of the cases, the patient was treated for a long time in a hospital or as an OPD patient.

D. **Medical history:** Nothing significant. No history of drug allergy.

E. **Surgical history:** There may be history of therapeutic keratoplasty and/or vitrectomy for endophthalmitis in the past

F. **Personal history:** Nothing significant.

G. **Family history:** Nothing significant

H. **Systemic investigation:** Nutritional status; pulse; BP; and other vitals

I. **Ocular examination:**
   - **Vision:** No PL
   - **Eyeball:** Shrunken appearance of the globe as a whole; deep seated eyeball or enophthalmos.

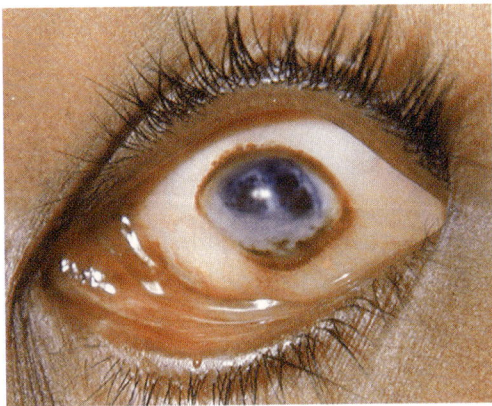

Fig. 2.19: Phthisis bulbi.

- ❖ **Movements:** Full
- ❖ **Eye lids:**
  - ➢ Deepening of the supratarsal sulcus.
  - ➢ Absence of the lid creases.
  - ➢ Narrow palpebral aperture (pseudoptosis).

  On separating the lids:
  - ➢ Small and distorted eyeball **(Fig. 2.19).**
  - ➢ Quadrilateral shape of the eyeball with depressions or furrows on it in different places.
- ❖ **Cornea:** Flat, irregular opacity with some white fibrous bands. There may be area of deep vascularization.
- ❖ **Sclera:** Normal
- ❖ **Anterior chamber, iris, pupil and lens:** Normal anatomy is lost and difficult to identify them separately.
- ❖ **Digital tension:** Low (soft as water bag).
- ❖ **Lacrimal sac:** Normal.
- ❖ **Head and face:** Nothing abnormal.
- J. **Provisional diagnosis:** Phthisis bulbi of RE or LE.

Self-assessment Questionnaire

1. **Points in favor of diagnosis:**
   - ➢ Shrunken appearance of the eyeball with quadrilateral shape,
   - ➢ Complete loss of vision with No PL and
   - ➢ On palpation—it is very soft.
2. **Differential diagnosis:** Total leucoma; total adherent leucoma; atrophic bulbi
3. **Causes of phthisis bulbi:**
   - ➢ Perforated corneal ulcer.
   - ➢ Large open globe injury.
   - ➢ Endophthalmitis.
   - ➢ Keratomalacia following vitamin A deficiency.
   - ➢ Chronic iridocyclitis and long-standing retinal detachment.
   - ➢ Absolute glaucoma → Ciliary body atrophy → Phthisis bulbi.
4. **Mechanism of phthisis bulbi:**
   - ➢ *Following perforation in infection:* Exudates or cyclitic membrane organizes on the ciliary body surface. The ciliary processes are then gradually destroyed. Then, there is decrease or cessation of aqueous production resulting in ocular hypotony **(phthisis bulbi)**.
   - ➢ Long-standing chronic IOP—rise gives pressure on the ciliary body in uncontrolled primary/secondary glaucoma, resulting in ciliary body atrophy or ciliary shock. Thereby, there is reduction or stoppage of aqueous formation—leading to ocular hypotony **(atrophic bulbi)**.

   [*Quadrilateral shape of the eyeball is due to the action of four recti muscles on a hypotonic eye—resulting in four depressions or furrows on the sclera.*]
5. **Differences between phthisis bulbi and atrophic bulbi (Table 2.7):**

TABLE 2.7: Differences between phthisis bulbi and atrophic bulbi.

Phthisis bulbi	Atrophic bulbi
1. More of quadrilateral shape	1. Relatively irregular shape
2. Occurs following severe open globe injury, panophthalmitis or endophthalmitis	2. Occurs following atrophy of the ciliary body, as in iridocyclitis or long-standing absolute glaucoma, etc.
3. Cornea, sclera or other structures are disorganized, so they cannot be distinguished separately	3. Internal structures are not disorganized, so they can be distinguished separately
4. Chances of calcification	4. No such chances

6. **Treatment of phthisis bulbi:** Mainly for cosmetic reason
   - Enucleation with intraorbital acrylic ball implant (*phthisis bulbi* is a relative indication for enucleation).
   - Scleral cosmetic shell—it gives a good cosmetic appearance.
7. **Complications of long-standing phthisis bulbi:**
   - *Bone formation:* The eyeball becomes stony hard. The structure involved in bone formation is choroid as it is highly vascular.
   - Recurrent red eye and uveitis.
   - Very rarely malignant changes may occur.

CHALAZION (OP 2.2)

A. **Patient's particulars:**

B. **Chief complaints:** Painless small nodular swelling of the right or left upper/lower lid for .... months

C. **History of present illness:** Patient was fine without any problem about a year back. She develops this swelling in the upper lid which is increasing in size very slowly. There is no pain, redness or watering from that eye. There is no history of trauma in that eye.

D. **Medical history:** Nothing significant

E. **Past history:** Any history of similar swelling in the past in the same eye or other eye. Nature of treatment at that time (medical or any surgical intervention).

F. **Family history:** Nothing significant

G. **Personal history:** Using spectacles.

H. **Systemic examination:** Nutrition status; built—normal. BP, pulse—normal. Other vitals—normal

I. **Ocular examination:**
- **Visual acuity:** May be 6/6 or may be with some refractive errors.
- **Near vision:** Normal (N6)
- **Ocular movements:** Normal.
- **Lids:**
  - A small pea-size nodular swelling in the middle of the upper eye lid, which is situated .... mm away from the lid margin (**Fig. 2.20A**).
  - It is firm with smooth surface, tense and non-tender on palpation.
  - Skin over the swelling is normal and free from the swelling.
- **Conjunctiva:** Bulbar part is normal. On eversion of the lid, corresponding circular area of palpebral conjunctiva is velvety red in color and slightly elevated.
- **Cornea:** Normal
- **Sclera:** Normal
- **Iris:** Normal
- **Pupil:** 3 mm. Normal reaction.
- **Intraocular pressure:** Normal
- **Lacrimal sac:** No regurgitation on pressure
- **Preauricular lymph node:** Not palpable.

J. **Provisional diagnosis:** Chalazion of RE/LE upper/lower lid (if more than one *chalazion*—the diagnosis is *multiple chalazion*).

Self-assessment Questionnaires

1. **Points favor of diagnosis:**
   - Small, firm, nodular swelling of the lid which is non-tender.
   - The swelling is away from the lid margin
   - It is slowly progressive
   - On eversion of lid, tarsal conjunctiva over the swelling—is velvety red in color and slightly elevated.
2. **Differential diagnosis:**
   - Stye (*see* page 51)
   - Internal hordeolum (*see* page 53).
   - Meibomian gland carcinoma
   - Foreign body granuloma
3. **What is a chalazion? (means—a hailstone):** It is a chronic nonspecific inflammatory granuloma of the meibomian gland. The glandular tissue becomes replaced by granulation tissue containing giant cells, probably as a result of chronic inflammation by a low virulence organism.
   Meibomian glands are modified sebaceous glands situated in the substance of tarsal plates in both lids. The meibomian ducts open at the corresponding lid margin
   The numbers of meibomian gland are more in the upper lid (30–40) than the

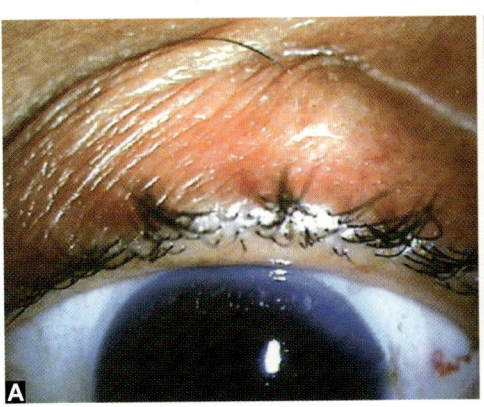 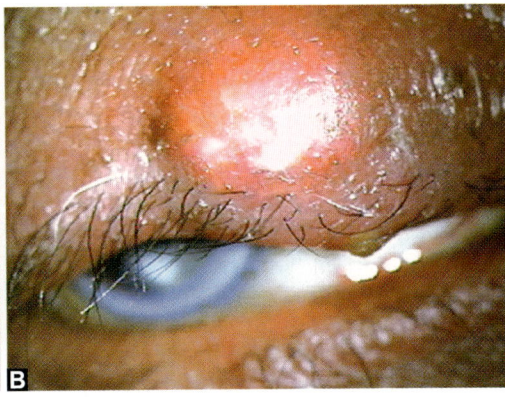

Figs. 2.20A and B: (A) Chalazion; (B) Infected chalazion (hordeolum internum).

lower (20–30). *That is why chalazion is more common in upper eye lid*

4. **Histopathology of a chalazion:**
   - Centrally, cheesy sebaceous material.
   - Surrounded by granulation tissue, having lymphocytes, epithelioid cells, foreign body type of giant cell and fine blood vessels.
   - All are enclosed by a fibrous capsule.
5. **Differences between chalazion and stye:** *See* Table 2.8

6. **Predisposing factors of chalazion:**
   - Young adults and children with poor lid hygiene
   - Chronic blepharitis
   - *Refractive error:* Excessive rubbing → Chronic inflammation → Meibomitis → Obstruction of the ducts of meibomian gland.
   - Chronic conjunctivitis, e.g., as in trachoma.
   - Diabetes mellitus in adults.
7. **Fate of untreated chalazion:**
   - Spontaneous resolution (smaller chalazion).
   - Remains as such.
   - Increase in size leading to mechanical ptosis.
   - Secondary bacterial infection with pain and acute inflammation—called '*Hordeolum internum*' **(Fig. 2.20B)**.
   - It may burst out through the palpebral conjunctiva (as a fungating mass of granulation tissue) or rarely, through the skin.
   - It may turn into a *'Marginal chalazion'* (i.e., the granulation tissue formed in the duct of the gland, projects as a reddish-gray nodule on the intermarginal strip).
   - It may be calcified.
   - Very rarely malignant changes may be seen, especially in old age with a history of recurrence (so, a histopathological examination should be done in such cases).

TABLE 2.8: Differences between chalazion and stye.

Chalazion	Stye
1. Chronic nonspecific granulomatous inflammation of meibomian gland	1. Acute suppurative infection of gland of Zeis/hair follicle
2. No symptoms and signs of inflammation unless secondarily infected	2. Pain, swelling, tenderness, etc.—all are present
3. Usually away from the lid-margin	3. At the lid-margin
4. No pus-point at the root of eyelash	4. Pus-point at the root of an eyelash
5. No preauricular lymphadenopathy	5. Preauricular or submandibular lymphadenopathy may be present
6. Treatment is surgical (incision and curettage)	6. Treatment is conservative and epilation of the involved eyelash

8. **Treatment of chalazion:**
   - *In case of small chalazion:*
     - Hot compress—3 times daily.
     - Steroid—antibiotic ointment with lid massage for a few days.
   - *For large chalazion:* Incision and curettage or scooping. Steps of operation (*see* page 185).
   - In case of *marginal chalazion:* After local anesthesia—just press out the material with thumb and index finger, or electrocoagulation by passing 20–30 m Amp current for few seconds.
   - *Intra-lesional (intra-chalazion) injection of depot steroid*: Triamcinolone acetonide, fortnightly for 3–4 such. This is more useful in chalazion near punctum. It may cause hypopigmentation and atrophy of the tarsal plate.
   - *In case of hordeolum internum:*
     - First, treat acute inflammation by:
       - Hot compress—3 times daily.
       - Systemic analgesics with antacids.
     - Topical antibiotic drops and ointment.
     - Systemic antibiotic (doxycycline).
   - After the acute phase subsides—treat it like a chalazion, i.e., by incision and curettage or scooping.

STYE (HORDEOLUM EXTERNUM) *(OP 2.2)*

A. **Chief complaints:** Acute pain and swelling of right or left upper/lower lid for ...

B. **Past history:** Similar swelling with pain in the past.

C. **Personal history:** Chronic illness, malnutrition or diabetes.

D. **Ocular examination:**
   - **Vision:** Normal or less.
   - **Ocular motility:** Normal.
   - **Eye lids:**
     - Edema of the whole lid margin
     - Redness of the lid.
     - Local temperature raised.
     - A swollen area, more at the lid margin and it has a whitish, round, raised pus point, at the root of the corresponding eyelash **(Figs. 2.21A and B).**
     - The swelling is tender.
     - Matting of few eyelashes may be present.
   - **Conjunctiva:** There may be mild conjunctival congestion and chemosis, and sometimes with discharge.
   - **Cornea and other structures:** Normal.
   - **Preauricular and sometimes submandibular lymph nodes:** May be enlarged and tender.

E. **Provisional diagnosis:** Stye *(hordeolum externum)* of the right or left upper/lower eyelid.

Self-assessment Questionnaires

1. **Points favor of diagnosis:**
   - Acute pain and swelling of the lid
   - Edema of the whole lid with matting of few eyelashes

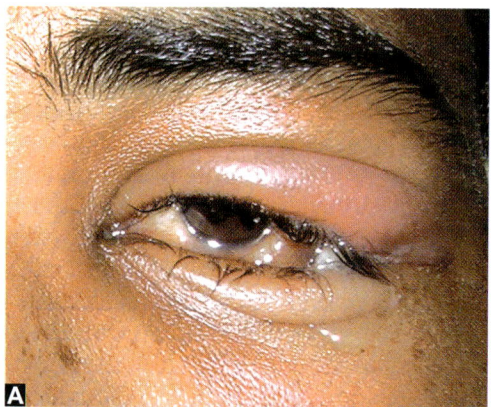
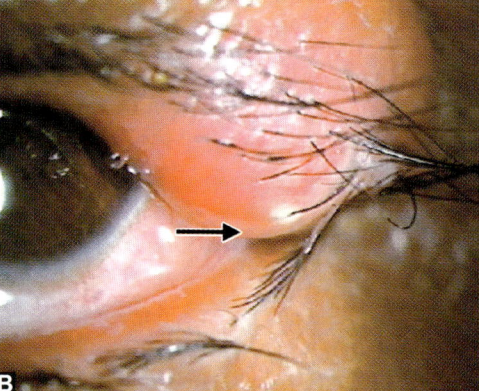

Figs. 2.21A and B: (A) Stye (hordeolum externum); (B) Pus point with eyelash.

- Localized swelling of lid margin with a raised pus point at eyelash root
- The swelling is tender with raised local temperature
2. **Differential diagnosis:**
   - *Hordeolum internum* (infected chalazion)
   - Chalazion
3. **Define stye (also called 'Hordeolum externum'):** It is an acute suppurative inflammation of one of the glands of Zeis.
4. **Differences between hordeolum externum and hordeolum internum (Table 2.9):**
5. **Predisposing factors of stye:**
   - Common in young adults and children; but may occur at any age, in debilitated person.
   - Organism—*Staphylococcus aureus* or *epidermidis*.
   - Errors of refraction.
   - Diabetes or other chronic illness with low body resistance.
6. **Complications, if untreated:**
   - Ulcerative blepharitis.
   - Lid abscess and cellulitis.
   - Facial cellulitis.
   - Rarely, orbital cellulitis.
7. **Treatment:**
   - Post-prandial blood sugar to exclude diabetes.
   - *Hot compress*—3 times daily.
   - *Evacuation of pus*—by pulling out the affected eyelash.
   - Alternately, it is incised with a sharp knife (e.g., 15-degree blade) which is momentarily painful (horizontal incision.
   - *Systemic analgesics* with antacids.
   - *Local antibiotics* drop or ointment (ciprofloxacin or gatifloxacin)—4-6 times daily for 2 weeks.
   - In multiple stye 'Stye in crops'—in addition to local treatment, a course of systemic doxycycline for 7–14 days or tablet azithromycin for 5 days is to be given to prevent recurrence.

TABLE 2.9: Differences between hordeolum externum and hordeolum internum.

Hordeolum externum (stye)	Hordeolum internum (infected chalazion)
1. Acute suppurative inflammation of gland of Zeis	1. Acute suppurative inflammation of meibomian gland
2. Pus-point at the lid margin, and root of an eyelash is involved	2. Pus-point away from lid margin, and eyelash is not involved
3. Maximum tenderness and swelling at the lid margin	3. Maximum swelling and tenderness away from the lid margin
4. No history of previous swelling of the lid	4. History of previous swelling of the lid
5. Conservative treatment and epilation of involved cilia is important	5. Conservative treatment and later on incision and curettage of chalazion

BITOT'S SPOT AND CONJUNCTIVAL XEROSIS (OP 4.4)

A. **Patient's particular:** Usually a child
B. **Chief complaints:**
   - Fish-scale like silvery white foamy opacity in both eyes for .....
   - Difficulty in night vision for ....
C. **Past history:** Acute diarrheal disease, measles, whooping cough or any acute illness in the recent past.
D. **Personal history:** Dietary habit of the child.
E. **General survey:** Nutritional status:........ Overall built:.........
Anemia: Chest: GI system: Skin: Hair:
F. **Ocular examination:**
   - **Vision:** Noted by fixation, following movements, identification of objects or toys, and counting finger, E-chart, etc.
   - **Movements:** Normal
   - **Lids:** Normal.
   - **Conjunctiva:**
     - Dry lusterless conjunctiva.
     - Wrinkling on the bulbar conjunctiva in horizontal meridian.
     - A triangular, silvery white, foamy or cheesy dry area away from the limbus on

the bulbar conjunctiva on the temporal side. The base of the triangle is towards the limbus. This area is not wetted by the tear film.
- Conjunctival pigmentation adjacent to the spot—may be present.
- **Cornea:** Normal or may be dull and lusterless. Window reflex may be distorted.
- **Sclera, anterior chamber, iris and pupil, lens, lacrimal sac:** All within normal limits.

G. **Provisional diagnosis:**
- Bitot's spot or
- Bitot's spot with conjunctival xerosis of both eyes.

Self-assessment Questionnaire

1. **Points favor of diagnosis:**
   - C/o white foamy opacity in both eyes following acute diarrheal diseases or measles
   - History of night blindness
   - Dry lusterless conjunctiva.
   - A triangular, foamy or cheesy silvery-white opacity on temporal side of the bulbar conjunctiva away from the limbus. The base of the triangle is towards the limbus.
   - This area is not wetted by the tear film.
2. **Types of xerosis (xerosis means dryness):**
   - *Xerosis epithelialis* is due to vitamin A deficiency and associated protein-energy malnutrition.
   - *Xerosis parenchymatous* is due to:
     - Sequalae of local ocular effect, e.g., trachoma, chemical burns, diphtheria, ocular cicatricial pemphigoid (OCP), Stevens-Johnson syndrome (SJS), etc.
     - Chronic exposure of the eye, e.g., ectropion, proptosis, lagophthalmos where the eye is not properly covered by the lids.
3. **Pathogenesis of Bitot's spot:**
   - The foamy Bitot's spot is due to horny epithelium which is cast off into the conjunctival sac and collected into the lower fornix initially. Then they accumulate on the temporal bulbar conjunctiva in a triangular fashion **(Fig. 2.22A)**.
   - Vicarious activity of the meibomian glands, with their fatty secretion, covers the dry surface so that the watery tears fail to moisten that area.
   - Profuse growth of the bacteria '*Corynebacterium xerosis*' which is responsible for foamy appearance **(Fig. 2.22B)**.
4. **Causes of night blindness:** (*See* page 5).
5. **Causes of vitamin A deficiency:**
   a. *Excessive demand but deficient supply* during the growing period (faulty dietary habits).
   b. *Defective utilization* (due to digestive problems), e.g., chronic diarrhea, worm infestation, malabsorption syndrome, etc.

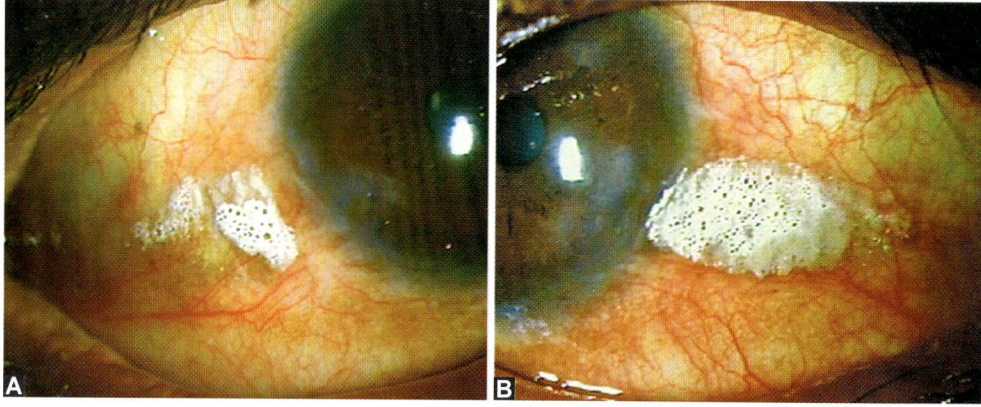

Figs. 2.22A and B: Bilateral Bitot's spot.

c. *Defective synthesis and storage* (*mainly in adults,* due to liver diseases), e.g., hepatitis, chronic alcoholism, cirrhosis of liver, etc.
6. **Clinical features of vitamin A deficiency** (*see* page 105).
7. **Define keratoconjunctivitis sicca or Sjogren's syndrome:** It is an autoimmune disease of middle-aged woman with polyarthritis, dryness of eyes (hyposecretion of tears due to lacrimal gland involvement) and dryness of mouth (xerostomia) due to hyposecretion of salivary glands.
8. **Treatment of Bitot's spot and conjunctival xerosis:** (*see* page 106).
9. **Features of hypervitaminosis A:** It may be acute or chronic.
   - *Acute hypervitaminosis A* (usually due to high dose of vitamin A (more than 3,00,000 IU at a time)—headache, nausea, seizures, dizziness, sign of increased intracranial tension (bulging of the fontanelle in children or *pseudotumor cerebri* in adults).
   - *Chronic hypervitaminosis A:*
     - General: Anorexia, nausea, vomiting, insomnia, tiredness, irritability.
     - Eyes: Papilledema, diplopia.
     - Skin: Desquamation, loss of hair, pruritus.
     - Hepatomegaly.
     - Skeletal system: Hyperosteosis of long bones, premature closure of the epiphyses.
10. **Special tests in dry eye:**
    - *Slit lamp examination* to find out tear-meniscus height, filaments, mucus debris and also lid margins.
    - *Tear-film break up time (TBUT)*—normally more than 10 sec. If it is less than 10 sec, it is abnormal.
    - *Schirmer's test* (to see the wettability of a filter paper after 5 minutes). Normal value: >10 mm
    - *Rose-Bengal staining* (to stain the devitalised epithelium).
    - *Lissamine green staining:* Similar to Rose Bengal test but with less irritation of the eye.
    - *Fluorescein stain* (to stain tear meniscus height, filaments and epithelial defect).
    - *Conjunctival impression cytology (CIC).*

ACUTE IRIDOCYCLITIS (RED EYE) (OP 6.1 AND 6.2)

A. **Patient's particulars:**
B. **Chief complaints:**
   - Acute pain, redness and watering for ...
   - Associated photophobia with dimness of vision for ....
C. **History of present illness:** Patient complains of sudden onset pain, redness in the RE or LE for 5–7 days. The pain is dull in nature with radiation towards forehead. There is associated watering and photophobia. All the symptoms are increasing with time.
   They may also complain of dimness of vision in the same eye for last few days. No history of colored halos. There was no history of ocular trauma or intraocular surgery.
D. **Past history:** Similar attack in the same or opposite eye may be present.
E. **Medical history:** History of joint pain (rheumatoid arthritis), neck pain (ankylosing spondylitis), etc., for last 2–3 years. No history of diabetes or hypertension. Sometimes history of fever or respiratory problem may be present.
F. **Personal history:** Nothing significant
G. **Family history:** Nothing significant
H. **Systemic examination:** Normal built, BP, pulse and other vitals normal. There may be some changes in hands and feet, or neck.
I. **Ocular examination:**
   - **Visual acuity:** May be normal or reduced.
   - **Ocular movements:** Normal.
   - **Eye lids:** There may be mild edema.
   - **Conjunctiva:** Circumciliary congestion; Chemosis may be present.
   - **Cornea:** Normal or mild haze; KPs are found on the posterior surface of the lower part of cornea. They may be—fine, medium or large (mutton fat) (seen with torch and loupe, or preferably with slit lamp) **(Fig. 2.23A).**

- ❖ **Sclera:** Congested. Tenderness present over the ciliary region *('ciliary tenderness')*
- ❖ **Anterior chamber:** Clear or turbid (due to aqueous cells and flare). Mild hypopyon may be present in severe cases.
- ❖ **Iris:** Muddy iris, i.e., normal pattern is lost.
- ❖ **Pupil:** Smaller, irregular; light reaction is present but sluggish.
  It may be dilated (atropinised) and then, light reaction is absent.
- ❖ **Lens:** Pigments over anterior lens surface, there may be presence of posterior synechiae.
- ❖ **Digital (finger) tension:** Normal/lower/higher.
- ❖ **Lacrimal sac:** Normal.

J. **Provisional diagnosis:** Acute iridocyclitis in RE or LE.

CHRONIC IRIDOCYCLITIS (OP 6.1 AND 6.2)

A. **Chief complaints:** Dimness of vision in the eye for ...

B. **History of present illness:** Almost same as acute iridocyclitis, except the symptoms are chronic in nature. The dimness of vision is more profound.

C. **Past history:**
- ❖ Acute attack of pain, redness and watering, and may be with dimness of vision.
- ❖ History of more than one attack.

D. **Personal history:** Joint pain, rheumatoid arthritis, ankylosing spondylitis, tuberculosis or syphilis.

E. **Ocular examination:**
- ❖ **Vision acuity:** Diminished.
- ❖ **Ocular movements:** Normal.
- ❖ **Eye lids:** Normal.
- ❖ **Conjunctiva:** Normal. There may be ciliary congestion.
- ❖ **Cornea:** Normal; old KPs (medium or large) may be present (seen with torch and loupe, or with slit lamp).
- ❖ **Sclera:** Normal.
- ❖ **Anterior chamber:** May be irregular due to posterior synechiae or iris bombe
- ❖ **Iris:** Pattern may be lost. Patchy areas of iris atrophy are seen. There may be *ectropion uveae.*
- ❖ **Pupil:** Irregular, may be smaller, at places there are posterior synechiae (*Festooned pupil*) **(Fig. 2.23B).**
- ❖ **Lens:** May be normal or cataractous. Pigments over the anterior lens surface. Presence of posterior synechiae (please note the extent of synechiae with a line diagram).
- ❖ **Digital (finger) tension:** Normal or higher.
- ❖ **Lacrimal sac:** Normal.

F. **Provisional diagnosis:** Chronic iridocyclitis.

Self-assessment Questionnaire

1. **Differential diagnosis in this case:**
   - ➢ Acute conjunctivitis
   - ➢ Acute angle-closure glaucoma

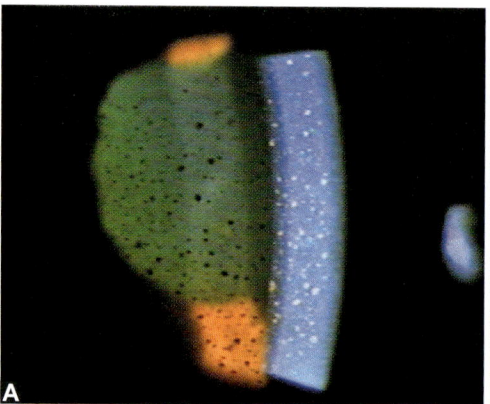 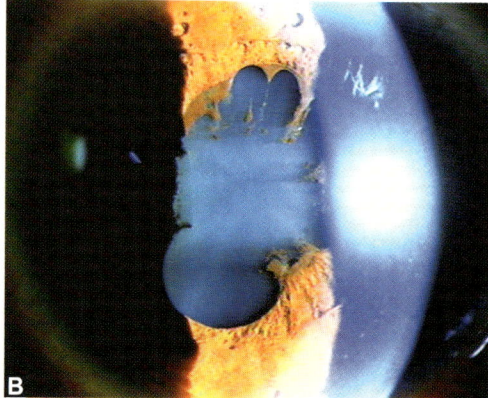

Figs. 2.23A and B: (A) Acute iridocyclitis; (B) Chronic iridocyclitis.

2. **Points favor of acute iridocyclitis:**
   - Sudden onset pain, redness, watering and photophobia
   - Ciliary congestion
   - Ciliary tenderness
   - Muddy iris
   - Pupil—small, irregular with sluggish reaction
   - Anterior chamber haziness with mild hypopyon
3. **Points against of acute conjunctivitis:**
   - Pain is very mild in conjunctivitis, only discomfort
   - No mucopurulent discharge
   - No conjunctival congestion
   - Cornea—KPs are absent
   - Iris, pupil and anterior chamber—normal in conjunctivitis
4. **Points against of acute angle-closure glaucoma:**
   - Colored halos not present
   - Visual loss is severe in ACG
   - Corneal edema
   - Shallow anterior chamber
   - Pupil mid-dilated and oval
   - IOP is very high in ACG
5. **Causes of iridocyclitis:**
   - *Idiopathic:* Difficult to find out the cause.
   - *Allergic:* Bacterial allergy (from septic focus), lens protein (as in ECCE), sympathetic ophthalmia, etc.
   - *Endogenous:* Tuberculosis, syphilis, toxoplasmosis, etc.
   - *Exogenous:* Penetrating injury.
   - *Secondary infection:* Spread from infection of cornea or sclera.
   - *Autoimmune:* Due to hypersensitivity to autologous tissue components, as in rheumatoid arthritis, ankylosing spondylitis, Still's disease, Behcet's disease, Reiter's disease, SLE, etc.
     - HLA-B27 is present in iritis patient with ankylosing spondylitis, psoriatic arthritis, Reiter's syndrome, etc.
     - HLA-B5 in Behcet's disease.
     - HLA-DW-22J in VKH syndrome.

   [*Systemic disease associated with anterior uveitis:*
   - *Non-infective:* All autoimmune diseases as above.
   - *Infective:* Herpes simplex, herpes zoster, tuberculosis, syphilis, etc.]
6. **Classification of uveitis (Table 2.10):**
   Pathologically: Non-granulomatous and granulomatous type.
   - *Non-granulomatous type:* Is due to allergic reaction (e.g., to *Streptococci, Staphylococci* or autoimmune).
   - *Granulomatous type:* Is due to tuberculosis, sarcoidosis or leprosy, etc.
7. **Non-granulomatous and granulomatous uveitis differences (Table 2.11):**
8. **Anatomical peculiarity with the pathology of iridocyclitis and explanation of different findings:**
   - Iris is a diaphragm of network of blood vessels and unstriped muscles.

TABLE 2.10: Anatomical standardize uveitis nomenclature (SUN) classification.

Type of uveitis	Primary site	Includes
1. Anterior	Anterior chamber	• Iritis • Anterior cyclitis • Iridocyclitis
2. Intermediate	Vitreous	• Pars planitis
3. Posterior	Choroid or retina	• Different choroiditis • Chorioretinitis • Retino-choroiditis • Retinitis • Neuroretinitis
4. Panuveitis	Anterior chamber, vitreous and choroid or retina	All parts including retina

TABLE 2.11: Non-granulomatous and granulomatous uveitis differences.

	Non-granulomatous uveitis	Granulomatous uveitis
Onset	Acute and short course	Insidious and chronic course
Severity	Severe and red eye	Relative mild and white eye
Nodules	No such nodules on the iris	Koeppe's/Bussaca's nodules on the iris
KPs	Fine to small KPs	Medium to large "Mutton-fat" KPs
Flare	Intense flare, often heavy fibrinous exudate; hypopyon	Mild to moderate flare
Parts involved	Mainly limited to the anterior uvea	Anterior uvea and retina—choroid are equally involved
Causes	Mostly idiopathic and immunogenic in nature	TB, sarcoidosis, leprosy, etc.

- The iris stroma is loose and spongy.
- Pupillary margin slides over the anterior surface of the lens.

Dilatation of the blood vessels allows large amount of exudation of plasma within loose and spongy stroma of the iris, causing it to be waterlogged and swollen. Sticky fibrin-rich fluid and inflammatory cells are responsible for producing aqueous flare and cells respectively, and very rarely mild hypopyon.

Explanations:
- *Ciliary congestion* is due to inflammation of the ciliary body.
- *Constriction of the pupil is due to:*
  - Waterlogging of the iris tissue.
  - Toxin acts both on the sphincter and dilator muscles, but sphincter muscle is stronger.
  - Radial arrangement of the iris vasculature.
- *Sluggish pupillary reaction is due to:*
  - Edema of the iris, and
  - Posterior synechiae.
- *Muddy iris is* due to accumulation of fluid and exudates over the surface of the iris. Crypts and furrows of iris become obliterated, and pattern is thus lost.
- *"Irregular pupil"* is due to posterior synechiae formation.

9. **KPs and their importance:**
   - KPs mean 'Keratic precipitates'. It is a sign of Iridocyclitis (specially of cyclitis). Actually, they are the clumps of leukocytes adherent to the corneal endothelium in iridocyclitis.
   - The inflammatory cells are wandering in the aqueous by the convection current and stick to the edematous endothelial layer of the cornea. They arrange in a triangular area at the lower part of the cornea *(Arlt's triangle)* due to gravitation. The smaller ones are above and the bigger ones are below.
   - The KPs may be fine, coarse (lymphocytes and plasma cells) or mutton fat type (macrophage and epithelioid cells). The fine KPs are found in allergic or acute type of iridocyclitis; the mutton-fat types are found in granulomatous uveitis, as in tuberculosis or sarcoidosis.
   - The KPs may be fresh, old or pigmented. The fresh KPs are solid, three dimensional in appearance; but the old KPs are shrunken, having crenated border, and a halo is seen in the surrounding endothelium.

The fate of KPs:
- They coalesce to form large KPs.
- They may be pigmented.
- They may be absorbed.

Presence of KPs on the corneal endothelium indicates that there is at least some iridocyclitis in active or healed form.

10. **Investigations in a case of anterior uveitis (iridocyclitis):**
    - **Blood:** Routine hemogram.

- *For arthritis:* Rheumatoid factor, ANF, ANA, HLA–typing (HLA B27)
- *For syphilis:* VDRL, FTABS.
  - *For tuberculosis:* Mantoux test, X-ray chest (PA), QuantiFERON Gold Test
  - Serum ACE, Kveim test (for sarcoidosis).
  - ELISA test for TB, toxoplasmosis, etc.
11. **Complications of iridocyclitis:**
   - *Posterior synechiae.*
   - *Seclusio pupillae* (due to 360° ring synechiae).
   - *Iris bombe:* Forward bowing of the peripheral iris, as aqueous gets blocked by *seclusio pupillae.* Anterior chamber becomes funnel shaped.
   - *Occlusio pupillae:* Pupil is occluded or covered by organized fibrinous exudates.
   - *Secondary glaucoma:* Due to albuminous aqueous blocking the anterior chamber angle.
   - *Posterior synechiae.*
   - Associated *trabeculitis and trabecular edema.*
   - Ring synechiae and *occlusio pupillae* leading to pupillary block.
   - *Peripheral anterior synechiae.*
   - *Total posterior synechiae:* Plastering of the whole iris with the anterior surface of the lens.
   - *Cyclitic membrane:* Behind the lens, more in cyclitis.
   - *Complicated cataract:* Typical breadcrumb appearance with polychromatic lusture.
   - Pseudoglioma due to vitreous exudation.
   - *Cystoid macular edema (CME):* Due to liberation of toxin, leading to macular edema.
   - *Phthisis (atrophic) bulbi:* Due to prolonged cyclitis → there is ciliary shock (atrophy) → less formation of aqueous → atrophic bulbi.
   - *Band-shaped keratopathy:* This is most commonly seen in young children with juvenile rheumatoid arthritis (IRA).
   - *Tractional RD:* Due to traction caused by cyclitic membrane—leading to retinal detachment.
12. **Treatment of iridocyclitis:**
A. **Local:**
   1. Hot compress—2–4 times daily.
   2. Use dark glasses.
   3. *Atropine (1%) eye drop or ointment*—3 times daily. Atropine acts in three ways:
      i. Keeping the iris and ciliary body at rest.
      ii. Diminishing hyperemia.
      iii. Preventing the formation of posterior synechiae and breaking down if any already formed.
      Combined mydriatic—cycloplegics (e.g., tropicamide and phenylephrine) may also be given instead of atropine.
      Atropine or other cycloplegic should be continued for at least 10–14 days after the eye appears to be quiet, otherwise a relapse is likely to occur.
   4. *Corticosteroids:* Local drops, ointment, or as sub-conjunctival or sub-Tenon injection. Local drops like dexamethasone, prednisolone acetate, etc. '1 hourly to 6 hourly' depending upon the severity of inflammation. *Sub-Tenon* injection of long-acting steroids (e.g., triamcinolone acetonide) along with injection atropine is very helpful in many cases.
   5. *Nonsteroidal anti-inflammatory drugs (NSAIDs):* Like, flurbiprofen, diclofenac, ketorolac, bromfenac, nepafenac, etc., are helpful to reduce pain and inflammation. These drugs are important in patients who are steroid responders (rise in IOP after application of topical steroids).
B. **Systemic:**
   1. Anti-inflammatory drugs—like, indomethacin.
   2. Oral steroids (prednisolone) in tapering doses in severe cases
   3. Antitubercular (AT) drugs in selected case.

4. Rarely, systemic immunosuppressive agents.
C. **Treatment of complications:**
   1. *Secondary glaucoma:* Tablet acetazolamide 250 mg 3–4 times daily, and/or timolol maleate eye drop (0.5%) twice daily.
   2. *Annular (ring) synechia:* Iridectomy
   3. *Iris bombe:* YAG laser iridotomy or '4 point iridotomy' (quadri-puncture) is done with a von Graefe cataract knife.
   4. *Removal of cataract:* When the eye becomes quiet, and it should be under the umbrella of systemic corticosteroids and atropine.

CHRONIC DACRYOCYSTITIS *(OP2.2)*

A. **Patient's particular:** Usually, young female; mostly left side is involved.
B. **Chief complaints:**
   ❖ Persistent watering from the left or right eye for …
   ❖ Accumulation of pus on the inner angle of the eye for …
C. **History of present illness:** Patients complains of constant watering from the left eye for last 1–2 years. She gives the history of mucoid or mucopurulent discharge with redness time to time. She also complains of periodic swelling below the inner canthus which is reduces by giving pressure over that region with regurgitation of pus or muco-pus.
   She has history of chronic rhinitis. No history of trauma, surgery or other problems.
D. **Past history:** Any operation or investigative procedure in the past. Any history of pain and swelling in the same eye.
E. **Medical history:** No history of diabetes, hypertension, etc.
F. **Personal history:** Nothing significant
G. **Family history:** Nothing significant
H. **Systemic investigations:** Normal built. Pulse, BP, other vitals, etc.
I. **Nasal examination:** Grossly look for:
   ❖ Deviated nasal septum (DNS).
   ❖ Hypertrophied inferior turbinate.
   ❖ Nasal polyp.
   ❖ Atrophic rhinitis.
J. **Ocular examination:**
   ❖ **Vision:** Normal.
   ❖ **Ocular movements:** Normal.
   ❖ **Lids:** Normal or mild matting of the eyelashes. Excoriation of the skin in the lower lid around lacrimal sac region. Normal lid closure.
   ❖ **Conjunctiva:**
      ➢ Mild to moderate conjunctival congestion—especially near the inner canthus.
      ➢ Accumulation of tears, pus or muco-pus in the inner canthus.
   ❖ **Cornea, iris and pupil, and lens:** Normal.
   ❖ **Lacrimal sac area:**
      ➢ A small globular swelling may be present over the sac region.
         [If it is large as in mucocele—describe the swelling **(Figs. 2.24A and B)**. The swelling is … mm in diameter. It is

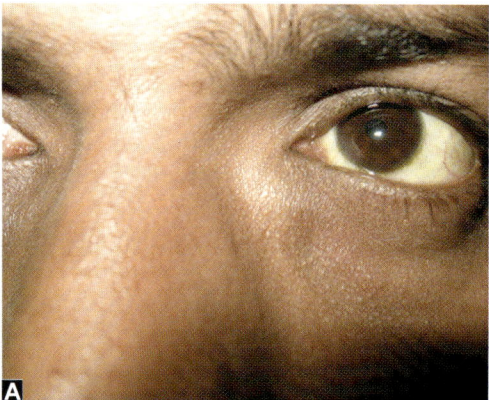 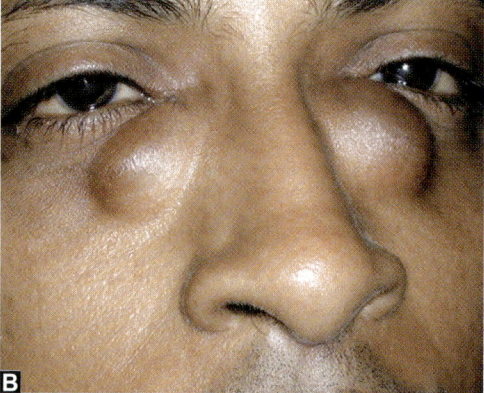

Figs. 2.24A and B: (A) Chronic dacryocystitis; (B) With mucocele (bilateral).

round, soft/moderately tense, smoother, non-tender and local temperature not raised. No pulsation, no bruit.]
- No tenderness or redness of the swollen area.
- *On pressure over the sac area,* there is regurgitation of mucus (mucocele) or pus (pyocele) or mucopus through the lower as well as upper punctum. (**ROPLAS: +ve** *means* **R**egugitation **O**n **P**ressure over **LA**crimal **S**ac is positive)
- Sometimes, this mucopus evacuates inside the nasopharynx (as the patient complains) on giving pressure over the sac region.
- In some cases, there may not be any swelling or 'ROPLAS: negative' (as the patient herself evacuated out the pus or mucopus by giving pressure over sac region before clinical examination).

K. **Provisional diagnosis:** Chronic dacryocystitis of left/right side.
   If a mucocele is present—diagnosis is *chronic dacryocystitis with mucocele.*

ACUTE DACRYOCYSTITIS (OP 2.2)

A. **Chief complaints:**
   ❖ Acute painful swelling over the sac region for …
   ❖ Watering for …

B. **History of present illness:** History of swelling around the medial angle of lower lid with severe pain radiating towards the frontal region. There may be associated fever and malaise.

C. **Past history:** Similar acute attack in the past may be present. History of watering from the same eye for … months/years.

D. **Ocular examination:**
   ❖ **Vision:** Normal.
   ❖ **Ocular movements:** Normal.
   ❖ **Lids:** Marked swelling of the lids, especially, the lower lid.
   ❖ **Conjunctiva:** Mild to moderate conjunctival congestion and may be with chemosis.
   ❖ **Cornea, iris, pupil and lens:** Normal.
   ❖ **Lacrimal sac:**
      - Marked swelling and redness of the skin over the sac region.
      - The swelling is extremely tender.
      - Local temperature is raised.
      - Edema at the root of the nose with surrounding cellulitis.
      - When lacrimal abscess is formed—the area is less tender and fluctuation may be positive.
      - It is better not to press over the sac region to elicit the presence of regurgitation. In fact, there is no regurgitation at this stage due to edema of the surrounding tissue blocking the canaliculi.
      - A fistula may be seen just below the medial canthal ligament.

F. **Provisional diagnosis:** Acute dacryocystitis (**Fig. 2.25A**) or lacrimal abscess (**Fig. 2.25B**) (with fistula) of left or right side.

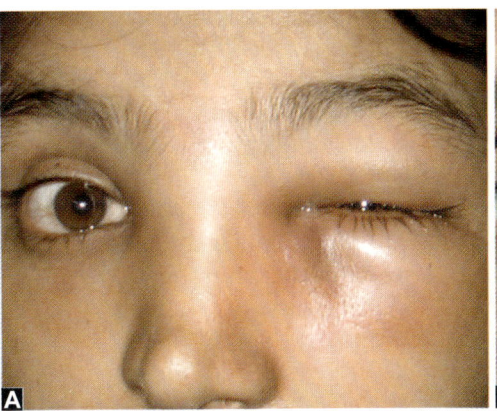 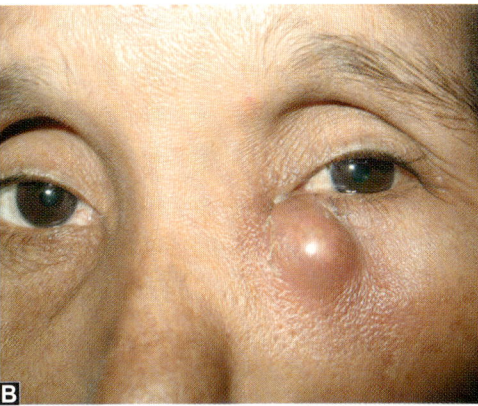

Figs. 2.25A and B: (A) Acute dacryocystitis; (B) Lacrimal abscess.

Self-assessment Questionnaire

1. **Eitiology of chronic dacryocystitis:**
   - Middle aged—more in female (male: female = 1:4).
   - Left eye more commonly affected (right: left = 1:7).
   - Lower socioeconomic status.
   - *Causes:*
     - Sac proper: Blockage of nasolacrimal duct due to narrowness or chronic inflammation.
     - Nasal factors: DNS, hypertrophied inferior turbinate, nasal polyp, chronic rhinitis, etc.
     - Organisms responsible: *Pneumococcus* (commonest); *Streptococcus, Staphylococcus, M. tuberculosis, M. leprae, Chlamydia*, etc.

2. **Epiphora and lacrimation—definition and causes:**
   - *Epiphora:* Overflow of tears due to defect, anywhere in lacrimal drainage system (tear secretion is normal), e.g.,
     - Ectropion.
     - Punctal stenosis or occlusion.
     - Canalicular block.
     - Nasolacrimal duct (NLD) block.

     The changes in lacrimal sac regurgitate in chronic dacryocystitis are; first watery → then mucoid (due to secretion from goblet cells in the sac) → mucopurulent → then purulent (frank pus).
   - *Lacrimation:* Here, there is oversecretion of tears without any defect in the drainage system, e.g.,
     - Emotional or psychological (commonest).
     - Irritation of conjunctiva or cornea by dust, fumes, etc.
     - Any superficial infection of the eyes.
     - Nasal irritation by any chemical (e.g., during chopping an onion).

3. **Complications of chronic dacryocystitis:**
   - Acute exacerbation of chronic dacryocystitis.
   - From acute dacryocystitis → there may be:
     - Lacrimal abscess.
     - Lacrimal fistula formation.
     - Orbital or facial cellulitis.
     - Lacrimal osteomyelitis,
     - Rarely, cavernous sinus thrombosis, etc.
   - Chronic conjunctivitis.
   - Recurrent acute conjunctivitis.
   - *Hypopyon corneal ulcer:* Chronic dacryocystitis, is in fact a constant menace to the eye surgeon or to the patient— as mild corneal abrasion due to any reason may be turned into hypopyon corneal ulcer because of *Pneumococcus.* (If there is foreign body in eye in presence of chronic dacryocystitis—after removal of foreign body it is better to block the puncta temporarily by cautery. The same procedure is also true for corneal ulcer with chronic dacryocystitis).

4. **Types of dacryocystitis:**
   - Congenital dacryocystitis (due to congenital non-formation of nasolacrimal duct).
   - Chronic dacryocystitis.
   - Acute dacryocystitis (acute exacerbation of chronic dacryocystitis).

5. **Investigations in case of chronic dacryocystitis:**
   - *To establish the diagnosis:*
     - Syringing or patency test (*see* page 164).
     - Fluorescein dye test: To find out functional or organic block.
     - chloramphenicol eye drop test (one eye at a time).
     - Radiography (dacryocystography).
   - *To prepare for operation:*
     - Blood for TLC, DLC, ESR and Hb.
     - Blood pressure and blood sugar (PP)
     - Bleeding time and clotting time.
     - ENT check up to exclude any contraindication for DCR (absolute contraindication is 'atrophic rhinitis').
     - General anesthesia fitness, if necessary.

6. **Treatment:**
   - *Dacryocystorhinostomy (DCR):* Here the communication is made between lacrimal sac and middle meatus of the

nose by an anastomosis between wall of lacrimal sac with the nasal mucosa. So, there will be no epiphora.
(Normally, *the nasolacrimal duct is directed downwards, backwards and laterally and opens into inferior meatus of the nose*).
Ideally, in all cases, DCR is the choice of surgery if not contraindicated. The contraindications are:
- Extreme old age.
- Atrophic rhinitis.
- Any growth in the sac.
- Nasal polyps.

› *Dacryocystectomy (DCT):* Here, the diseased lacrimal sac is removed totally. The main idea is to remove the reservoir of infection, but the watering will still persist.
  Indications:
  - Extreme old age.
  - Any growth in the sac.
  - Atrophic rhinitis.
  - Tuberculosis of the lacrimal sac.
  - Technical difficulties while performing DCR operation.

› *Conservative treatment for acute dacryocystitis:*
  - Hot compress—3–4 times daily.
  - Systemic broad-spectrum antibiotics.
  - Analgesics and antacid.
  - Local antibiotic drops.
  - In lacrimal abscess: Drainage of pus (dacryocystostomy).
  - After everything subsides: DCT or DCR operation may be planned in future.

› *Congenital dacryocystitis:*
  - Sac massage and giving hydrostatic pressure to open the nasolacrimal duct.
  - If it fails, probing and syringing under GA.
  - If it fails, DCR operation when the child is little older.

› In Emergency situations (e.g., with corneal ulcer, with lens-induced glaucoma or foreign body cornea, etc.): The puncta should be blocked temporarily by:
  - Thermocautery.
  - Electrocautery.
  - Silicone plug and stitching.
  - Cyanoacrylate glue.
  - Later, a planned surgery will be considered.

7. **Complications of DCR operation:**
   a. *Bleeding:* (i) Primary and (ii) Secondary.
   b. Wound gape.
   c. Fistula formation.
   d. Ugly scar or keloid formation.
   e. Closure of anastomosis channel (failed DCR).
   f. Osteomyelitis.

   And in DCT operation:
   a. All of the above except No. (e).
   b. Incomplete removal: Retained part of sac especially near fundus, which may lead to recurrent chronic dacryocystitis with some regurgitation and discharge.

8. **Disadvantages of external DCR**
   External DCR is the gold-standard treatment in chronic dacryocystitis for more than 100 years. Long-term results are always better.
   But it has the following *disadvantages:*
   › Intraoperative bleeding
   › Increased risk of postoperative nasal bleeding
   › Increased secondary infection
   › Prolonged recovery time
   › Hypertrophic scar—a cosmetic blemish, especially in young subjects

9. **Endonasal or transcanalicular laser DCR:**
   › *Endolaser DCR:* It has gained popularity following introduction of laser and better nasal endoscope. Endolaser DCR may be with silicone tube intubation. It is mainly performed by ENT surgeons. It can avoid ugly cutaneous scar formation. Success rate is approximately 70–80%.
   › *Transcanalicular DCR:* Transcanalicular diode laser assisted DCR with or without intubation is another good option with better results. There is no visible scar;

no intra- or postoperative bleeding; less surgical time; very fast recovery. Diode laser has the additional advantage of coagulation effect over all other types of available lasers. Long-term results with this procedure are still under evaluation.

EPISCLERITIS (OP 5.1)

A. **Chief complaints:**
- Localized redness of the eye for ....
- Pain or discomfort in the same eye for same duration.

B. **History of present illness:** No history of photophobia or discharge. History of recurrence may be present.

C. **Personal history:** Gout, rheumatoid arthritis or any other collagen disorder is important.

D. **Ocular examination:**
- **Vision:** Usually normal.
- **Movements:** Normal.
- **Conjunctiva:**
  - Localized congestion around a nodular swelling.
  - Conjunctiva overlying the nodule is freely mobile.
- **Cornea, anterior chamber, lens, iris and pupil:** Usually normal.
- **Sclera:**
  - A circumscribed episcleral nodule, purple in color, about 2–3 mm diameter.
  - It is 1–3 mm away from the limbus mainly at the palpebral area **(Fig. 2.26)**.
  - The nodule is immobile.
  - It is tender on giving pressure through the lid.
  - An old lesion may have slate grey in appearance on which the conjunctiva is often adherent.
- **Digital tension:** Normal.
- **Lacrimal sac:** Normal.

E. **Provisional diagnosis:** Episcleritis.

Self-assessment Questionnaire

1. **Define episcleritis:** It is a benign inflammatory process affecting the episcleral

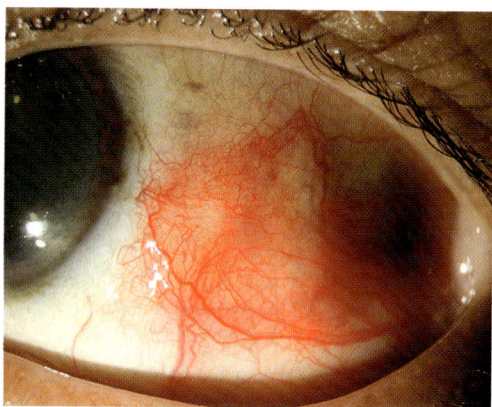

Fig. 2.26: Episcleritis.

tissue that lies between the conjunctiva and the sclera.

2. **Causes of episcleritis:**
   - 2/3rd cases are idiopathic
   - Rheumatoid arthritis or other collagen vascular diseases.
   - Allergic reaction to an endogenous toxin, e.g., streptococcal or tubercular.
   - *Infectious:* Herpes zoster, herpes simplex, syphilis, etc.

3. **Complications of episcleritis:**
   - Recurrent attack: When the attacks are fleeting but frequently repeated, it is called *episcleritis periodica fugax.*
   - Chronic episcleritis.
   - Deeper extension into the sclera may lead to scleritis.

4. **Differential diagnosis of episcleritis:**
   a. Phlyctenular conjunctivitis.
   b. Inflamed pinguecula.
   c. Scleritis.

5. **Differences between episcleritis and scleritis:** (*See* page 111).

6. **Treatment:**
   - NSAID eye drop, e.g., indomethacin, flurbiprofen, ketarolac or nepafenac eye drop—3–4 times daily.
   - Oral anti-inflammatory agents e.g., ibuprofen, indomethacin, diclofenac, etc.
   - Rarely, weak steroids eye drop (fluorometholone or loteprednol)—4 times daily in selective cases.

TRICHIASIS *(OP 2.3)*

A. Chief complaints:
- Irritation and foreign body sensation in the eye for ...
- Watering from the same eye for ...

B. History of present illness (Special point): No history of fall of foreign body in the eye.

C. Past history: Removal of eyelash (self or by doctor).

D. Ocular examination:
- **Vision:** Normal
- **Movements:** Normal
- **Lids:**
  - Blepharospasm, may be associated entropion
  - One or more distorted eyelash(es)—directed backwards towards the globe and touching the cornea or conjunctiva.
- **Conjunctiva:** Localized conjunctival congestion.
- **Cornea:**
  - Adjacent superficial punctate keratitis.
  - Fluorescein stain may be positive
  - Adjacent superficial corneal opacity maybe present.
  - Superficial vascularization.
- **Other structures:** Normal.

E. Provisional diagnosis: Trichiasis of upper/lower lid of RE/LE.

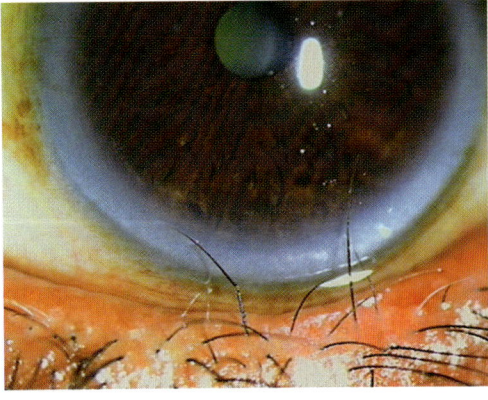

Fig. 2.27: Trichiasis.

Self-assessment Questionnaire

1. **Define trichiasis:** This is the distortion of the cilia or eyelash which are directed backwards and rub against the globe specially the cornea **(Fig. 2.27)**.
   Distichiasis: A rare congenital condition in which there is an extra posterior row of cilia, occasionally in four lids. The posterior row occupies the position of the meibomian glands, and the eyelashes may irritate the cornea.
2. **Causes of trichiasis:**
   a. *Congenital:* Distichiasis.
   b. *Acquired:*
      - Blepharitis
      - Membranous conjunctivitis
      - Trachoma
      - External hordeolum
      - Burns—thermal or chemical
      - Stevens-Johnson syndrome
      - Operations on the lid margins, e.g., tarsorrhaphy.
      - Lid injuries.
3. **Complications:**
   - Recurrent punctate corneal erosions.
   - Superficial corneal opacities.
   - Vascularization of the cornea.
   - Recurrent corneal ulcers.
   - Non-healing corneal ulcer.
4. **Treatment:**
   - *Temporary:* Epilation of the offending eyelashes. (*See* page 90, 162)
   - Permanent treatment (*see* page 163).

BLEPHARITIS

A. Chief complaints:
- Itching of the eyelids for ....
- Falling of eyelashes even on simple rubbing of the eyelids ...

B. History of present illness (special points):
- History of seborrhea or dandruff of the scalp.
- History of using kajal, surma or other cosmetics.

C. Personal history: Parasitic infestation of the scalp or eyelash.

D. Ocular examination:
- **Vision:** Normal or less.
- **Ocular movements:** Normal.
- **Lids (more in upper lid):**
  - The lid margins are swollen and red.

- White dandruff-like small scales at the roots of the eyelash.
- Cylindrical dandruff or sleeves around eyelashes (*Demodex folliculorum*)
- At few places, matting of the eyelashes.
- Fall of eyelashes on slight pulling or rubbing.
- In ulcerative form, there may be ulceration or bleeding following removal of crust.
- Lid margin may be distorted.
- Hyperemia of palpebral conjunctiva adjacent to the lid margins.

❖ **Conjunctiva:** May show conjunctival congestion.
❖ **Cornea:** Superficial punctate keratitis may be seen in lower part of the cornea.
❖ **Sclera and other structures:** Normal.
E. **Provisional diagnosis:** Blepharitis.

Self-assessment Questionnaire

1. **Causal factors for blepharitis:**
   - Staphylococcal infection.
   - Refractive errors.
   - Chronic conjunctivitis.
   - Unhygienic lid conditions.
   - *Using cosmetics:* Kajal, surma, mascara, etc.
   - Dandruff of the scalp or seborrhea
   - *Demodex infestation* of eyelashes with chronic blepharitis in 30%

2. **Types of blepharitis:**
   - *Anterior blepharitis:* Squamous type and ulcerative type **(Fig. 2.28A)**.
   - Posterior blepharitis or meibomianitis (meibomitis) **(Fig. 2.28B)**.

3. **Differences between squamous and ulcerative blepharitis (Table 2.12):**

TABLE 2.12: Differences between squamous and ulcerative blepharitis.

Squamous blepharitis	Ulcerative blepharitis
1. Hyperemic lid margin and white scales at the root of eyelashes	1. Yellowish crusts at the root of the eyelashes
2. On removing the scales—no bleeding or no raw surfaces	2. On removal of crust—there is raw area which may bleed
3. Eyelashes are normal	3. Eyelashes—glued together, may be lacking, or may be distorted
4. Lid margin is little swollen, but normal	4. Lid margin is thickened and distorted

4. **Complications or sequalae of blepharitis:**
   - Trichiasis.
   - Madarosis (loss or scanty eyelashes).
   - Chronic conjunctivitis.
   - Superficial punctate keratitis or SPK (in lower 1/3 of the cornea)
   - Entropion.

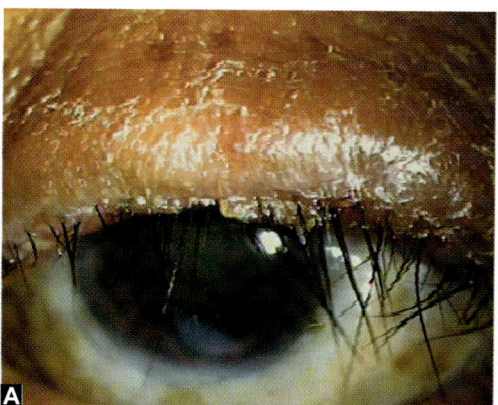 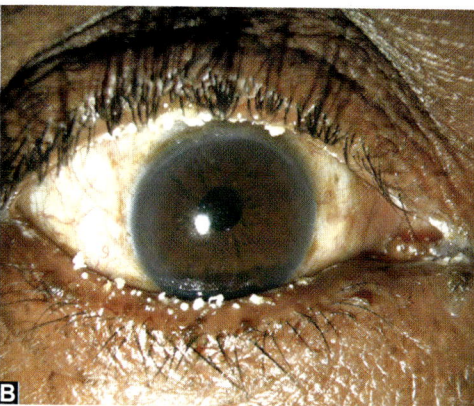

Figs. 2.28A and B: (A) Blepharitis; (B) Meibomianitis (tooth paste sign).

- Tylosis (hypertrophied lid margins with consequent drooping due to its weight).
- Ectropion of the lower lid and epiphora.

5. **Treatment:**
   a. *Local:*
      - Warm sodium bicarbonate lotion (3%) is applied with cotton bud to the lid margin to soak the crusts or scales—3 times daily. Alternately, baby shampoo may be applied.
      - Removal of crusts or scale by a cotton swab.
      - Loose and diseased eyelashes are to be epilated.
      - Tea-tree oil for *Demodex* infestations
      - Antibiotic ointment or antibiotic-steroid ointment is to be applied by rubbing the lid margins 3 times daily.
      - An antibiotic drop may also be added if the infection seems to be more acute in nature.
   b. *Systemic:* A course of systemic doxycycline for 2–4 weeks is useful in severe ulcerative form of blepharitis.
   c. *General:*
      - Ocular hygiene. Avoid mascara, kajal, or any cosmetics, etc.
      - Use medicated shampoo for dandruff.
      - Vitamins including vitamin A.
      - Correction of refractive errors.
      - Treatment of louse infestation of the body.

6. **Posterior blepharitis (*Meibomianitis*) and its treatment:** It is chronic inflammation of the meibomian glands, occurs in middle-aged, mainly due to *Staphylococcus epidermidis* infection. It may be associated with rosacea.
   - *Symptoms:* Watering; Frothy discharge, mainly at the outer canthi; and foreign body sensation.
   - *Signs:* White frothy discharge, thick meibomian secretion like toothpaste (*tooth paste sign*), blocked meibomian openings, and on eversion of lids vertical yellow streaks shining through the conjunctiva.
   - *Treatment:* Hot fomentation—2-3 times daily; vertical lid massage (tarsal massage) and removal of secretion with a moist cotton applicator; azithromycin eye ointment—2-3 times daily; tear substitutes—4 times daily and systemic doxycycline for 4-6 weeks.

CHAPTER 3

Brief Theories and Viva

OCULAR ANATOMY (AN 41.1)

Gross Anatomy of the Eyeball

Three concentric layers of eyeball:
1. **Outer supporting layer:** It consists of transparent cornea (1/6th) and opaque sclera (5/6th), and their junction, the limbus.
2. **Middle vascular layer:** It is called uvea. It consists of choroid, ciliary body and the iris.
3. **Inner neural layer:** Retina

Conventionally, eyeball is divided into *two segments*: Anterior and posterior.
1. **Anterior segment:** It is the anterior one-third of the eyeball in front of the anterior vitreous face.
   It includes: Crystalline lens (suspended from ciliary body by fine zonules) and the structures anterior to it, i.e., iris, cornea and two aqueous-field chambers—anterior and posterior.
   Anterior chamber: Bounded anteriorly by the posterior surface of the cornea, and posteriorly, by the iris, part of ciliary body and part of the anterior surface of the lens which is exposed at the pupil.
   Central anterior chamber depth: 2.5 mm and *volume*—0.25 mL.
   Posterior chamber: It is a small triangular space, bounded anteriorly by back of the iris and part of ciliary body, and posteriorly, by the lens and zonules and laterally by the ciliary body. Volume—0.06 mL. It communicates with the anterior chamber through the pupil.
   Aqueous humor fills these chambers within the anterior segment and provides nutrients to the surrounding structures.

   [Some ophthalmologists specialize in the management of anterior segment diseases and they called **anterior segment surgeons**.]
2. **Posterior segment:** It comprises the posterior two-thirds of the eyeball behind the crystalline lens. *It includes* anterior hyaloid face, vitreous humor, retina, choroid and the optic nerve head.
   [Similarly, some ophthalmologists specialize in the management of posterior segment diseases and they called **posterior segment surgeons**.]

Ophthalmic Measurements
- Orbital volume: 30 mL
- Globe volume: 6.5 mL
- Vitreous volume: 4-4.5 mL
- Anterior chamber volume: 250 µL
- Conjunctival sac volume: 35 µL
- Eyedrop volume: 50 µL
- Lens diameter: 9.5 mm
- Anterior capsule thickness: 14 µm
- Posterior capsule thickness: 2–4 µm
- **Distance from the limbus:**
  - Superior rectus (S): 7.7 mm
  - Lateral rectus (L): 6.9 mm
  - Inferior rectus (I): 6.5 mm
  - Medial rectus (M): 5.5 mm
  - Ciliary body: 1 mm
  - Ora serata: 7–8 mm
- Optic disc: 1.5 mm
- Fovea: 1.5 mm
- Foveolar avascular zone (FAZ): 500 micron
- Rod photoreceptor cells: 120 million
- Cone photoreceptor cells: 6 million
- **Visual field:**
  - Superior: 60°
  - Inferior: 70°
  - Nasal: 60°
  - Temporal: 100°

Anatomy of the Eyelid

Structures (Anterior to Posterior)

- **Cutaneous layer:** Having creases, and without any long hair.
- **Subcutaneous tissue:** Loose areolar tissue *devoid of fat.*
- **Muscular layer:**
  - Orbicularis oculi
  - Levator palpebrae superioris (LPS) in upper lid only
  - Muller's muscle
- **Fibrous layer:**
  - Orbital septum—towards orbital margin.
  - Tarsal plate—towards lid margin. Different glands of eyelid (i.e., Meibomian glands, gland of Zeis, glands of Moll, glands of Krause and Wolfring) lie in this plane.
- **Palpebral conjunctival layer:** Innermost layer of the eye lid.

Muscles of the Eyelid

- **Orbicularis oculi:**
  - *Action:* Lid closure, blinking, winking, squeezing helps in drainage of tears.
  - *Nerve supply:* Zygomatic branch of facial (7th cranial) nerve.
  - *In case of its paralysis:* There will be lagophthalmos (leading to exposure keratitis), and also epiphora due to orbicularis (lacrimal) pump failure.
- **Levator palpebrae superioris (LPS):** Present only in upper lid.
  - *Origin:* From the apex of the orbit, above the annulus of Zinn.
  - *Insertion:* In 5 parts:
    - Main tendinous slip—into upper margin and anterior surface of the tarsal plate.
    - Anterior slip—to under surface of the lid skin.
    - Posterior slip—to upper fornix with superior rectus sheath.
    - Medial and lateral slips—to medial and lateral palpebral ligaments.
  - *Action:* Elevates the upper eyelid including upper fornix and helps in the formation of upper lid crease.
  - *Nerve supply:* Upper division of oculomotor nerve (3rd cranial).
  - *Paralysis of LPS*—causes ptosis.
- **Muller's muscle (unstriped):**
  - *Upper Muller's muscle:* Arises from the striped fibers of LPS, and is inserted into upper border of the tarsal plate.
  - *Action:* Elevates the upper lid.
  - *Lower Muller's muscle:* Arises from inferior rectus muscle, and inserted into the lower tarsal plate.
  - *Action:* Elevates the lower lid to some extent.
  - *Nerve supply:* Cervical sympathetic nerve.
  - Paralysis of cervical sympathetic nerve causes *Horner's syndrome* (ptosis, miosis, ipsilateral anhydrosis of the face).

Glands of the Eyelid

- **Meibomian glands:** These are modified tubular sebaceous glands, secrete the lipid layer of the tear film. They are situated within tarsal plate, arranged vertically, and opens by a single duct onto the margin of the lids. *Number:* 30–40 in upper lid and 20–30 in lower lid.
- **Glands of Zeis:** These are sebaceous glands lie in the lid margin and open in the follicle of eyelashes.
- **Glands of Moll:** Modified sweat gland, situated immediately behind the hair follicles.
- **Glands of Krause and Wolfring:** These are accessory lacrimal glands, situated on the palpebral conjunctival side.

Inter-marginal strip: Is the free edge of the lid. It is lined by stratified epithelium which forms a transition between the skin and conjunctiva. It has the following anatomical landmarks (the anterior to posterior):

- Anterior round border
- Eye lashes
- Grey line
- Orifices of the ducts of Meibomian glands
- Posterior sharp border.

Gray line is a landmark for lid splitting surgery, as it indicates the position of loose fibrous tissue between orbicularis oculi and the tarsus.

Functions of the Eyelids
- Protect the eyeball proper from external injuries—sunlight, dust, fumes, foreign body, etc.
- Maintain the precorneal tear film (by sharp posterior border of the lid margin) by the natural act of blinking.
- Drainage of tears by lacrimal pump system.
- Interrupt and limit the amount of light entering the eye.
- Emotional expressions, like winking.

Anatomy of the Conjunctiva

It is a mucous membrane covering inner surface of the lids and reflected to cover the anterior part of the eyeball over sclera, up to limbus.

Parts
- **Palpebral part:** Consists of marginal, tarsal and orbital part. It is firmly adherent to the deeper tissue.
- **Bulbar part:** Over the sclera and freely mobile.
- **Fornix:** It is the cul-de-sac at the junction of palpebral and bulbar conjunctiva.
- **Limbal:** Conjunctiva at the corneal junction (adherent).

Microscopic Appearance
- **Epithelium:**
  - Two layers of epithelium over the palpebral conjunctiva and the transitional stratified squamous epithelium at the intermarginal strip.
  - From fornices to the limbus—the epithelium is gradually thicker (4-6 layers) and it is stratified epithelium at the limbus.
  - *Goblet cells* (mucin secreting cells) are present throughout the epithelium, especially more near the fornices.
- **Subepithelial layer:** Of loose connective tissue containing leukocytes.
- **Fibrous layer:** Much dense and blended with deeper structures (e.g., episclera or tarsus).

Nerve supply: Ophthalmic division of trigeminal (5th cranial) nerve.

Anatomy of the Lacrimal Apparatus

The lacrimal apparatus consists of two parts:
1. Secretory portion
2. Collecting portion.

A. **Parts of the secretory portion:**
Lacrimal gland: A tubuloalveolar gland, lies in the anterolateral portion of the roof of orbit. It has two parts—orbital and palpebral. Its ducts open separately onto the superior temporal fornix.
Nerve supply: Via facial nerve, parasympathetic from salivatory nucleus.
Accessory lacrimal glands of Krause and Wolfring: These are located deep in the conjunctiva, near the fornixes, especially on the temporal side.

B. **Parts of the drainage portion (lacrimal passage):**
- **Two lacrimal puncta:** Two small openings—situated near the posterior lid margin about 6 mm from the inner canthus. Punctum is situated upon a slight elevation (seen in elderly people), called *lacrimal papilla*.
- **Two canaliculi:** Pass from the punctum to the lacrimal sac. They first directed vertically for 1-2 mm, then horizontally into the lacrimal sac. Sometimes, they join together to from a common canaliculus before opening into the sac.
- **Lacrimal sac:** Lies on the lacrimal fossa formed by the lacrimal bone. When distended, it is about 15 mm long and 5-6 mm wide. The upper portion, called fundus, lies slightly above medial palpebral ligament. Sac itself is covered by orbicularis muscles and loose fibrous tissues.
- **Nasolacrimal duct:** It is the continuation of lacrimal sac. It is 12-24 mm long and 3-6 mm in width. It has two parts—*intra-osseous* and *intra-meatal*. It passes downwards, slightly out-wards and backwards *to open into the anterior part of the inferior meatus of the nose*.
  Upper end of nasolacrimal duct is the narrowest part. Mucous lining forms an

imperfect valve at the orifice into the nose (valve of Hasner).
In case of dacryocystorhinostomy (DCR)—the new opening opens at the middle meatus of the nose, after making an anastomosis between the lacrimal sac and nasal mucosa of the middle meatus.

Anatomy of the Cornea

A. Structures of the cornea (five layers): From anterior to posterior or superficial to deep.
1. **Stratified epithelium** (continuous with the epithelium of the conjunctiva, 5–6 cells deep.
2. **Bowman's membrane** (once eroded, never regenerates, leaves behind a superficial corneal scar).
3. **Stroma or substantia propria** (90% of total corneal thickness and continuous with the sclera).
4. **Descemet's membrane** is the basement membrane of the corneal endothelium. It has poor potential to regenerate.
5. **Endothelium** (single layered flattened cells) never regenerates in human after any injury/loss.

> **Note**
> **Pre-Descemet's layer (Dua's layer):** A new layer was described by Harminder S Dua, from India, in 2013. It is hypothetically 15 µ thick, the fourth corneal layer from top, and located between the corneal stroma and Descemet's membrane.

B. Nerve supply of the cornea: Ophthalmic division of 5th cranial nerve via nasociliary branch. The nerve fibrils are non-myelinated. The corneal nerves do not carry proprioceptive sensation.

C. Measurements:
- **Diameter** of cornea is 11 mm vertically and 12 mm horizontally.
- **Central corneal thickness (CCT)** is about 500 µ; and peripherally 800 µ.
- **Refractive index** of the cornea is 1.34
- **Dioptric power** is about +43.0D to +45.0D.
- **Radius of curvature:** anterior surface = 7.8 mm; posterior = 6.5 mm.

D. Nutrition of the cornea (cornea does not have any blood vessel).
- Oxygen from atmosphere via tear film.
- Perilimbal plexus of blood vessels
- Aqueous humor.

E. Cornea is transparent and it is maintained by:
- Regular arrangement of stromal collagen fibrils (Lattice theory).
- Absence of blood vessels.
- Absence of myelinated nerve fibers.
- Relative dehydration by active transport of fluid outwards (maintained mainly by endothelial Na-K ATPase pump system).
- Special intercellular junction controls the fluid traffic.
- Optimum intraocular pressure to control fluid transport.

F. Corneal endothelium is the most important layer for maintaining the function of the cornea. It is examined grossly by slit lamp and best seen *by a specular microscope* at a magnification of 500 times. The cells can be counted, and cellular morphology can be studied.

The average endothelial cell count in young adult is 2500–3000 cells/sq mm and decreases with the age.

Anatomy of the Uvea

The uveal tract consists of three parts (*uvea* means 'grape'):
A. **Anterior:** Iris, a free circular diaphragm, with a central opening, called pupil.
B. **Intermediate:** Ciliary body.
C. **Posterior:** Choroid.

A. Structures of the iris: Consists of four layers (anterior to posterior)
1. **Anterior endothelium:** Continuous with the corneal endothelium.
2. **Stroma:** It consists of spongy connective tissue with radial blood vessels forming the minor circle of iris; nerves and smooth muscles.
3. **Smooth muscles:** They are two in number.
   i. *Sphincter pupillae:* A circular bundle of smooth muscles running around the

pupillary margin—causes constriction of the pupil.
   ii. *Dilator pupillae:* Arranged radially near the root of the iris—causes dilation of the pupil.
4. **Posterior two layers of epithelium:** Both layers are pigmented and developmentally share the same origin with the retina.
   Nerve supply of the iris:
   > *Sensory:* Nasociliary nerve, branch of 1st division of 5th cranial nerve.
   > *Sphincter pupillae:* Oculomotor nerve (3rd cranial nerve).
   > *Dilator pupillae:* Nerves derived from cervical sympathetic chain.

B. **Structures of the ciliary body:** In antero-posterior section, it is roughly an isosceles triangle, with base forwards. Iris is attached at the middle of its base. It is covered by two layers of epithelium, continuous with the iris anteriorly and retina posteriorly.
❖ The chief mass of the ciliary body is composed of unstriped muscle fibers, called *ciliary muscles.*
❖ The inner surface of ciliary body is divided into two regions:
   1. *Pars plicata:* Anterior part; about 70 plications. They have *ciliary processes* responsible for the production of the aqueous.
   2. *Pars plana:* Posterior part ('*safe zone*' of the eye) a relatively safe and avascular zone for pars plana lensectomy or vitrectomy operation and for intravitreal injection.
   Ciliary body extends backwards as far as the ora serrata. At this point the retina proper begins abruptly.

Nerve supply of the ciliary body:
❖ **Sensory:** Via nasociliary branch of 5th cranial nerve.
❖ **Ciliary muscles:** Oculomotor and sympathetic nerves.

Functions of ciliary body:
❖ Formation of aqueous humor by the ciliary processes.

❖ Ciliary muscles help in accommodation for near work.
❖ Ciliary muscles also help in opening up Schlemm's canal and thus facilitate in aqueous out flow.

C. **Structures of the choroid:** Consists of *three layers of blood vessels*, having supporting structures on either side.
1. Larger outer vessels layer (of Haller)
2. Medium middle vessels layer (of Sattler)
3. Choriocapillaries.

Blood supply of the choroid:
❖ **Short posterior ciliary arteries:** Branches of ophthalmic artery, 10–20 in number.
❖ **Long posterior ciliary arteries:** Each divide into two branches that extend circumferentially to form '*major arterial circle*' of the iris.
❖ **Anterior ciliary arteries:** Terminal branches of two muscular arteries of each rectus muscle (except the lateral rectus, which has one). They send branches to the '*major arterial circle*' of the iris.

Venous blood of the uvea is collected by a series of veins into the *vortex veins* (4 in number) located behind the equator of the globe. The vortex veins drain into the superior and inferior ophthalmic veins.

LAYERS AND REGIONS OF RETINA

A. Retina consists of ten layers. From outside (choroid-side) to inwards:
1. Retinal pigment epithelium (RPE).
2. Layer of rods and cones.
3. External limiting membrane.
4. Outer nuclear layer.
5. Outer plexiform layer.
6. Inner nuclear layer.
7. Inner plexiform layer.
8. Ganglion cell layer.
9. (Optic) nerve fiber layer.
10. Internal limiting membrane.

Rods are about 125 million in number, but the cones are about 7 million. Cones are responsible for acuity of vision and color vision in photopic condition. Rods are for scotopic vision (i.e., vision in dim light).

B. **Regions of the retina:**
- ❖ **Ora serrata:** It is the anterior termination of retina, located 7.5–8 mm from the limbus.
- ❖ **Central retina:** Is 4.5 mm in diameter. Central part of this region is called macula leutea which contains yellow pigment, xanthophyll.
  Fovea centralis is a depressed area at its center, about 3 mm (2 disc diameter) temporal to the disc and 0.8 mm below the horizontal meridian. It measures about 1.5 mm (1500 µm). Its central depression is called *foveola*, measuring about 0.5 mm (500 µm).
  Foveola is nourished solely by the choriocapillaries of the choroid and does not contain any vessels, and hence, called *foveolar avascular zone (FAZ)*. The photoreceptors in the fovea are exclusively cones.
- ❖ **Peripheral retina:** Here, photoreceptors are predominantly rods.
- ❖ **Functionally,** retina is divided into temporal and nasal portion, by a line drawn vertically through the center of the fovea. Temporal nerve fibers pass to the lateral geniculate body of the same side.
- ❖ **Ophthalmoscopically,** optic nerve serves as a landmark to divide the retina into superior and inferior temporal portions, superior and inferior nasal portions, and a central retina.

Anatomy of the Extraocular Muscles

They are six in number. Four rectus muscles and two oblique muscles.
- ❖ **Origin of the rectus muscles:** Common origin from annular tendon of Zinn around the optic foramen at the apex of the orbit.
  Insertion: They are inserted onto the sclera after piercing the Tenon's capsule. The distance from limbus are as follows:
  Superior rectus (S) = 7.7 mm
  Lateral rectus (L) = 6.9 mm
  Inferior rectus (I) = 6.6 mm
  Medial rectus (M) = 5.5 mm
- ❖ **Origin of superior oblique:** Common origin at the apex of the orbit from annular tendon of Zinn → runs to the trochlea, at the upper and inner angle of orbit → becomes tendinous → reflected backwards under the superior rectus muscle.
  Insertion: On the sclera at superolateral part of posterior pole.
- ❖ **Origin of inferior oblique:** Arises anteriorly from the lower and inner orbital walls near the lacrimal fossa. It is the only muscle, not arising from the apex of the orbit.
  Insertion: It is inserted on the sclera at inferolateral part of the posterior pole of the globe (corresponds to the area near macula).
- ❖ **Nerve supply:** All the muscles are supplied by 3rd cranial (oculomotor) nerve except, lateral rectus—by 6th (abducens) nerve and superior oblique—by 4th (trochlear) nerve.
- ❖ **Actions of the extraocular muscles:** (Remember mnemonic SINRAD superior intorsion, recti adduction)

Muscle	Primary action	Secondary action	Tertiary action
Medial rectus	Adduction	–	–
Lateral rectus	Abduction	–	–
Superior rectus	Elevation	Intorsion	Adduction
Inferior rectus	Depression	Extorsion	Adduction
Superior oblique	Intorsion	Depression	Abduction
Inferior oblique	Extorsion	Elevation	Abduction

Grades of Binocular Vision

- ❖ **1st:** *Simultaneous macular perception (SMP)*—ability to see images of two dissimilar objects simultaneously
- ❖ **2nd:** *Fusion*—ability to fuse two similar but incomplete images
- ❖ **3rd:** *Stereopsis*—ability to recognize the depth of an object correctly

The Bony Orbit

The orbits are pear-shaped cavities. Their medial walls are parallel, but lateral walls diverge at an angle of 45°. The orbit is roughly 40 mm in height, width and depth, its volume is about 30 mL. The ratio of eyeball volume with the orbital volume is 1:4.5.

Bony orbit is formed by the parts of seven bones:
1. Frontal
2. Maxillary
3. Zygomatic
4. Sphenoid
5. Lacrimal
6. Ethmoidal
7. Palatine.

Contents of the orbit:
- Eyeball with intraorbital part of the optic nerve
- Retrobulbar fat.
- Extraocular muscles.
- Ophthalmic arteries and veins.
- 3rd, 4th, 5th (first two division) and 6th cranial nerves, and ciliary ganglion.
- Lymphatic vessels and sympathetic plexus.
- Tenon's capsule and orbital fascia.
- Lacrimal glands and lacrimal sac.

Surgical Spaces of Orbit

From the surgical point of view there are **four spaces** within the orbit. They are relatively self-contained.
1. **Subperiosteal space:** Between the bones of orbital wall and the periorbita (periosteum).
2. **Peripheral (peribulbar) space:** Between the periorbita and the extraocular muscles which are joined by fascial connections.
3. **Central space:** A cone-shaped area enclosed by the muscles (the 'muscle-cone').
4. **Tenon's space:** Around the globe.

OCULAR PHARMACOLOGY (PH 1.58)

Routes of Administration of Ocular Medicine

- **Systemic:** Oral (e.g., tablet acetazolamide), intravenous (e.g., methyl prednisolone), intramuscular (e.g., antibiotics for severe periocular infections)
- **Local:**
  a. Topical—eye drops, gel and ointments
  b. Injection:
     Periocular
     - Subconjunctival (e.g., dexamethasone, atropine, etc.)
     - Posterior sub-Tenon (e.g., triamcinolone, lignocaine, etc.)
     - Retrobulbar (e.g., lignocaine, bupivacaine, etc.)
     - Peribulbar (e.g., lignocaine, bupivacaine, etc.)
     Intraocular
     - Intracameral (into anterior chamber) (e.g., adrenaline, pilocarpine, lignocaine, viscoelastic agents, trypan blue, etc.)
     - Intravitreal (into the vitreous cavity) (Table 3.1)

Antibiotics Used in Ophthalmology

- **Broad-spectrum:** Ciprofloxacin (0.3%), moxifloxacin (0.5%), gatifloxacin (0.3%; 0.5%), chloramphenicol (0.5%), tetracycline (1%)
- **Effective against gram-positive organisms:** Moxifloxacin, gatifloxacin, vancomycin, ceftazidime, and cefazoline

TABLE 3.1: Intravitreal injections.

Drug group	Indications	Drug used
Antibiotic	Endophthalmitis	Vancomycin, ceftazidime, amikacin
Antifungals	Endophthalmitis	Amphotericin-B, voriconazole
Antivirals	Viral retinal necrosis or retinopathy	Ganciclovir, foscarnet
Anti-VGEF	DR, Wet-AMD, ROP	Ranibizumab, bevacizumab, aflibercept
Steroids	Macular edema in RVO, chronic uveitis	Triamcinolone, dexamethasone

- **Effective against gram-negative organisms:** Gentamycin (0.3%), ciprofloxacin (0.3%), amikacin, tobramycin (1%), and polymyxin-B

Antifungals Used in Ophthalmology

They are fungistatic in nature. They are mainly used in fungal keratitis and fungal endophthalmitis.

Three groups of agents are used:
1. **Polyenes:** Natamycin (5%) and amphotericin B (0.15–0.25%) eye drops
2. **Azoles:** Voriconazole, ketoconazole, econazole, fluconazole, itraconazole, etc.
3. **Flucytosine:** 5-fluorocytosine.

Antivirals Used in Ophthalmology

- **Acyclovir:** Both oral and ointment (for herpes simplex or zoster ocular infection)
- **Valacyclovir:** Oral (for herpes simplex or zoster ocular infection)
- **Gancyclovir:** As ointment or IV injection in herpes simplex or CMV ocular infection
- **Oral valgancyclovir:** CMV infection

Steroids in Ophthalmology

The corticosteroids reduce the inflammatory responses of the ocular tissues by—decreasing capillary permeability, limiting exudation and inhibiting the formation of new vessels and granulation tissue.

Indications:
- **Sterile inflammations:** Uveitis, scleritis, optic neuritis, chemical injury, disciform keratitis, etc.
- **Allergic problems:** Phlycten, allergic conjunctivitis, contact dermatitis, vernal keratoconjunctivitis, etc.
- **Postoperative:** Following cataract surgery, keratoplasty, vitrectomy, trabeculectomy, etc.
- **Miscellaneous:** Corneal graft rejection, thyroid exophthalmos, temporal arteritis, optic neuritis, etc.

Route of administration: Local and systemic

Local: Three types—(1) topical, (2) periocular, and (3) intraocular.
1. **Topical preparation:** Mostly available as drops and also as ointment, sometimes with antibiotic combination.
   - Hydrocortisone acetate: 0.5%
   - Prednisolone acetate: 1.0%
   - Dexamethasone phosphate: 0.1%
   - Betamethasone: 0.5%
   - Fluorometholone: 0.1%
   - Loteprednol etabonate: 0.5% and 0.2%
   - Difluprednate: 0.05% (a precursor of prednisolone).
2. **Periocular:**
   - *Subconjunctival:* Mainly, injection dexamethasone and combination with gentamycin—at the end of surgery
   - *Posterior sub-Tenon's:* Injection triamcinolone as in postoperative cystoid macular edema (CME)
   - *Peribulbar:* In thyroid ophthalmopathy, cornea graft rejection.
3. **Intraocular:** Intravitreal injection—triamcinolone acetonide or dexamethasone implants in uveitic CME, diabetic macular edema (DME)

Systemic: Oral and intravenous.
Oral: Prednisolone is the most commonly used oral corticosteroid.
Intravenous: Methylprednisolone (500 mg to 1 g) or dexamethasone

Ocular side effects/complications:
- Steroid-induced glaucoma
- Steroid-induced cataract
- Delayed wound healing
- Increased risk of superinfection (bacterial/fungal)

Nonsteroidal Anti-inflammatory Drugs (NSAIDs)

Nonsteroidal anti-inflammatory agents are used to avoid side effects of steroids. They are as follows:
- Flurbiprofen
- Ketorolac

- Bromfenac
- *Nepafenac:* It has the best corneal and intraocular penetration
- Indomethacin (oral route)

Uses

Mainly used as eye drops except oral indomethacin.
- Prevent intraoperative miosis during intraocular surgery.
- As prophylactic and therapeutic agent in cystoid macular edema (CME).
- Reduce ocular inflammation when steroids are contraindicated; as in vernal conjunctivitis; scleritis, allergic conjunctivitis, mild iridocyclitis and postoperative cases.

Ophthalmic Viscosurgical Device (OVD)

Simply called as viscoelastics. These are tissue-protective viscoelastic gels with higher molecular weight.

The Types

- **Dispersive OVD:** Hydroxypropyl methylcellulose (HPMC) 2% and chondroitin sulphate (Viscoat). It provides excellent coating of the corneal endothelium and protect it.
- **Cohesive OVD:** Sodium hyaluronate (1% and 1.4%). These agents maintain anterior chamber space and push the iris-lens diaphragm.
- **Visco-adaptive OVD:** Sodium hyaluronate (2.3%). It displays different behaviors during different stage of surgery. Higher cohesiveness with some pseudo-dispersive property.
- **Combination OVD:** Combination of 4% chondroitin sulphate and sodium hyaluronate (Discovisc). It behaves like a highly cohesive OVD with endothelial protection similar to a dispersive substance.

Uses

- Creates and maintains depth of the anterior chamber during surgery—mainly during capsulorrhexis, IOL implantation in-the-bag, etc.
- Protects the corneal endothelium throughout the surgery from mechanical trauma
- Acts as a soft instrument for gentle maneuver of intraocular tissue.
- It is used during foldable-IOL loading within the IOL-cartridge.

Antivascular Endothelial Growth Factors

Vascular endothelial growth factor (VEGF) is a naturally occurring signal protein which is responsible for angiogenesis or growth of new blood vessels.

The anti-VEGF agents block the VEGF molecules and thus benefit the patients by decreasing the abnormal and harmful new blood vessels formation, and by decreasing the leakage and macular edema.

The Anti-VEGF Agents

- Bevacizumab (Avastin)—off label use
- Ranibizumab (Lucentis/Accentrix)
- Pegaptanib (Macugen)—not available now
- Aflibercept (Eylea)
- Brolucizumzb (Pagenex)

Indications

- Wet age-related macular degeneration (AMD)
- Choroidal neovascular membrane (CNVM)
- CRVO/BRVO with macular edema
- Diabetic macular edema (DME)
- Eales disease and Coats' disease
- Post-surgical refractory CME
- Neovascular glaucoma (NVG) and/or neovascularization of iris (NVI)

Tear Substitutes (Artificial Tears)

These are lubricating eye drops or gel used to relieve dryness and irritation in ocular surface diseases. They are also used to moisten contact lenses and to treat irregular corneal surface.

They are:
- **Cellulose polymers:** Carboxy methyl cellulose (CMC), hydroxypropyl methyl cellulose (HPMC)

- Polyvinyl alcohol (PVA); polyvinyl pyrrolidine
- Polyethylene glycol (PEG) and HP Guar
- Carbomer
- Sodium hyaluronate
- Ointment—petroleum gel, lanolin, etc. for night application.

Miotics

Miotics are the drugs which cause meiosis or pupillary constriction. Systemically used drug e.g., morphine is a strong miotic, but it is not used as a miotic.

Local Miotics
- **Cholinergic miotics:** Three types:
  1. *Direct stimulant:* Acetylcholine (miochol); pilocarpine (1–4%)
  2. *Indirect stimulant, i.e., anticholinestrase:* Eserine (0.25–1%) neostigmine, phospholine iodide (0.06–0.25%), etc.
  3. *Combination of direct and indirect action:* Carbachol (Miostat)
- **Sympathetic miotics:** Rarely used. Thymoxamine (0.5%) solution is a powerful miotic—used as an antidote of phenylephrine.

Pilocarpine is the only miotic which is used widely. Acetylcholine and carbachol are available in western world for intraocular use.

All miotics also stimulate the ciliary muscles to contract, so that the eye assumes a state of accommodation (or *accommodative spasm*).

Uses of Miotics
- Almost in all cases of glaucoma including primary angle-closure or primary open-angle glaucoma.
- **Intraocular use:**
  - During cataract surgery after implantation of PC IOL (with dilute pilocarpine directly into the anterior chamber).
  - During cataract surgery, before insertion of AC IOL (primary or secondary).
  - Before penetrating keratoplasty procedure.
  - In endothelial keratoplasty procedures, e.g., DSEK or DMEK
- In the treatment of accommodative convergent squint.
- May be useful in accommodative failure.

Mydriatics and Cycloplegics

Pupil dilating drugs are called *mydriatics*. All drugs which dilate the pupil also paralyze accommodation in greater or lesser degree due to paralysis of the ciliary muscles *(cycloplegia)*. Systemically used atropine causes pupillary dilatation.

Local Mydriatics
- **Parasympatholytic mydriatics:** Abolish the action of acetylcholine and paralyze the *sphincter pupillae*—atropine (1%), homatropine (1–2%), cyclopentolate (0.5–1%), tropicamide (0.5–1%)
- **Sympathomimetic mydriatics:** Directly acts on *dilator pupillae*—adrenaline (1 in 10,000) as intracameral (into A/C) injection, and phenylephrine drop (5–10%)
- Intracameral lignocaine (xylocaine) also causes mydriasis.

Phenylephrine is a rapidly acting mydriatic and its effect lasts for 12 hours. It has little effect on ciliary muscles and not considered as cycloplegic.

But all other *parasympatholytic drugs* are cycloplegics. Among these, *atropine is the strongest cycloplegic and its effect lasts for 10–15 days*. Homatropine is moderately effective, and its effect lasts for 48–72 hours.

Cyclopentolate and tropicamide are very rapidly acting drugs and their cycloplegic effects last for 12–24 hours.

Uses of Mydriatics
- To check dilatation before cataract surgery—to evaluate type and grade of cataract, any zonular problem, subluxation, etc.
- For fundus examination and posterior segment procedure, e.g., FFA, retinal laser, etc.
- During ECCE with or without PCIOL or posterior segment surgery.

- After cataract surgery—to check IOL status/position and PCO
- To test any posterior synechia is present or not.
- To break posterior synechia (along with cycloplegic) in iridocyclitis.

Uses of Cycloplegics

- For refraction in children and in hypermetropic subjects.
- Refraction in cases where the pupil is very small.
- In case of iridocyclitis, keratitis and endophthalmitis.
- In accommodative convergent squint.
- In case of accommodative spasm.
- As *'Penalization'* treatment in amblyopia (only with Atropine).
- Long-term use to prevent progression of myopia (diluted atropine—0.01%)

NSAIDs (flurbiprofen, ketorolac or nepafenac) eye drops are used along with mydriatics for prolonging their action during intraocular surgery.

Combination of mydriatic—cycloplegic is *always better* before cataract or retinal surgeries, e.g., homatropine and phenylephrine; tropicamide and phenylephrine.

Mydriatics should be used with caution in angle-closure glaucoma and in patients with very shallow anterior chamber.

ANTIGLAUCOMA MEDICATIONS (OP 6.9)

Antiglaucoma drugs (ocular hypotensive) are used to lower intraocular pressure.

Two types: *(1) Systemic and (2) Topical*

1. Systemic:
   a. **Carbonic anhydrase inhibitors:** Tablet acetazolamide (Diamox) 250 mg 1–2 tablets 4 times daily.
      Adverse events: Hypokalemia (a potassium supplement is necessary), tingling of the hands and feet, stomach upset, frequent urination.
   b. **Hyperosmotic agents:**
      - Injection mannitol—20% solution used intravenously.
        Adverse events: Fluid and electrolyte imbalance, acidosis, marked diuresis, pulmonary congestion, headache, blurred vision.
      - Oral glycerol—50% solution used (30 mL pure glycerin with 30 mL of lemon juice)—3 times daily.
        Adverse events: Bloating, nausea, vomiting, thirst, headaches, dizziness and diarrhea.

2. Topical:
   a. **Parasympathomimetic:** Pilocarpine (1–4%) eye drop 3 time daily. 2% solution is commonly used.
      Adverse events: Spasm of accommodation, headache, myopia, increase iridocyclitis
   b. **Beta-blockers:**
      - Timolol maleate (0.25–0.50%)—twice daily.
        Adverse events: Hypotension, bradycardia, fatigue, shortness of breath; rarely depression. *Not to be given in COPD, asthma and heart block patients.*
      - Betaxolol (0.50%) a cardio-selective, β-blocker—twice daily. A safer drug.
   c. **Topical carbonic anhydrase inhibitors:** Dorzolamide (2%) or brinzolamide (1%) eye drop—thrice daily.
      Adverse events: Stinging, burning, hyperemia
   d. **Alpha$_2$ agonist:** Brimonidine (0.2%)—twice daily.
      Adverse events: Stinging, fatigue, headache, drowsiness, dry mouth and nose, higher allergic reaction.
   e. **Prostaglandin analogues (PGAs):** Latanoprost (0.005%), bimatoprost (0.03% or 0.01%), or travoprost (0.004%) or tafluprost (0.0015%) eye drop once daily.
      Adverse events: Stinging, redness, itching, darkening of the eyelid, eyelash growth, droopy eyelids
   f. **Rho-kinase inhibitors:** *Ripasudil or netarsudil (0.02%)*—twice daily.
      Adverse events: Redness, stinging and corneal deposits and corneal microcysts

Antiglaucoma drugs may be used alone or in combination (topical and systemic; or fixed-dose combination of topical preparation)—depending upon the height of intraocular pressure.

Systemic Complications/Reactions to Important Eye Drops

Atropine: Raised body temperature, dry mouth, swallowing problem
Cyclopentolate: Hallucination, behavioral changes, vertigo or syncope
Pilocarpine: Headache, sweating, bradycardia
Timolol: Respiratory distress in COPD or asthma patient, arrhythmia in heart block patients
Phenylephrine: High BP, tachycardia or extra-systole

Ocular Complications of Important Systemic Medications

- **Steroids:** Cataract and glaucoma
- **Chloroquine/hydroxychloroquine:** Triad of—keratopathy, myopathy (accommodation failure) and retinopathy (Bull's eye maculopathy)
- **Quinine:** Impaired dark adaptation, amblyopia
- **Ethambutol:** Toxic optic neuropathy
- **Chlorpromazine:** Cataract
- **Sulphonamides/phenytoin/allopurinol:** Stevens-Johnson syndrome
- **Amantadine:** Corneal edema
- **Amiodarone:** Vortex keratopathy
- **Sildenafil:** Blue vision, photophobia, permanent vision loss due to anterior ischemic optic neuropathy (AION).

PHYSIOLOGY OF VISION (OP 1.1 AND PY 10.17)

- When light falls upon the retina, two essential reactions occur in the photoreceptors (cones and rods)—*photochemical* and *electrical*.
- **Cones:** Higher threshold receptors for day-light vision *(photopic vision)* and color vision
- **Rods:** Low threshold receptors for night vision *(scotopic vision)*. It contains visual pigment (Rhodopsin).
- The rods are much more sensitive to low illumination than the cones.
  Mesopic vision is a combination of photopic and scotopic vision in low-light situations. Most of the night-time outdoor activities are in the mesopic vision range.

Photochemical reaction: It triggers the cascade of biochemical reactions and generates of electrical impulses (via *Rhodopsin cycle*).

Electrical reaction: By a complex process of photo-transduction, i.e., phenomenon of conversion of light energy into nerve impulses. Then the processing and transmission of visual sensation to visual perception

A battery of **electrodiagnostic tests** is now in clinical uses for assessing the integrity of the retina and its central connections.

Electrooculography (EOG): It measures the average amplitude of resting potential of eye in light- and dark-adapted states, to evaluate the condition of the retinal pigment epithelium (RPE). Abnormal in RPE diseases.

Electroretinography (ERG): Means a gross record of electrical potential changes in the retina after stimulation with light.

ERG is a useful in diagnosis and prognosis of certain retinal disorders (e.g., retinitis pigmentosa, rod-cone dystrophy, etc.); in siderosis bulbi (earliest sign); cortical blindness or hysterical blindness; assessing retinal functions in presence of media opacity (e.g., cataract, corneal opacity, or vitreous hemorrhage).

Visual-evoked potential (VEP): The VEP is the electroretinography (EEG), recorded at the occipital pole. It tells the integrity of the afferent visual pathways. It is important in assessing the optic nerve or macular functions in presence of opacities in the media.

Visual perceptions: Four types of sensation result from stimulation of retina by light:
1. **Light sense:** Faculty to perceive light in all gradations of intensity. Light minimum is

the minimum amount of light energy which causes a visual sensation.

Dark adaptation: The increase in sensitivity of the eye for detection of light that occurs in the dark is called dark adaptation. Delayed dark adaptation occurs in diseases of rods, e.g., retinitis pigmentosa and in vitamin A deficiency.

Light adaptation: It refers to the fall in the visual threshold on moving from darkness into a well-lit room.

2. **Form sense:** To perceive the shape of object in outer world. Cones play a major role, therefore form sense is most acute at fovea. Visual acuity is a measure of form sense.
3. **Contrast sense:** Ability to perceive slight changes in luminance between regions not separated by sharp borders. *Contrast sensitivity* is reduced in many ocular diseases, e.g., in glaucoma, cataract, macular diseases or refractive errors. Sometimes, it is more important than the loss of visual acuity. Contrast sensitivity is also important in old age and after cataract surgery. Several test systems are available (both for distance and near)—Pelli-Robson chart, Regan chart, functional acuity contrast test (FACT), etc.
4. **Color sense:** Ability to distinguish between different colors as excited by light of different wavelengths. *The theories of color vision:*

   Trichromatic theory (Young-Helmholtz): Three kinds of cones: One is more sensitive to long wavelength (red—570 nm), One to medium wavelength (green—535 nm). One to short wavelength (blue—440 nm). All other colors are perceived by combination of this.

   The opponent color theory (Herrings): Three sets of receptor system—red-green, blue-yellow and black-white. Each system found as an antagonist pair. Stimulation of one of an opponent pair produces excitation of that receptor system and inhibition on other, e.g., red light stimulates red receptors and simultaneously inhibits green.

It is now accepted that both the theories are important to understand the mechanism of color vision.

Color Blindness

Two types: (1) Congenital and (2) Acquired
1. **Congenital:** Most common and inherited as an X-linked recessive anomaly. Male 7% and female only 0.7%, have congenitally defective color vision. Visual acuity is normal, and fundus appears normal. The defect is present at birth and stationery. A *protanope* has (protan means first) the red sensation missing, a *deuteranope* (deutan means second) has the green, and *a tritanope* (tritan means third) has the blue sensation missing. *Red-green blindness is most common in congenital type.*
   Achromatopsia: Means the individual born with severely deficient color perception, where there is absence of all three cones, and thus visual acuity is also very much reduced, and nystagmus is present.
2. **Acquired:** Occurs as a result of diseases of the cones, macular diseases, nuclear sclerosis, optic nerve disease, and drug-induced (e.g., ethambutol, chloroquine).

OPTICS AND REFRACTION OF THE EYE *(PY 10.17)*

But for all practical purposes, refraction by the eye, takes place at two structures: The anterior corneal surface and the lens.
- Optical power of cornea = + 43D (40–45D)
- Optical power of the lens = +17D (16–20D)

Reduced Eye of Donder

For all practical purposes, the optical system of the eye is being treated as a single ideal refracting surface (or single lens system). This is the reduced eye (of Donder).

The optical center (Nodal point) of this lens lies 7.08 mm behind the anterior corneal surface, just in front of the posterior pole of the lens. Rays which pass through nodal point, will not be appreciably refracted.

Purkinje-Sanson Images

Four types:
- **1st image (P1):** It derives from the anterior corneal surface. It is the brightest and erect image and moves in the same direction.
- **2nd image (P2):** It derives from the posterior corneal surface; it lies adjacent to 1st image. It is faint but erect image.
- **3rd image (P3):** It derives from the anterior lens surface. It is largest, dim, and erect image.
- **4th image (P4):** It derives from the posterior lens surface. It is small, dim and inverted, as the posterior lens surface is concave. The image lies at the pupillary plane and moves in the opposite direction.

REFRACTIVE ERRORS OF THE EYE (OP 1.2)

Emmetropia: It is the normal condition in which the incident parallel rays come to a perfect focus upon the light-sensitive layer of retina, when accommodation is at rest.

Ametropia (refractive errors): It is the condition where the incident parallel rays do not come to a focus upon the light-sensitive layer of retina. Ametropia may be due to one or more of the following conditions:

1. **Abnormal length of the globe (axial ametropia):** Too long in myopia, too short in hypermetropia. 1 mm enlargement causes—3.0D myopia and 1 mm shortening will cause +3.0D hypermetropia.
2. **Abnormal curvature of the refractive surfaces of the cornea or lens (curvature ametropia):** Too strong or steep curvature in myopia, too weak or flat in hypermetropia. 1 mm steepening causes −6.0D myopia and 1 mm flattening causes +6.0D hypermetropia.
3. **Abnormal refractive indices of the media (index ametropia):** Myopia due to nuclear sclerosis.
4. **Abnormal position of the lens:** Displacement forwards in myopia, displacement backwards in hypermetropia.

Among these, axial ametropia is perhaps, the most common type.

There are three types of refractive errors: Myopia, hypermetropia and astigmatism.

Myopia

Definition: (*means* 'to shut the eye'). Here, the incident parallel rays come to a focus anterior to the light-sensitive part of the retina, when accommodation is at rest.

Types
1. **Developmental myopia:** Very rare, myopia may be —10D at birth.
2. **Simple myopia:** Usually up to −5D to −6D and without any degenerative change in the fundus.
3. **Pathological myopia:** Degenerative and essentially progressive, may be up to −20D to −30D.

It may be:
- **Axial myopia:** When the axial length is more.
- **Curvature myopia:** Typically seen in keratoconus.
- **Index myopia:** In nuclear sclerosis of the lens in old age.

If a myopia is more than −6.0D, it is called *high myopia.*

Problems with Myopic Eyes
- More incidence of peripheral retinal degeneration, e.g., lattice degeneration
- Retinal break with or without vitreous hemorrhage
- Retinal detachment
- Liquefaction of the vitreous gel
- Posterior cortical cataract and more nuclear sclerosis
- Higher incidence of open angle glaucoma
- Divergent squint (exophoria or exotropia)
- Scleral collapse during surgery due to low scleral rigidity

Treatment
- **Spectacle correction:** With appropriate minus lenses. Myopia must not be overcorrected, and in practice, high myopia is always slightly under corrected.

- ❖ Contact lens correction.
- ❖ Surgery:
  - ➤ Radial keratotomy (RK)—obsolete now-a-days.
  - ➤ Photorefractive keratoplasty (PRK) by excimer laser.
  - ➤ Laser-assisted *in situ* keratomileusis (LASIK)—most popular.
  - ➤ Small incision lenticule extraction (SMILE)—with femtolaser.
  - ➤ 'Minus' power PC IOL implantation, even in presence of clear crystalline lens (called *phakic IOL or pIOL implantation*)
  - ➤ Removal of clear crystalline lens with PCIOL implantation—if the myopia is –15 D or more.
  - ➤ Intracorneal implantation of a minus power lenticule.
- ❖ General nutrition and ocular hygiene.
- ❖ Genetic counseling in case of high progressive myopia.
- ❖ Low concentration atropine eye drops (0.01%) to slow progression in case of younger children.

Hypermetropia

Definition: Here, the incident parallel rays come to a focus posterior to the light-sensitive layer of the retina, when accommodation is at rest.

In fact, all newborn are almost always hypermetropic (by *average* +2.5D)

Types of Hypermetropia

- ❖ **Axial hypermetropia:** When the axial length of eyeball is smaller (1 mm shortening will cause +3D hypermetropia).
- ❖ **Curvature hypermetropia:** If the cornea or lens is flatter (1 mm flattening causes +6D hypermetropia).
- ❖ **Index hypermetropia:** Due to increase in refractive index of the cortex of the lens in old age.

Aphakia is an example of high degree of hypermetropia.

Depending upon the act of accommodation, total hypermetropia (tH) may be divided into:
- ❖ **Latent hypermetropia (lH):** Which is corrected by the physiological. Tone of the ciliary muscle.
- ❖ **Manifest hypermetropia (mH):** It is made up of two components:
  1. *Facultative hypermetropia (fH):* It is that part of hypermetropia which can be corrected by the effort of accommodation.
  2. *Absolute hypermetropia (aH):* Which cannot be overcome by the effort of accommodation.

  tH = lH + mH (fH + aH).

Problem with Hypermetropic Eyes

- ❖ Accommodative asthenopia or eye strain
- ❖ Amblyopia—more common with uniocular high hypermetropia
- ❖ Young patient tends to develop latent convergent squint (esophoria)
- ❖ Higher incidence of angle-closure glaucoma
- ❖ Early onset of presbyopia
- ❖ Choroidal effusion and vitreous upthrust during cataract surgery

Treatment

- ❖ Spectacles correction with convex lenses. Full cycloplegic refraction is a must for hypermetropia with full correction
- ❖ Contact lenses
- ❖ **Hyperopic LASIK:** Up to +6.0D of hypermetropia
- ❖ Excimer laser PRK
- ❖ **Clear lens extraction with IOL implantation:** If the patient is in the presbyopic age >45 years.
- ❖ **Secondary IOL implantation:** In aphakia induced hypermetropia

Astigmatism

Definition: It is condition, the incident parallel rays do not come to a point focus upon the retina instead they may form line, due to refraction varies in different meridians of the eye [etymology—a (without) + stigma (a point)]

Types of Astigmatism

Theoretically, no eye is 'stigmatic' as the vertical curvature of the cornea is greater than the horizontal by 0.25D owing to pressure of the upper eyelid on the globe. This is 'astigmatism with the rule' (called WTR). As the age advances, it tends to disappear or even reverse, i.e., horizontal curvature is greater than vertical. This is 'astigmatism against the rule (called ATR).

The common cause of 'astigmatism against the rule' is surgical aphakia or ECCE (plus cylinder at 180° or minus cylinder at 90°) due to limbal scarring.

Astigmatism may be **regular** or **irregular**.

Regular astigmatism: When the two principal meridians of greatest and least curvature are at right-angle to each other.

If the two meridians do not lie the principal plane but remain at right angle to each other—then it is termed *oblique astigmatism*. Occasionally, the axes are not right-angled but crossed obliquely, called *bi-oblique astigmatism*.

Regular astigmatism may be:
- **Simple:** Where one meridian is emmetropic and the other is myopic or hypermetropic (simple myopic/hypermetropic astigmatism).
- **Compound:** Where both the principal meridians are either myopic or hypermetropic (compound myopic/hypermetropic astigmatism).
- **Mixed:** Where one meridian is myopic and other one is hypermetropic. Vision is not impaired much in mixed astigmatism.

Asthenopia or headache is the main symptom of astigmatism. Visual acuity is affected more only with high astigmatism.

Irregular astigmatism is due to irregularities in the curvature of the meridians—which cannot be corrected fully by spectacle lenses.

Causes of Irregular Astigmatism
- Scarring of the cornea (more with nebula)
- Keratoconus
- Corneal epithelial dystrophies
- After penetrating keratoplasty
- Lenticonus

Treatment
- Regular astigmatism—spectacles correction by sphero-cylindrical lens with correct axis.
- Irregular astigmatism—by contact lens.
- Refractive corneal surgery may be helpful in high corneal astigmatism, e.g., astigmatic keratotomy (AK), limbal relaxing incision (LRI), etc.
- Removal of sutures in astigmatism following ECCE or keratoplasty
- Phacoemulsification with toric IOL implantation in cataract surgery—if preoperative astigmatism is >1.0D.

Presbyopia

Definition
This is a physiological aging process in which the near point gradually recedes beyond a distance at which the individual is accustomed to read or to work. Truly speaking, it is not a refractive error.

This is due to advancing age where the tone of the ciliary muscle is decreased, as well as due to loss of plasticity of the crystalline lens.

Symptoms
Gradual difficulty in reading small prints especially, in the evening or in dim light. Inability to perform near work meticulously—sewing, threading a needle, etc. Later eye strain or headache develops while performing near task.

Treatment
To provide the patient spectacles with appropriate convex lenses so that his accommodation is reinforced, and his near point is brought within a useful distance. It is better to under-correct than to over-correct.

The rough rule: Usually, +1.00 Dsph at 40 years; +1.50 Dsph at 45 years; +2.00 Dsph at

50 years; +2.50 Dsph at 55 years; or +3.00 Dsph at 60 years or more.

The glasses may be unifocal (in the form of half-eye spectacle) or bifocals (in the form of Kryptok or executive bifocal glasses) or it may be progressive lens.

Anisometropia

This is a condition in which the refractive error between the two eyes show a considerable difference.

A minor difference of refraction is not uncommon, but it seldom gives rise to symptom. Binocular vision is usually maintained if the difference does not exceed more than 2.5D. But if it is more, the effort of fusion may give rise to symptoms of eyestrain.

Eitiology

- Usually, congenital.
- Unequal rates of change in refraction between two eyes.
- Corneal diseases and cataract.
- Following surgical and non-surgical trauma.

Problems of Anisometropia

- Imperfect binocular vision with an effort to fuse the images leads to symptom of eyestrain.
- Uniocular vision and the worse eye will become amblyopic, especially in children.
- Development of squint—convergent in children and divergent in adults.
- Diplopia—due to unequal image sizes.

Treatment

- Contact lenses are most suitable.
- Iseikonic glasses.
- If the patient is amblyopic—the better eye is to be patched (occlusion treatment) and later orthoptic exercises should be given to develop binocularity. This is to be done within 6 years of age.
- Excimer laser PRK or LASIK procedure.

Visual Acuity Assessment, Pin Hole test, Menace Reflex and Blink Reflex *(OP 1.3)*

See page 8

INDICATIONS AND PRINCIPLES OF REFRACTIVE SURGERY *(OP 1.4)*

- Refractive surgery is a type (essential or non-essential) of eye surgery to correct refractive status of the eye and to decrease or eliminate dependency on spectacles or contact lenses.
- These include various methods of *surgical remodeling of the cornea* (keratomileusis or incision-based), *lens implantation*, *lens replacement* or some time in combination.
- The most widely performed type of refractive surgery is LASIK (*laser-assisted in situ keratomileusis*), where excimer laser is used to reshape the cornea.

The indications for refractive surgery:

- Myopia (commonest)
- Hypermetropia
- Astigmatism
- Presbyopia

Successful refractive eye surgery can cure or reduce these common vision disorders.

Types and Principles of Refractive Surgery

Corneal Incision Procedures

- **Radial keratotomy (RK):** To reduce myopia or astigmatism. Now-a-days mostly replaced by other refractive procedures.
- **Arcuate keratotomy (AK):** Also known as astigmatic keratotomy. It uses curvilinear incisions at the peripheral cornea to correct high astigmatism, e.g., post-keratoplasty astigmatism.
- **Limbal relaxing incision (LRI):** Incision at the peripheral cornea to reshape it and to correct minor astigmatism (typically 2D or less). LRI is often performed with modern cataract surgery with femto laser.

AK and LRI are the procedures to reshape (flatten) the cornea in a selective meridian, depending upon the axis of the astigmatism.

Flap Procedures

- **LASIK:** Here, the surgeon first makes a corneal flap (anterior lamellar at 100–180 micron depth) using either an automated

microkeratome or femtosecond laser. Then, targeted amount of the stromal bed is ablated with excimer laser as calculated by the machine. The flap is subsequently replaced. The main aim is to flatten the corneal dome in myopia.
- **Refractive lenticule extraction (ReLEx):** instead of ablation, with femto laser a thin lenticule of stroma is cut and removed.
- **Small incision lenticule extraction (SMILE):** A newer technique without a flap. Femto laser cuts the lenticule within corneal stroma, then same laser is used to create a small incision at the periphery. Special instruments are used to separate and remove the lenticule.

Surface Procedures
- **Photorefractive keratectomy (PRK):** The difference from LASIK is that the top layer of the epithelium is removed (and a bandage contact lens is used), so no flap is created.
- **Subepithelial surface procedures:** LASEK, Epi-LASIK, etc. The main idea is to protect corneal epithelium.

Lens-based Refractive Procedures
- **Phakic intraocular lens (pIOL):** pIOL is designed for high degree of refractive error that cannot be safely corrected with corneal-based refractive surgery. This IOL is also called—implantable collamer lens, or ICL, which is surgically implanted in front of the crystalline lens. As the crystalline lens is not removed, patients can accommodate their eyes.
- **Refractive lens exchange (RLE):** Also called *clear lens extraction or CLE*—an intraocular lens (IOL) is used to replace crystalline lens in order to improve vision. The procedure is same as cataract surgery. RLE can be performed by implanting monofocal IOL (for very high myopia or hyperopia) for whom LASIK is not recommended. Multifocal IOLs may be an option for low hypermetropia in presbyopic age.

Bioptics: This is a combination of a lens implant procedure (ICL or RLE) with a corneal laser procedure (LASIK or PRK).

Other refractive procedures:
- **Conductive keratoplasty (CK):** CK is a non-invasive, thermal refractive surgery procedure used to correct mild to moderate hyperopia and presbyopia in people over age 40. It uses a tiny probe with radiofrequency (RF) energy (instead of a laser), to apply heat to the peripheral cornea. The heat shrinks the peripheral cornea. This increases the steepness of the central cornea and improves the optical power. This is an obsolete procedure now.
- **Intrastromal corneal ring segments (INTACS):** After making small incisions in the cornea, two crescent ring segments are implanted between the layers of the corneal stroma. It is used to flatten the central cornea to treat myopic astigmatism in keratoconus.
- **Corneal inlay:** A corneal inlay consists of a porous black disc (2–3 mm) with a pin-hole. It is implanted within the cornea after making stromal pocket. Its principle is just like pin-hole. It is used for presbyopia.
- **Scleral procedures:** Different scleral surgical procedures are used to treat presbyopia. These include—*scleral microincisions* by Erbium laser, *scleral micro-implants*, etc., in ciliary body zone. The principle is to restore true physiological accommodation combined with pseudo-accommodation, as well as improving the effective range of focus in presbyopia.

AMBLYOPIA (OP 1.5)

Definition
Amblyopia denotes a unilateral or bilateral reduction in best corrected vision, without any detectable organic ocular lesion.

This is either due to formed-vision deprivation or abnormal binocular vision, or both.

The most sensitive period of developing amblyopia is in the first 6 months of life; and after 6 years of age, amblyopia does not usually develop.

Characteristics of an Amblyopic Eye
- Reduction in visual acuity.
- **Crowding phenomenon:** Visual acuity is better when the test letters are viewed singly (optotype), rather than in groups
- **Neutral density filter test:** Amblyopic eye shows no change in visual acuity with a neutral density filter.
- **Color vision:** Not affected.
- **Eccentric (extrafoveal) fixation:** Degree of amblyopia is proportionate to the distance of the eccentric point from the fovea.

Types
- **Strabismic amblyopia:** Develops in a squinting eye, as a result of continued suppression, and it persists even when the deviated eye is forced to fixate. It is the most common cause.
- **Anisometropic amblyopia:** Occurs in the more ametropic eye, as a result of constantly blurred image. This is more with high aniso-hypermetropia and aniso-astigmatism than with aniso-myopia.
- **Iso-ametropic amblyopia:** It is bilateral and associated with almost equally high refractive error in both eyes. It is also more with bilateral high hypermetropia.
- **Meridional amblyopia:** Amblyopia caused by uncorrected significant astigmatism
- **Strabismic anisometropia amblyopia:** This eye has strabismus associated with anisometropia.
- **Stimulus deprivation amblyopia** (*amblyopia ex anopsia*): Results from the non-use of one eye in infancy or early childhood and is caused by opacity in the media (cataract or leukoma) and ptosis.
- **Reverse amblyopia:** Reverse amblyopia is a result of penalization of the sound eye with patching or atropine during amblyopia treatment of the original amblyopic eye.

Mechanism of Strabismic Amblyopia
- Strabismic eye prevents the normal process of fusion. This can result in **suppression** of the deviating eye, diminishing the visual acuity and loss of binocularity.
- Retinal image blur in strabismic eye can **inhibit cortical activity**, preventing normal visual development.
- Long-standing inhibition of visual input to the retinocortical pathways causes a **restructuring of the visual cortical circuits in the visual cortex**. This in turn causes deep amblyopia.
- Degree and incidence of amblyopia is greater in esotropia than in exotropia.

Treatment
- **Removal of opacity** in the media (e.g., congenital cataract)
- **Full correction of refractive errors**
- **Occlusion therapy:** The treatment should be started as early as possible. The aim is to occlude the sound eye, and to force to use the amblyopic eye.
- **Surgical correction of congenital strabismus or severe ptosis**
- Other modes of therapy:
  - *Atropine penalization:* An alternative to occlusion, atropine is used to blur the sound eye only
  - *Pleoptics:* They are the methods of re-establishment of foveal fixation and may be helpful in older children.
  - *CAM stimulator therapy*

LID AND ADNEXAL CONDITIONS (OP 2.1; 2.2 AND 2,3)

Hordeolum Extremum and Internum
See page 53

Blepharitis
Blepharitis is the subacute or chronic inflammation of the eyelid.
Associated with—uncorrected refractive errors, dandruff and parasitic infestation (*Demodex folliculorum* and *Phthiriasis palpebrum*)

Types
Anterior: Squamous and ulcerative blepharitis
Posterior: Meibomianitis (meibomitis)

Symptoms
Anterior: Itching, irritation, watering and loss of eyelashes
Meibomitis: Watering, frothy discharge and foreign body sensation

Signs
Anterior: Dandruff-like scales, yellow crust, madarosis and matting of eyelashes
Meibomitis: Meibomian seborrhea, blocked meibomian orifices, meibomian secretion is expressed as toothpaste (tooth-paste sign)
Complications: Madarosis, trichiasis, marginal keratitis and instability of tear-film.

Management
- Lid hygiene and lid scrub
- Hot compress and lid massage
- Erythromycin or tetracycline eye ointment (may be combined with steroid).
- Systemic doxycycline for 2–4 weeks or tablet azithromycin in case of children
- Tea-tree oil for *Demodex folliculorum*

Preseptal Cellulitis

It is a type of orbital cellulitis anterior to the orbital septum. Occurs in younger children. Causative organisms: *Strept pneumoniae, Staph aureus* and *H. influenzae*

Clinical Features
- Presents with lid swelling, pain and watering
- Acute periorbital swelling and redness.
- Increased warmth and tenderness of the eyelids.
- Conjunctival chemosis.
- Sometimes, fever with leukocytosis.
- A fluctuating mass signifies **lid abscess** formation.

Treatment
- Hot compress,
- Oral antibiotics and analgesics.
- Topical antibiotics.
- Drainage of the lid abscess (*see* page 186)

Dacryocystitis

See page 60–63

Hemangioma of Lids

- Cavernous hemangiomas are common in children
- Hemangioma often follows the distribution of the 1st and 2nd divisions of the fifth nerve.
- Sometimes, it is associated with hemangioma of the choroid (may be with glaucoma), and hemangioma of the leptomeninges, called *Sturge-Weber syndrome.*
- Hemangiomas appear bluish when seen through skin, and form swellings which increase in size on crying, or lowering the head.
- **Treatment:** Small hemangiomas may well be left alone. But large hemangiomas require treatment by intralesional steroid injection, or by superficial radiotherapy.

Dermoid Cyst

A dermoid cyst is a congenital non-malignant tumor that can occur on ocular surface or periocular area. Dermoid contains fat, sebaceous material, skin and/or hair.

Types
Orbital dermoid: It is typically found under the skin, near the bony orbit, at end of the eyebrow or medial canthus. It is smooth, firm, non-tender mass. It may gradually increase in size and often require removal.

Epibulbar dermoid: May be of two types:
1. **Posterior epibulbar dermoid:** It is a usually found under the temporal upper eyelid and sometimes are visible only when lifting the eyelid. It does not cause visual problem.
2. **Limbal dermoid:** It is found at the limbus. It may be large enough to cause high astigmatism and affect vision. Child develops amblyopia.
In some cases of epibulbar dermoid, they are associated with **Goldenhar's syndrome**, i.e., with preauricular skin tags, vertebral anomalies and hemifacial hypoplasia.

Treatment

Surgical excision with a lamellar sclero-corneal patch graft at an early age to prevent amblyopia.

Ptosis

It means drooping of the upper eyelid, which may be unilateral or bilateral, and partial or complete.

Types

Congenital

Acquired

- **Neurogenic:** 3rd nerve palsy, Horner's syndrome
- **Myogenic:** Myasthenia gravis, senile ptosis
- **Mechanical:** Large upper lid mass
- **Traumatic:** Trauma to levator muscles, post-surgical
- **Pseudoptosis:** As seen in enophthalmos, phthisis bulbi

Clinical Evaluation

History, degree of ptosis (mild, moderate, or severe), ptosis measurement, assessment of levator (LPS) function, jaw-winking phenomenon, Bell's phenomenon, clinical photographs and tensilon test (to exclude myasthenia gravis).

Treatment

Mostly surgical.
- **Congenital severe ptosis**—should be operated before 6 months to prevent amblyopia
- **Fasanella-Servet** operation for—mild ptosis (as in Horner's syndrome)
- **LPS resection**—via skin or conjunctival approach
- **Frontalis suspension**—when the LPS action is poor.

Entropion

Entropion is an inward turning of the eyelid with rubbing of the eyelashes on the conjunctiva and/or cornea.

Types

- Involutional (senile)—most common
- Cicatricial
- Acute spastic
- Congenital—rare

Symptoms

Foreign body sensation, pain, lacrimation and discharge.

Signs

- In turning of the lower eyelid or some cases upper lid
- Conjunctival congestion
- Discharge with matting of the eyelashes
- Blepharospasm
- Superficial corneal opacities and distortion of the window reflex
- Sometimes, corneal ulceration

Treatment

- Various kind of plastic surgery of lids
- Temporary relieve—by pulling the skin outward with a strip of *adhesive tape.*

Ectropion

It is an outward turning of the eyelid away from the globe.

Types

- Involutional (senile)—most common
- Cicatricial
- Paralytic
- Congenital—rare

Clinical Features

- In case of lower lid involvement → inferior punctum is not in contact with the globe → epiphora and excoriation of the skin around the lid.
- Chronic exposure of the conjunctiva → secondary infection and keratinization → keratitis or frank corneal ulcer.

Treatment

Always surgical correction.

Lid Lag

Lid lag is the static situation in which the eyelid is higher than normal with the downgaze movement of the eye.

Causes
- Thyroid eye diseases (most common)
- Cicatricial eyelid diseases
- Congenital ptosis.

Lagophthalmos

Inability to close the eyes completely, leading to exposure of the eye.

Minor degree of *nocturnal lagophthalmos* is not uncommon and does not require any treatment.

Causes
- Facial nerve palsy
- Leprosy
- Severe proptosis and thyroid exophthalmos
- Comatose patient
- Skin disorder—ichthyosis
- Overcorrection of ptosis surgery

Sequalae
- Eye is red, irritable and watery
- Dryness of the lower part of the bulbar conjunctiva and cornea.
- Exposure keratitis → corneal ulceration → corneal perforation.

Treatment
- Instillation of artificial tears at daytime, and antibiotic ointment at night—to prevent corneal drying.
- Temporary closure of the lids by adhesive tapes.
- **Tarsorrhaphy:** A temporary or permanent lateral or paracentral tarsorrhaphy
- **Lid (upper) load operation with gold plate**—useful in facial palsy.
- **Treatment of the cause**—as in proptosis due to orbital tumor or thyroid exophthalmos.

HOW TO GIVE LACRIMAL SAC MASSAGE IN CONGENITAL DACRYOCYSTITIS *(OP 2.3 AND 9.1)*

This is indicated in congenital dacryocystitis. First line of treatment is conservative with sac massage by the parents.

The procedure is as follows (**Fig. 3.1**):
- The parent's nail of the index finger that will be used for the massage must be clipped.
- The hands must be washed before and after the sac massage.
- Vaseline or baby oil may be applied to the finger as a lubricant
- Place the tip of index finger at the medial canthus of the affected eye (over the medial palpebral ligament)
- The massage is begun by giving pressure at the medial canthus (which is effective in blocking the common canaliculus thus preventing reflux backward through the canaliculi).
- Press firmly and move the index finger in short downward strokes for 5–10 times.
- This downward pressure with increasing hydrostatic pressure within the sac, will cause rupture of the membrane.
- Put a drop of antibiotic eye drop as prescribed.

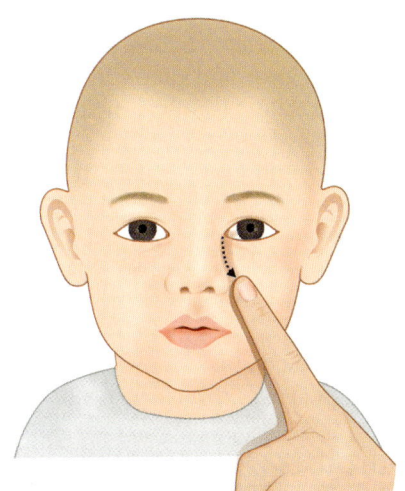

Fig. 3.1: Sac massage.

- ❖ Repeat these steps 3–4 times a day for 3 months.

TRICHIATIC CILIA (EYELASH) REMOVAL BY EPILATION (OP 2.3)

Indications
To remove ingrowing eyelashes (trichiasis).

Goal
To prevent corneal abrasion and further to prevent corneal ulcer.

Requirement
- ❖ Magnification (magnifying loupe)
- ❖ Torchlight
- ❖ Gauze piece
- ❖ Local anesthetic eye drops
- ❖ Epilation forceps (*see* page 162)

Procedure
- ❖ Topical anesthetic drop is not mandatory
- ❖ Using magnification and identify the eyelashes which need epilating
- ❖ **For lower eyelashes:**
  - ➢ Ask the patient to look upward, fix his/her gaze, and keep still
  - ➢ With an index finger, gently hold down the lower eyelid
- ❖ **For upper eyelashes:**
  - ➢ Ask the patient to look downward, fix his/her gaze, and keep still
  - ➢ With a thumb, gently ease upper eyelid up against the orbital rim
- ❖ With the epilation forceps in the other hand, hold the ingrowing eyelash close to its base and pull gently forward to pluck it out
- ❖ Repeat until all in growing lashes are epilated
- ❖ Between each epilation, wipe the eyelash off the forceps with a clean swab

ORBITAL CELLULITIS (OP 2.4)

Etiology
- ❖ **Age:** Usually child or young adult.
- ❖ **Sinus infections:** From the frontal, maxillary or ethmoidal sinusitis (most common cause).
- ❖ **Penetrating orbital injury:** It may be with retained intraorbital foreign body.
- ❖ **Thrombophlebitis:** From a focus in the adjacent skin, dental or nasopharyngeal infection
- ❖ **Postoperative:** Following enucleation of the globe.
- ❖ **Causative organisms:** *Strep. pneumoniae, Staph. aureus, Strepto. pyogenes* and *H. influenzae* in children under 5 years of age.

Types
The orbital septum, the dense fascia (which separates the anterior structures from the orbit), divides the cellulitis into two types: (1) **Pre-septal cellulitis** (*see* page 87) and (2) **Orbital cellulitis.**

Symptoms
- ❖ A sudden onset of unilateral severe pain and swelling of the lids associated with fever.
- ❖ Diplopia due to limitation of movements.
- ❖ Lacrimation and photophobia.
- ❖ Impairment of vision lately.

Signs
- ❖ Lid marked edema and tenderness.
- ❖ Conjunctiva chemosis and congestion.
- ❖ Proptosis commonly the eyeball is displaced laterally and downwards.
- ❖ Limitation of ocular movements.
- ❖ Ophthalmoscopy may show features of optic neuritis in severe cases.

Course and Complications
- ❖ Subsides completely with prompt treatment.
- ❖ Orbital abscess formation, which may point and burst on the skin near the orbital margin.
- ❖ Meningitis, brain abscess, and cavernous sinus thrombosis, which may be fatal.
- ❖ Central retinal arterial occlusion, optic neuritis and optic atrophy may lead to blindness.

Management

- Patient should be admitted immediately.
- Intravenous (IV) broad-spectrum antibiotics should be started immediately
- **In children under 5 years of age:** The antibiotics should cover *H. influenzae*. choice of IV antibiotics are—ceftriaxone, cefotaxime and ceftazidime.
- **In adult or older children:** Cefuroxime or Piperacillin-tazobactam is given every 4 hourly.
- If MRSA is suspected, add IV vancomycin (15 mg/kg) twice daily to the above regimen.
- IV metronidazole may be required along with antibiotics.
- Once the improvement is documented within 48-72 hours, switch to oral antibiotics for 5-7 days.
- A multidisciplinary approach is usually required for patients with orbital cellulitis—under the care of pediatrician, ENT surgeon, ophthalmologist and general physician.
- Hot compress and analgesics to relieve pain.
- **Simultaneously, the patient should be investigated for etiological factors:**
  - Nasal and conjunctival swab culture.
  - X-ray of the paranasal sinuses (PNS).
  - Complete hemogram
  - Ultrasonography B scans to detect an orbital abscess.
  - Cerebrospinal fluid study and CT scan of the brain, if intracranial spread is suspected.
- **Surgery:**
  - Drainage of the orbital abscess.
  - Incision and drainage of the lid abscess.
  - In most cases, it is necessary to drain the infected sinuses as well.

Cavernous Sinus Thrombosis *(OP 2.5)*

This is an acute thrombophlebitis that originates from a purulent infection of the face, paranasal sinuses (PNS), ear or orbit that drains through the veins into the cavernous sinus.

Most cases occur in otherwise healthy individual. Patients with chronic sinusitis or uncontrolled diabetes, or patients on oral contraceptives may be the risk factor.

The causative agent is generally *Staph aureus,* although *Streptococci, Pneumococci,* and fungi may be implicated in rare cases.

Clinical Features

- Onset is usually violent with severe pain along the ophthalmic division of 5th nerve
- High fever and prostration.
- These are rapidly followed by proptosis, with congestion and edema of the lids and conjunctiva.
- Ophthalmoplegia occurs, and the lateral rectus is the first muscle to be affected.
- Edema of the mastoid region (a pathognomonic sign) indicating back-pressure in the mastoid emissary vein.
- There may be papilledema and visual loss.
- Other eye becomes similarly affected within few hours, due to inter-cavernous communication.
- Death may occur from meningitis or pulmonary infarction.

Investigations

- Imaging-contrast-enhanced CT scan and MRI of the orbit and/or paranasal sinuses.
- Complete hemogram, ESR, blood cultures, and sinus cultures help to establish and identify primary source of infection.
- Lumbar puncture is necessary to rule out meningitis.

Treatment

- Intensive intravenous antibiotic is necessary to control infection.
- Anticoagulants to prevent extension of the clot.
- Corticosteroids may also be used to reduce swelling.
- Surgery may be needed to drain the site of primary infection.

PROPTOSIS AND ORBITAL TUMORS *(OP 2.6, 2.7 AND 2.8)*

Forward protrusion of the eyeball beyond the orbital margin is called proptosis or exophthalmos.

Exophthalmos means an active or dynamic protrusion of the eyeball (usually bilateral). Classically seen in thyroid ophthalmopathy.

Proptosis means a passive protrusion of the eyeball, classically seen in space occupying lesion in the orbit and hence, usually unilateral.

Enophthalmos: Inward displacement of the globe. *The causes are:* Microphthalmos, phthisis bulbi, Horner's syndrome and blow-out fracture of the orbital floor.

Causes of Unilateral Proptosis

- **Inflammatory:** Orbital cellulitis, panophthalmitis. orbital pseudotumor
- **Neoplastic:** Benign—hemangioma, dermoid, lymphangioma, glioma of the optic nerve; malignant—rhabdomyosarcoma, meningioma and retinoblastoma
- **Vascular:** Retrobulbar hemorrhage (RBH) and orbital varices
- **Parasitic:** Cysticercosis
- **Systemic diseases:** Thyroid ophthalmopathy, leukemic deposits in leukemia (chloroma)
- **Orbital mucormycosis:** This is a recent complication in post COVID-19 patients (mostly among uncontrolled diabetics) who has survived and received steroids, immunosuppressants and oxygen therapy for few days. The organism responsible—is mucor (also called black fungus). It also affects the paranasal sinuses and brain (rhino-orbito-cerebral mucormycosis). The patient may have complete loss of vision and may require multidisciplinary approach. Exenteration may require in severe cases.

Causes of Bilateral Proptosis (Exophthalmos)

- **Congenital:** Craniosynostosis
- **Endocrine:** Thyroid ophthalmopathy
- Cavernous sinus thrombosis
- **Metastatic:** Leukemia, neuroblastoma.

Investigations

- History taking in details
- Measurement of proptosis (exophthalmometry)
- Detailed ocular examination including palpation
- Look for pulsation
- Systemic evaluation
- Routine hemogram
- X-Ray orbit, CT scan and MRI of orbit
- USG B-scan orbit
- Fine needle aspiration cytology (FNAC) or incisional biopsy
- Lastly, excisional biopsy exact diagnosis in many orbital lesions can only be made by histopathological studies.

Management

- **Medical:** Orbital cellulitis; thyroid ophthalmopathy; orbital pseudotumor; antifungals (amphoterecin B and posaconazole) in rhino-orbito-cerebral mucormycosis.
- **Surgical:**
  - Lateral tarsorrhaphy
  - Anterior orbitotomy
  - Lateral orbitotomy
  - Orbitotomy via different routes (transconjunctival, transnasal or transcranial).
  - Exenteration in malignant lesions
  - *Radiotherapy*
- Stereotactic radiosurgery
- Chemotherapy or Immunotherapy in selective cases

Indications for Appropriate Referral in Orbital Tumors *(OP 2.8)*

- Orbital tumors are challenging even when they are very small and/or benign in nature.
- They can threaten vision, facial appearance and in some cases life-threatening.

- Primary physician may help by prescribing—tear supplement, antibiotic ointment at night and/or lid taping to prevent drying of cornea.
- These complicated cases are not for general ophthalmologist or secondary hospitals set up.
- They should be seen carefully and treated at a tertiary eye center by an experienced oculoplastic surgeon.
- **So, all cases are to be referred**

INTRAOCULAR TUMORS (OP 2.7)

Classification

Iris Tumors
- **Benign:** Iris nevus
- **Malignant:** Melanoma; metastatic carcinoma

Ciliary Body Tumors
- **Malignant:** Medullo-epithelioma (diktyoma); melanoma

Choroidal Tumors
- **Benign:** Nevus; hemangioma
- **Malignant:** Melanoma, metastatic carcinoma
- **Retinal tumor:** Retinoblastoma

Among these, the most important tumors are: **Retinoblastoma** and **choroidal melanoma**

Retinoblastoma

Clinical Features
- **Leukocoria or amaurotic cat's eye reflex:** Most common mode of presentation (60%)
- **Squinting of the eye:** Second most common (20%).
- Secondary glaucoma which may be associated with buphthalmos.
- Proptosis (due to orbital involvement)

Signs
- Unilateral dilated pupil with white pupillary reflex (leukocoria)
- Strabismus
- Intraocular tension is higher
- Heterochromia of the iris

Management
Investigations: X-ray of the orbit, ultrasonography: USG B-scan; CT scan of the orbit and brain, MRI imaging; *aqueous humor paracentesis*—for cytology and lactate dehydrogenase (LDH) enzyme assay. FNAC when other diagnostic tests are inconclusive.

Treatment
- **Enucleation:** Excision of the eye with long optic nerve stump. The treatment of the second eye depends on the size and location of the tumor.
- **Exenteration:** Exenteration of the orbit in case of orbital involvement
- **Radiotherapy:** It is done by external irradiation or by a Cobalt-60 scleral plaque.
- **Photocoagulation:** Xenon arc photocoagulation is useful for certain small retinoblastomas
- **Cryotherapy:** It is useful for small peripheral tumors. The tumor should be frozen by triple-freeze and thawing technique.
- **Chemotherapy:** It is indicated following enucleation in advanced cases and in presence of distant metastases. Cyclophosphamide and vincristine are used.
- **Combination of therapy:** To achieve best results.
- **Genetic counseling:** This is important in bilateral cases and if two or more cases of retinoblastomas occur in a family.
- **Follow-up:** It is extremely important in case of treated retinoblastoma.

Choroidal Melanoma

Clinical Features
Average age is 50 years and more common in males. Extremely rare among blacks.

Symptoms
- Symptoms result from exudative retinal detachment and secondary glaucoma caused by increase in choroidal volume.
- Patient may present with decreased visual acuity, or visual field defect, and ocular pain.

- In some cases, patient is asymptomatic, and the tumor is detected by a routine fundoscopy.

Ophthalmoscopically
- Tumor is invariably unilateral and solitary.
- A typical melanoma appears as a pigmented and elevated oval mass.
- The color is frequently brown, it may be mottled with black or dark-brown pigment or it may be amelanotic.
- As the tumor grows—a brown exudative detachment results owing to break in the Bruch's membrane.
- An accumulation of orange pigment (lipofuscin) in the RPE is commonly seen
- Other ocular features—choroidal folds, subretinal hemorrhage, vitreous hemorrhage, cataract and posterior uveitis.
- The lymph nodes are not affected, but distant metastasis in the liver and elsewhere are the common cause of death.

Management
- **First investigate to establish diagnosis:** Medical evaluation, indirect ophthalmoscopy, fluorescein angiography, USG B-scan, P-32 uptake test, CT scan and MRI
- Observation for slowly growing tumor
- **Enucleation:** It is indicated for very large melanomas
- Radioactive scleral plaques (Cobalt-60 or Iodine-125)
- Heavy-charged particle irradiation (protons or helium)
- Photocoagulation
- Chemotherapy and immunotherapy may be useful in cases with distant metastases.

RED EYE (CONJUNCTIVITIS) (OP 3.1 AND 3.3)

Etiological Classification
Infective Conjunctivitis
Acute
Bacterial:
- Mucopurulent conjunctivitis—*Staph. aureus, Streptococcus, Pneumococcus, H. influenzae*, etc.
- Purulent conjunctivitis—*N. gonorrhoeae*
- Membranous conjunctivitis—*C. diphtheriae*

Viral:
- Epidemic keratoconjunctivitis (adenoviral conjunctivitis)
- picoRNA viral conjunctivitis (hemorrhagic)

Subacute or chronic
- Nonspecific: Angular conjunctivitis—*Moraxella*
- Specific: Trachoma

Allergic Conjunctivitis
- Simple allergic conjunctivitis
- Phlyctenular conjunctivitis
- Vernal conjunctivitis (spring catarrh)
- Giant papillary conjunctivitis

Pathophysiology: Conjunctivitis is the inflammation of the conjunctiva. It is characterized by:
- Dilation of the conjunctival vessels
- Hyperemia (conjunctival congestion)
- Chemosis (edema of the conjunctiva)
- Cellular infiltration and exudation
- Various kinds of discharge

Clinical Features
Symptoms
- Redness of the eyes
- Serous, mucoid or mucopurulent, discharge
- Grittiness or foreign body sensation
- Stickiness of the eyelids
- Photophobia and colored halos around the light.

Signs
- One eye may be more affected than the other
- Lid edema, matting of the eyelashes
- Conjunctival congestion and chemosis
- Follicular reaction in viral conjunctivitis
- Papillary reaction in allergic conjunctivitis
- Mucopurulent discharge or flakes of mucopus
- Subconjunctival petechial hemorrhage in some cases

TABLE 3.2: Differential diagnosis of conjunctivitis.

Condition	Duration	Visual acuity	Discharge	Conjunctiva	Lymphadenopathy	Laterality	Associated features
Viral conjunctivitis	1–2 weeks	May be affected	Serous	follicular reactions	Pre-auricular	Unilateral, spreads bilateral	Viral URTI
Bacterial conjunctivitis	Few days	Unaffected	Mucopurulent or purulent	Mild papillary reactions	Occasional	Unilateral, spreads bilateral	None
Allergic conjunctivitis	Seasonal	Unaffected	Mucoid or Ropy	Moderate papillae	None	Bilateral	Atopy

- Preauricular lymphadenopathy in adenoviral conjunctivitis

Differential Diagnosis of Conjunctivitis (Table 3.2)

Complications

Complications of conjunctivitis are rare, but some of the problems may cause serious and include:
- New born conjunctivitis may be serious for general health
- Gonococcal conjunctivitis—may lead to corneal involvement leading to perforation
- Membranous conjunctivitis by C diphtheriae is life threatening
- Adenoviral conjunctivitis—punctate epithelial keratitis and permanent visual problems
- Allergic conjunctivitis—corneal problem including keratoconus and LSCD
- Trachoma can cause corneal blindness
- Psychological problems in atopic/vernal conjunctivitis

Management

Bacterial Conjunctivitis

- Frequent eye wash with lukewarm saline solution to clean crusts and discharge.
- Use dark glasses to prevent photophobia.
- A broad-spectrum antibiotic eye drop, e.g., chloramphenicol or ciprofloxacin is used frequently. Depending upon the severity, it may be four times daily to 1 hourly.
- An antibiotic eye ointment like tetracycline, gentamicin or chloramphenicol at bedtime.
- Other family members are to be treated simultaneously.
- To prevent contamination and further spread:
  - The patient must keep his hands clean.
  - The patient should lie on the affected side (to prevent its spread to the unaffected eye).
  - Personal belongings of the patient like towel, handkerchief, pillow, etc. should be kept separately.

Viral conjunctivitis: Frequent wash, tears substitutes, antibiotic drops to prevent secondary infection

Allergic conjunctivitis: As discussed in vernal conjunctivitis

Differential Diagnosis of RED Eye (Table 3.3)

"Red eye" is a layman's term, applied to any condition with dilatation of conjunctival and or ciliary blood vessels.

Red Eye (Acute Iridocyclitis)
(OP 3.2 and 6.1)

See page 55–57

TABLE 3.3: Differential diagnosis of red eye.

	Acute conjunctivitis	Acute iridocyclitis	Angle closure glaucoma	Episcleritis	Subconjunctival hemorrhage
Symptoms:					
Pain	Discomfort; irritation; itching in allergy	Moderate pain; more localized to eye	Severe radiating pain	Mild to moderate pain	Painless
Discharge	Watery, or mucopurulent	Watery	Watery	Nil or watery	Nil
Photophobia	Mild	Severe	Mild to severe	Nil	Nil
Visual problem	Nil	Mild	Marked	Nil	Nil
Onset	Gradual	Gradual.	Sudden.	Gradual	Sudden
Systemic feature	None	Malaise, joint pain.	Prostration often vomiting.	Usually none	Acute straining, e.g., cough; raised BP
Previous history	Possible previous attacks	Similar previous attacks.	Transient blurring, pain or halos.	Similar previous attacks	Usually none
Signs:					
Visual acuity	Normal	May be little less	May reduce to PL	Normal	Normal
Congestion	Conjunctival; superficial (pink)	Ciliary (brick-red)	Ciliary (purple)	Patch of dilated vessels (pink)	Patch of hemorrhage (bright-red)
Cornea	Normal	KPs	Steamy, epithelial edema	Normal	Normal
Anterior chamber	Normal	Cloudy, cells and flare	Clear; very shallow	Normal	Normal
Pupil and light reflex	Normal	Small irregular; sluggish reaction	Oval; mid dilated; sluggish	Normal	Normal
Iris	Normal	'Muddy iris'	Often edematous	Normal	Normal
IOP	Normal	High, low or normal	Very high (50 mm Hg)	Normal	Normal
Tenderness	Non-tender	Mild to moderate	Marked	Mild to moderate	Non-tender

Differences Between Conjunctival and Ciliary Congestion (Table 3.4)

TABLE 3.4: Differences between conjunctival and ciliary congestion.

Conjunctival congestion	Ciliary congestion
1. Bright red in color	1. Pinkish or dusky red in color
2. Mostly near the fornix	2. Around the limbus (circumcorneal)
3. Branched dichotomously	3. Radially arranged
4. Branches of posterior conjunctival vessels	4. Branches of anterior ciliary vessels
5. Easily blanched by pressure or Phenylephrine (10%) drop	5. No such blanching
6. Vessels fill up from the fornix	6. Vessels fill up from the limbus
7. Indicates superficial involvement, e.g., conjunctivitis, simple hyperemia	7. Indicates deeper tissue involvement e.g., iritis, keratitis or scleritis

TRACHOMA (OP 3.4)

Definition

(*Means 'rough' and 'swelling'*). It is a chronic inflammation of the conjunctiva and cornea, characterized by the presence of follicles, papillary hypertrophy of the conjunctiva, and growth of blood vessels over the cornea.

The specific agent is *Chlamydia trachomatis*. Trachoma was earlier known as *Egyptian ophthalmia*.

Etiological Factors

- Any age, more common among preschool children
- **Agent:** *Chlamydia trachomatis*
- Dry, dirty and sandy weather.
- Poor, unhygienic conditions.
- "Eye-seeking" flies *(Musca Sorbens)*
- Close person to person contacts.

Pathophysiology

- It is caused by *Chlamydia trachomatis* (subtypes—A, B, Ba, and C).
- It also causes genital infection (subtype D to K) and lymphogranuloma venereum (subtype L1, L2 and L3).
- Infection causes inflammation of the conjunctiva with lymphocytic infiltration, plasma cells and macrophages within the follicles. The follicles have typical germinal centers with islands of profuse B-cell proliferation surrounded by of T cells.
- Recurrent conjunctival infection causes prolonged inflammation that leads to conjunctival scarring.
- Scarring is associated with destruction of conjunctival epithelium, loss of goblet cells, and replacement of loose subepithelial stroma with thick compact bands of different collagen fibers.

Symptoms

- Foreign body sensation or grittiness and itching
- Watering, photophobia and redness
- Discharge is usually scanty but may be more in secondary infection.

[*Acute trachoma:* When a secondary infection, e.g., mucopurulent or purulent conjunctivitis is superimposed on a relatively mild chronic trachoma, it is called acute trachoma.]

Signs

- Bulbar congestion.
- Velvety papillary hypertrophy.
- **Follicles**—mostly in upper tarsal conjunctiva; on limbus (leading to Herbert's pit-pathognomonic), or on bulbar conjunctiva.
- **Pannus:** It is a characteristic sign. It is defined as fine subepithelial neovascularization, arranged vertically with round cell infiltration, mainly seen in the upper limbus and upper part of the cornea. **It is of two types:** Progressive and regressive. In *Progressive pannus*, the cellular infiltration extends beyond the terminal ends of neovascularization. *In regressive pannus*, the vessels extend a short distance beyond the area of cellular infiltration.

The above-mentioned signs are seen in active trachoma. Further signs are described later, in the healed stage or stage of sequelae.

WHO Classifications of Trachoma (FISTO) (Table 3.5)

Diagnostic criteria in field survey: Individual cases must have *at least two* of the following signs:
- Follicles at the upper tarsal conjunctiva.
- Limbal follicles or their sequelae, *Herbert's pits*.
- Typical upper tarsal conjunctival scarring (*stellate-shaped scar*).
- Vascular pannus, mostly at the upper limbus.

Herbert's pits are the only clinical signs unique to trachoma, but they do not occur in every case.

Differential Diagnosis
- Allergic conjunctivitis
- Ophthalmia neonatorum
- Viral conjunctivitis
- Bacterial conjunctivitis
- Toxic/chemical conjunctivitis
- Trichiasis

Complications/Sequelae of Trachoma

A. **Eye lids:**
- Trichiasis
- Ptosis (sleepy eyes).
- Scaphoid or boat-shaped lid.
- Cicatricial Entropion.
- Tylosis (rounding of the lid borders).
- Madarosis (loss of eyelashes).
- Chalazion.

B. **Conjunctiva:**
- Loss of fornices.
- Parenchymatous xerosis.
- Symblepharon.
- Pigmentation.
- Pseudo-pterygium.

C. **Cornea:**
- Herbert's pit.
- Healed pannus leading to hazy cornea.
- Different grades of corneal opacity.
- Trachomatous nodular keratopathy (nodular degneration).
- Loss of sensation.

D. **Lacrimal sac:** Chronic dacryocystitis.

Treatment

A. **Therapeutic:**
WHO recommends *two antibiotics* for trachoma control: Oral azithromycin and tetracycline (1%) eye ointment
1. **Systemic:** Oral azithromycin is the drug of choice, easy to administer as single dose.
2. **Local:**
   - Tetracycline ointment (1%)—twice daily for 4–6 weeks.
   - Sulphacetamide (10% or 20%) drop—4 times daily for 4–6 weeks,
   - Topical azithromycin is also helpful, but not easily available.

This is followed by 'intermittent treatment' with tetracycline ointment twice daily for 5 consecutive days, in each month for 6 months. This is especially important in epidemic or hyperendemic zone.

TABLE 3.5: WHO classifications of trachoma (FISTO).		
Trachomatous follicles (TF)	Active disease which needs treatment	5 or more follicles of 0.5 mm diameter—on the upper tarsal plate. Some papillae may also be present. If properly treated—there will be no or minimal scarring
Trachoma intense (TI)	Severe disease—needs urgent treatment	Numerous follicles. 50% area—papillae. High-risk of conjunctival scarring
Trachomatous scarring (TS)	Old, now inactive lesion	Tarsal conjunctival cicatrization with white fibrous bands
Trachomatous trichiasis (TT)	Needs corrective surgery	Presence of at least one trichiatic eyelash
Trachomatous opacities (TO)	From previous trachoma causing visual loss	Presence of corneal opacity covering part of the pupillary region

B. **Prophylactic:**
- Improvement of personal hygiene and sanitation.
- Avoid kajal, Surma, etc.
- Avoid person-to-person close contacts.
- Periodic tetracycline (1%) eye ointment as 'intermittent therapy'.
- Oral azithromycin—single dose 20 mg/kg body weight to a maximum of 1 gm. It should be repeated every 12 months in endemic areas.
- Health education.

C. **Treatment of complications:**
- Excision of the fornix
- Tarsectomy
- Surgery for trichiasis and entropion
- Pannus may be treated by cryoapplication or peritomy
- Corneal ulcers—as general outline.
- Mechanical expression of the follicles—by Roller forceps, silver nitrate painting or diathermy (may cause more scar formation).

D. **SAFE strategy for trachoma:** WHO-developed international efforts to eliminate trachoma as a blinding disease.
S–Surgery to correct—trichiasis (and/or entropion)
A–Antibiotics (oral azithromycin)—for *C. trachomatis* infection
F–Facial cleanliness—to reduce person-to-person transmission
E–Environmental improvement to reduce risk of community transmission

VERNAL CONJUNCTIVITIS (OP 3.5)

Vernal conjunctivitis (spring catarrh) is a bilateral, recurrent, seasonal allergic conjunctivitis in children caused by exogenous allergens.

Etiological Factors
- **Age:** 3–12 years.
- Boys are more affected than girls.
- Prevalent in summer months in India and subsides during winter.
- External allergens like dust, pollens and moulds in presence of dry, hot weather.
- Personal or family history of atopy or allergy.
- Self-limiting course (around 11–14 years of age).

Clinical Features
Symptoms
- Intense itching (due to alkaline nature of the discharge).
- Ropy discharge (due to fibrinous nature of the discharge).
- Photophobia burning and foreign body sensation.

Signs
Three types of vernal conjunctivitis—(1) palpebral, (2) bulbar and (3) mixed.
1. **Palpebral type** is the most common but bulbar type is more common among blacks.
2. **Palpebral type:** Cobble-stone appearance of papillary hypertrophy of the palpebral conjunctiva (due to dense fibrous tissue and pressure exerted by the adjacent hard papillae).
   The color of the papillae is bluish white (milky hue) due to hyaline degeneration. In severe cases, the connective tissue septae rupture, giving rise to giant papillae.
3. **Bulbar type:** Multiple, small, nodule-like gelatinous thickening around the limbus, mostly at the upper.
   Discrete superficial spots (Horner-Tranta's dots) are found scattered around the limbus.

Pathophysiology
- VKC is IgE-mediated hypersensitivity reaction via mast cell release.
- Activated eosinophils are thought to play a significant role
- Additional attention has been given to the CD4 T-helper-2 driven type IV hypersensitivity with immunomodulators such as IL-4, IL-5, and beta-FGF.
- A possible endocrine mechanism also play a role as there is a decrease in symptoms and prevalence after puberty

Differential Diagnosis

- Giant papillary conjunctivitis (as seen in soft contact lens wearer, nylon suture after surgery, or artificial eye user).
- Trachoma.
- Phlyctenulosis (multiple limbal phlycten).
- Follicular conjunctivitis (mainly in lower fornix, but no papilla and no seasonal variation).

Complications

Complications are mainly due to corneal involvement (vernal keratoconjunctivitis). The keratopathy changes are as follows:
- Punctate epithelial keratitis.
- Epithelial micro-erosions—leading to corneal ulceration (shield ulcer)
- Corneal plaque.
- Subepithelial scarring—usually in the form of a ring scar. Pseudo-gerontoxon resembles an arcus senilis with appearance of cupid's bow.
- Patients with vernal catarrh also have a higher incidence of keratoconus.

Treatment

- Cold compress (may be with ice-cube) which is soothing.
- **Topical steroids**—like, dexamethasone, fluorometholone, or loteprednol: 4–8 times daily depending upon the severity.
  Long-term use of topical steroids has problems like cataract and glaucoma. Dilute steroid (1:10) or weak steroid preparation can be used rather safely.
- **Disodium chromoglycate (2–4%)**—four times daily as drops. It can be used safely for a prolonged period. It mainly, prevents the fresh attack, as it is a mast-cell stabilizer.
- **Topical antihistaminics**—like azelastine, epinastine, bepotastine, olopatadine, etc., are helpful to give relief from severe itching.
- **Oral antihistaminics**—for 2–4 weeks to control severe itching
- **Topical nonsteroidal anti-inflammatory drugs**—like, ketorolac or flurbiprofen may be useful.
- **For giant papillae**—cryoapplication, or excision may be done.
- **For shield ulcer**—debridement with amniotic membrane transplantation
- **Acetylcysteine (10–20%) drop**—to prevent excessive mucus production.
- **Supratarsal injection of depot steroids** (i.e., triamcinolone 0.1 mL)—in severe recalcitrant cases.
- Protection from external allergens.

PTERYGIUM (OP 3.6)

See page 33

SYMBLEPHARON (OP 3.7)

This is a condition of adhesion of the lid to the globe, as a result of adhesion between the bulbar and palpebral conjunctiva.

Etiology

- Chemical burns (mostly alkali)
- Thermal burns including burn due to molten metal
- Membranous conjunctivitis
- Ocular cicatricial pemphigoid (OCP)
- Stevens-Johnson syndrome (SJS)
- Erythema multiforme major (EMM)
- Postoperative (e.g., pterygium surgery)
- Trachoma

Pathophysiology

- Any ocular surface insult which produces raw surfaces upon two opposed areas of bulbar and palpebral conjunctiva will lead to abnormal adhesion during the healing process.
- This healing process is abnormal.
- Bands of fibrous tissue are formed, and they stretch between the lid and the globe. The bands may be narrow or broad. The Immune-mediated inflammatory process continues to excite fibrous proliferation.
- Cornea is also involved in severe cases.

Types

There are three types of symblepharon are as follows:

1. **Anterior symblepharon:** Bands are limited to the anterior parts and not involving the fornix.
2. **Posterior symblepharon:** Bands are obliterating the fornix only.
3. **Total symblepharon:** The lids are completely plastered against the globe and leaving a small fixed palpebral aperture.

Symptoms
- Pain and redness—due to exposure
- Burning sensation
- Watering—due to inadequate lacrimal drainage.
- Photophobia
- Cosmetic disfigurement.

Signs
- Signs of exposure
- Restriction of ocular movement
- Visible fibrotic band
- Obliteration of the fornix at places.
- May be associated partial or total limbal stem cell deficiency (LSCD)

Differential Diagnosis
- Large recurrent pterygium
- Pseudo-pterygium
- Ankyloblepharon—adhesion of the edges of the upper eyelid with the lower eyelid.

Complications
- The adhesion encroaches the limbus and grow over the cornea, leading to vision loss
- Diplopia—due to limitation of the ocular movements resulting from pronounced adhesion.

Management

Prevention
- Sweeping a glass rod—well coated with ointment, around the upper and lower fornices, so that they are well packed with ointment. This procedure is to be repeated several times each day according to severity.
- Scleral contact shell (Conformer) fitting—to separate the two mucosal surfaces to prevent their adhesions.
- Treatment of the cause—as in OCP, need systemic immune-suppressants

When Established
- **If there is a small band:** Just excise the band.
- **If it is moderate:** Excise the band with intraoperative MMC (0.02%) and amniotic membrane transplantation
- **If it is extensive:** Radical excision of the scarred conjunctival tissues, and mucous membrane graft to cover the bare area (mucous membrane is taken from upper fornix of opposite eye, or from the buccal mucosa).
- May be combined with simple limbal epithelial transplantation (SLET) procedure, especially in chemical burn.

Prevention of Recurrence of Adhesion
- By therapeutic contact lens
- By scleral shell at least for 6 weeks.
- High dose of steroids is helpful to prevent formation of excessive granulation tissues).

TECHNIQUE OF REMOVAL OF FOREIGN BODY FROM EYE (OP 3.8 AND 4.8)

Correct steps for removal of foreign body from ocular surface:
1. Search for the foreign body with a good torch light and if necessary, with a loupe (a slit lamp is much better).
2. Surface foreign bodies are removed with irrigation and a moistened cotton-tipped applicator.
3. Evert the upper lid to find out any foreign body in the **subtarsal sulcus** *(commonest site of lodgment of a foreign body)*. If it is there, remove it with a sterile cotton swab or pellet, under topical anesthesia.
4. *If the foreign body is on the cornea,* put 4% lignocaine or 1% proparacaine drop to anaesthetize the ocular surface.

5. If it is superficial, remove the foreign body with a sterile cotton bud simply by touching it.
6. If it is not possible to remove it, take a disposable sterile hypodermic needle of any size and remove the foreign body by lifting. It will cause only a point damage. Do not scratch and cross the pupillary zone of the cornea.
7. If the foreign body is embedded into the deeper stroma of the cornea, take the patient to the OT and remove the foreign body with a needle under operative microscope.
8. In all cases apply antibiotic ointment and if necessary cycloplegic drop. Put a pad for few hours. Examine the patient on the next morning, and start frequent antibiotic drops for the next few days.
9. In case of old iron foreign body, there is formation of rust-ring around the foreign body. It is also to be removed carefully with a needle.
10. After successful removal, finally re-evaluate the area with fluorescein stain and cobalt blue filter.
11. *In all cases of corneal foreign body, always examine the lacrimal sac by giving pressure over the sac region to rule out any chronic dacryocystitis.*
12. If it is present, the lower punctum is temporarily occluded by thermocautery and antibiotic drops and ointment are to be applied frequently after removal of foreign body.
    If the foreign body is intraocular—refer the patient to a tertiary eye care center for proper investigation and then removal.

CORRECT TECHNIQUE OF INSTILLATION OF EYE DROPS *(OP 3.9)*

Instruction to the Patient

- **Step 0:** Always **check the expiry date** before installation of any eye drop.
- **Step 1:** Wash and dry your hands; **shake the bottle** vigorously if it contains a suspension
- **Step 2:** Remove the cap of the eye drop vial but **do not touch the dropper tip**. Place the dropper cap on a clean tissue paper.
- **Step 3:** Stand in front of the mirror for self-administration and tilt your head backwards. Gently pull the lower eyelid to form a pouch.
- **Step 4:** Hold the dropper above the selected eye for instillation of the drop. Squeeze **just one drop** into the pouch. **Try not to touch your eye, eyelashes, or anything else with the dropper tip in order to keep it sterile.**
- **Step 5:** Close your eyes and do not blink. Keep the eye closed for 1–2 minutes after application of eye drop.
- **Step 6:** Immediately after instillation of drops, press gently on the tear duct (inner corner of the eye) with index finger for a minute. This will prevent drainage of eye drops into the nostril and mouth.
- **Step 7:** Wipe away any liquid that falls on to your cheek with a tissue paper. And recap the bottle.
- **Step 8:** Repeat the above steps in the other eye if the drop is prescribed for both eyes.
- **Step 9:** Again, wash your hands to remove any medication.
- **Step 10:** When eye drops of two different drugs are prescribed—**give a gap of at least 5 minutes** between each eye drop. This will prevent the first drug from being diluted or washed away by second drug. When an eye drop and eye ointment are prescribed always instill the eye drop first and then the ointment.

Some Tips to Remember

- Use multidose vial eye drops for not more than 4 weeks from the date of first opening even if the dates are valid.
- Single use eye drops (minims) do not contain any preservatives and they should be discarded after first use.
- Eye drops are sterile products. Do not try to open it using safety pins.
- Each eye can hold only one drop. Additional drops will be a waste.

- Most eye drops sting or irritate the eye for few seconds. If symptoms persist, speak to your eye care practitioner.
- Store the eye drops at room temperature, away from heat and direct light.

CORNEA (OP 4)

Enumerate and Discuss the Types of Corneal Ulceration (OP 4.1)

Definition

A corneal ulcer is defined as a loss of corneal epithelium with underlying stromal infiltration and/or suppuration associated with signs of inflammation with or without hypopyon.

Etiological Classification

Microbial Keratitis

- Bacterial
- Fungal
- **Viral:** HSV and HZV
- **Parasitic:** Acanthamoebal and microsporidial

Non-infective Corneal Ulcer

Central

- Exposure keratitis/ulcer
- Neurotrophic keratitis/ulcer
- Atheromatous ulcer

Peripheral

- Marginal keratitis/ulcer
- Phlyctenular keratitis/ulcer
- Mooren's ulcer
- Corneal ulcer associated with collagen vascular diseases

Risk Factors for Corneal Ulcer

- Corneal foreign body with vegetable materials
- Corneal abrasion, injury or burn
- Contact lens wearers (overnight use, unhygienic CL)
- People with herpes infection
- Inappropriate use of steroid eye drops
- Chronic dry eye
- Uncontrolled diabetes, collagen vascular diseases
- **Eyelid disorders:** Lagophthalmos, trichiasis and entropion

Differential Diagnosis of Infective Keratitis (OP 4.2)

See page 39–41

Enumerate the Causes of Corneal Edema (OP 4.3)

- **Inflammatory:** Corneal ulcer, HSV endotheliitis, acute iridocyclitis (due to endothelial damage)
- **Traumatic:** Mechanical—due to endothelial damage, chemical burn
- **Postsurgical:** Post-cataract surgery corneal edema, failed corneal graft
- **Increased intraocular pressure:**
  - Acute edema in angle-closure glaucoma
  - Epidemic dropsy glaucoma.
  - Chronic edema in long-standing cases—as in absolute glaucoma and buphthalmos.
- **Corneal dystrophy:** Fuchs' endothelial dystrophy (FECD), posterior polymorphous dystrophy (PPCD) and congenital hereditary endothelial dystrophy (CHED)
- **Hypoxia of the cornea:** As in contact lens wearer due to epithelial edema, as a result of prolonged deprivation of atmospheric oxygen.
- **Acute hydrops in keratoconus:** Due to descemet membrane tear
- **ICE syndrome:** Mixed mechanism—due to high IOP and corneal endothelial problem

Causes and Management of Dry Eye (OP 4.4)

New definition of dry eye (DEWS II–2017): "Dry eye is a multifactorial disease of the ocular surface—characterized by a loss of homeostasis of the tear film, and accompanied by ocular symptoms, in which tear film instability and hyperosmolarity, ocular surface inflammation and damage, and neurosensory abnormalities play etiological roles."

Causes of Dry Eye (Table 3.6)

TABLE 3.6: Causes of dry eye.

Categories	Causes
Aqueous tear deficiency	• Keratoconjunctivitis sicca (Sjogren syndrome) • Secondary to collagen diseases (e.g., rheumatoid arthritis) • Surgical removal of lacrimal gland • Drug-induced, like antihistaminics, antipsychotic drug, etc. • Neuroparalytic hyposecretion
Mucin deficiency	• Goblet cell dysfunctions: Hypovitaminosis A • Goblet cell destruction: In alkali burn, trachoma, OCP, SJS • Drug-induced: Preservatives in eye drops, beta-blockers
Lipid abnormalities	• Various types of blepharitis including meibomianitis • Computer vision syndrome • Anhydrotic ectodermal dysplasia (congenital absence of meibomian gland)
Lid surfacing abnormalities	• Lagophthalmos • Exposure keratitis • Entropion, ectropion • Lid-notching • Coloboma of the lid
Epitheliopathies	• Recurrent erosions • Limbal lesions • Hard contact lens • Topical anesthesia

Levels of Severity of Dry Eye (DEWS Classification) (Table 3.7)

TABLE 3.7: Levels of severity of dry eye (DEWS classification)*.

Levels	Previous term	Clinical features
Level 1	Mild dry eye	Mild conjunctival signs; normal Schirmer; slightly lower TBUT; no other problems
Level 2	Moderate dry eye	Mild corneal signs, abnormal TBUT, abnormal Schirmer's value
Level 3	Severe dry eye	Marked conjunctival and corneal sign; abnormal TBUT and Schirmer; symptomatic
Level 4	Extremely severe dry eye	More visual symptoms; severe corneal erosions; constant features

*International Dry Eye Workshop (DEWS), 2007.
(TBUT: tear-film break-uptime)

Management Outline of Dry Eye (DEWS Recommendation)

A stepwise management approach is required at different levels of dry eye.

Step 1: In Level 1
- ❖ Patient education and counseling
- ❖ Dietary modification
- ❖ Tears substitute (any type) 4 times/day,
- ❖ Environmental management (e.g., air conditioner in room)
- ❖ Systemic medication review
- ❖ Control ocular allergy
- ❖ Address contact lens problems.

Step 2: In Level 2—steps to follow from step 1
- ❖ Tears substitute—preservative-free (6–8 times)
- ❖ Oral doxycycline in MGD
- ❖ Topical anti-inflammatory agents
- ❖ Topical cyclosporine (0.05%)—twice daily,
- ❖ Lid hygiene
- ❖ Nutritional support (omega-3 fatty acid).
- ❖ This also includes punctal plugs and other minor OPD procedures such as meibomian gland expression, vector thermal pulsation therapy, and intense pulsed light treatment.

Step 3: In Level 3—steps from level one and two
- ❖ Tears substitute (preservative-free) 1 hourly
- ❖ Autologous serum eye drop (20–50%)
- ❖ Bandage contact lens
- ❖ Oral secretagogues

Step 4: In Level 4—it is refractory dry eye. Steps from level one to three
- Tears supplement (preservative-free) —1/2 hourly to 1 hourly
- Oral immunosuppressants, e.g., oral cyclosporine
- Acetyl cysteine 20% eye drop
- Tarsorrhaphy or botulinum toxin
- Amniotic membrane grafting
- Limbal cell transplantation (auto/allograft).

CAUSES OF CORNEAL BLINDNESS (OP 4.5)

Corneal diseases are a major cause of blindness worldwide, second only to cataract. Recent survey by NPCB and VI (2015–2019) showed that *overall prevalence of corneal blindness is 7.4%, second only to cataract blindness.*

The major causes are *(importance wise)*:
1. **Infectious keratitis (corneal ulcer):** Bacterial, fungal, viral and protozoal
2. **Pseudophakic or aphakic bullous keratopathy:** As a complication of cataract surgery
3. **Corneal injury:** Open globe/chemical/thermal
4. **Hereditary dystrophies:** Stromal (macular and lattice) dystrophies, endothelial (FECD, CHED)
5. **Corneal ectasia:** Keratoconus, post-LASIK ectasia
6. **Trachoma:** Much less in India now
7. **Vitamin A deficiency:** Much lower incidence now
8. **Congenital conditions:** Sclerocornea, Peter's anomaly, dermoid, etc.
9. **Miscellaneous:** River blindness (onchocerciasis)—not in India

Vitamin A Deficiency

- Vitamin A deficiency (VAD) along with protein energy malnutrition (PEM) causes severe blinding corneal destruction.
- *Vitamin A deficiency is a systemic disease that affects cells and organs throughout the body.*
- The characteristic ocular manifestations of VAD ranging from night blindness to corneal melting are termed as xerophthalmia
- Approximately, one-fifth of preschool-age population of the world is estimated to be vitamin A deficient, with just less than 1% being night blind at any given time.

Major Clinical Features of Xerophthalmia (WHO Classification) (Table 3.8)

- **XN (night blindness):** It is usually the earliest manifestation of VAD; sometimes termed as chicken eyes (chicken lack rods and are thus night blind).
- **X1A and X1B (conjunctival xerosis and Bitot's spot):** The conjunctival epithelium in VAD, is transformed from normal columnar to stratified squamous with a resultant loss of goblet cells, formation of a granular cell layer and keratinization of the surface.
- **X2 (corneal xerosis):** A hazy, lustuerless dry appearance of the cornea, is first seen near the inferior limbus.
- **X3A and X3B (corneal ulceration/keratomalacia):** They indicate permanent destruction of a part, or all the corneal stroma, resulting in permanent structural alteration.
- **XS (xerophthalmic scar):** They are usually bilateral and indicate healed sequelae of prior corneal disease related to VAD.

TABLE 3.8: Major clinical features of xerophthalmia (WHO classification).

Types	Clinical picture
XN	Night blindness
X1A	Conjunctival xerosis
X1B	Bitot's spot
X2	Corneal xerosis
X3A	Corneal ulceration/keratomalacia (<1/3 corneal surface)
X3B	Corneal ulceration/keratomalacia (>1/3 corneal surface)
XS	Corneal scar
XF	Xerophthalmic fundus

- **XF [xerophthalmic (uyemura's) fundus]:** Small white lesions on the retina, seen in some cases of VAD, are only of academic interest. They may be associated with constriction of the visual fields.

Treatment

Xerophthalmia is a medical emergency as it carries a high risk of corneal destruction and blindness and/or sepsis and death.

Treatment Schedule for Xerophthalmia

Vitamin A (WHO recommendation):
- **Immediately upon diagnosis:** 200,000 IU vitamin A orally.
- **Next day:** 200,000 IU vitamin A orally.
- **Within 1-4 weeks:** 200,000 IU orally.
  Children between 6 and 11 months, or less than 8 kg- half the above dose.
  Children less than 6 months old-one-quarter of the above dose.

IM injection vitamin A (water-soluble) 100,000 IU is given, when:
- The child cannot swallow
- In case of persistent vomiting
- In severe malabsorption
- Where the compliance is poor.

Oral administration is preferred, as it is safe, cheap and highly effective even in presence of mild diarrhea (as it is also helpful for the intestinal epithelium).

Eye care: In case of corneal involvement
- **Board-spectrum antibiotic ointment:** Moxifloxacin or ciprofloxacin—4 times daily.
- **Atropine eye ointment:** 2 times daily.
- **If secondary infection is present:** Second antibiotic is added.
- **Tears substitute eye drop:** 4 to 8 times daily.

Preventing recurrence: This is for the vulnerable children.
- By inexpensive, readily available vitamin A rich diet.
- Periodic administration of a large dose of vitamin A at an interval of 6 months.

Vitamin A Prophylaxis

Three main intervention strategies are as:
1. Increasing the dietary intake of foods rich in vitamin A and provitamin A.
2. Periodic administration of large doses of oral vitamin A.
3. Administration of commonly consumable fortified food items (vitamin A fortification).

Sources of Vitamin A
- **Vegetable sources:** Dark-green leafy vegetables, spinach, carrot, tomato, pumpkin, etc.
- **Animal sources:** Liver, meat, cod-liver oil, shark-liver oil, egg-yolk, etc.
- **Fortified food items:** Vitamin A enriched commercially available food items.

Daily Requirements
- School children, adolescent and adults: 2,250 IU (750 µg)
- Children (0-4 years): 1,000-2,000 IU (300-400 µg)
- Pregnancy and lactation: 3,000 IU (750 + 300 µg)

Target Group
- **Infants 6-11 months (including HIV+):** 100,000 IU vitamin A once.
- **Children 12-59 months (including HIV+):** 200,000 IU vitamin A every 6 months

Target group is determined by:
Where vitamin A deficiency is a public health problem—prevalence of night blindness is 1% or higher in children 24-59 months of age or lower serum vitamin A level.

This prophylaxis may be for entire neighborhood *(mass prophylaxis)*, or for high-risk group *(selective prophylaxis)*.

The high-risk conditions are as follows:
- Children with severe PEM
- Children with measles
- Children with diarrhea, lower RTI, or other acute infection (e.g., malaria, chickenpox, etc.).

They should receive a dose of 200,000 IU vitamin A orally at the time of diagnosis by the pediatrician.
Children below 1 year should receive half dose.

INDICATIONS AND TYPES OF KERATOPLASTY (OP 4.6)

Overall Indications of Keratoplasty

- Infective keratitis—most common
- Corneal scar (healed ulcer)
- Pseudophakic corneal edema/bullous keratopathy
- Fuchs' endothelial dystrophy
- Non-Fuchs' corneal dystrophies—lattice, macular
- Keratoconus
- Failed graft

Types of Keratoplasty

Morphological Types

- Full thickness or penetrating keratoplasty (PK)
- Partial thickness or lamellar keratoplasty (LK)

Anterior lamellar keratoplasty (ALK):
- Superficial anterior lamellar keratoplasty (SALK)
- Deep anterior lamellar keratoplasty (DALK)

Posterior lamellar keratoplasty (PLK):
- Descemet stripping (automated) endothelial keratoplasty (DSEK/DSAEK)
- Descemet membrane endothelial keratoplasty (DMEK)
- **Keratoprosthesis** (artificial cornea transplantation)

Types—According to Purpose

- **Optical:** Primary purpose is being the improvement of vision (e.g., leucoma, keratoconus, etc.).
- **Tectonic:** Restoration of altered corneal structure (e.g., thinning, perforation, etc.).
- **Therapeutic:** Tissue substitution for refractory corneal diseases (e.g., nonhealing or perforated corneal ulcer, limbal dermoid, etc.).
- **Cosmetic:** Replacement, without the hope for visual improvement.

Frequently, several purposes are addressed when a keratoplasty is performed.

According to Type of Surgery

- **Simple keratoplasty:** Keratoplasty is performed alone.
- **Combined keratoplasty:** When combined with:
  - Cataract extraction (ICCE/ECCE)
  - ECCE/SICS/phaco with PCIOL implantation (triple procedure)
  - Vitrectomy
  - Glaucoma surgery

Indications and Methods of Tarsorrhaphy (OP 4.7)

See page 185

Eye Donation and Eye Banking (OP 4.9 and 4.10)

- Corneal blindness in India—approximately 1.2 million (bilateral—60%)
- Only 8–10% cases will be benefitted by a corneal transplantation
- Addition of new patients in India is >50,000/year
- As per vision-2020 India, we need to perform 100,000 corneal transplants every year
- With an utilization rate of 50% in keratoplasty, we need 200,000 cornea/year to meet this goal.
- This donor corneas come from eye donation after death of an individual via eye banking.
- Cornea cannot be collected from any living person.

Eye Donation: Two Types

1. **Voluntary eye donation (VED):** It is the result of realization of one's social responsibility towards people with corneal blindness. Among all collections, 70–75% of eye donation is from voluntary aged

donors who die in their homes, hospitals, or nursing homes. Only 35–40% of the eyes from voluntary donation are utilized for transplantation.

The reasons for low utilization are:
- Age of the donor
- Longer death-to-enucleation time
- Non-availability of donor's complete medical history.

2. **Hospital cornea retrieval program (HCRP):**
   - Here, an eye donation counsellor (EDC, or previously called grief counsellor) makes timely and sensitive request to the near relatives of the bereaved in a hospital set up to make an eye donation. With several leaflets and close intimate education, he or she wins the heart of the relatives of the deceased.
   - If the consent is given, he organizes quick collection of donor tissue (whole eyeball or in situ corneoscleral rim) so that the family is not inconvenienced.
   - The overall conversion (request by EDC versus actual donation) is between 5% and 45% in different hospitals. The donor cornea collection through HCRP is around 25–30% of total collection in last few years in India.

Advantages of HCRP
- Access to younger and healthier tissues.
- Availability of donor medical history.
- Reduce death-to-enucleation time.
- Blood sample collection much easier
- Higher tissue utilization rate (65% or more).
- More scope of training and future research.
- Cost effective.

Choice of Hospitals
- Large multispecialty hospitals with 500 beds or more.
- Death rate = 3–4 deaths/day or >10 deaths/week.
- Centralized death reporting system
- Should be close vicinity (within 5–15 km) to the linked eye bank.
- Should have signed memorandum of understanding (MoU) between both.

- Help and active support is required from all levels of the staff of the hospital.

Instructions to the family member by the Doctor/Eye Bank Personnel before collection (during receiving a call):
- To cover both eyelids properly
- Place a moist cotton or ice cube over the closed eyelids
- To raise the head end of the deceased
- To switch off the fan of the room. If A/C is there, keep it on.
- Keep medical records and death certificate ready with xerox copies.

Collection (Retrieval)

- After getting information of death, and proper written consent from the next of kin, eye bank technician collects the eyes.
- The eyeballs should be collected with 4–6 hours of death (traditional postmortem time).
- 4–5 mL blood is also collected from deceased (from jugular or femoral vein) at the same time—for 4 serology tests of the donor (HIV, hepatitis B, hepatitis C and syphilis)
- It is important to know the age of the donor, time of death and cause of death before enucleation of the donor globe.
- Most eye banks accept eyes from donors between 6 months and 80 years of age.

Two types of collection:
1. **Whole globe:** After enucleation, whole eyeball is kept in a moist chamber for transportation
2. **In-situ corneoscleral (CS) button:** Excised *in-situ* and placed in MK medium or Cornisol or Optisol-GS medium with endothelial side up.

Contraindications:
- **Medical:** Death due to unknown cause, rabies, HIV, hepatitis B, hepatitis C, syphilis, leukemia, Creutzfeldt-Jacob disease, severe septicemia, COVID-19 disease, etc.
- **Ocular:** Corneal pathology, retinoblastoma, malignant melanoma, exposure keratitis, etc.

Functions of an Eye Bank

- Collection of donor eyes.
- Evaluate, process and storage of donor cornea.
- Distribution and utilization of the highest quality of donor tissue for transplantation.
- Provide for soliciting eye donation from potential donors.
- Provide and process eye tissue for teaching or research, as needed.
- To promote public education relation system.
- To promote HCRP to improve collection of donor eyes from hospital deaths.

Tissue Processing

- Torch light examination
- Slit lamp evaluation
- **Serology testing:** HIV, hepatitis B, hepatitis C and syphilis
- C/S button preparation (for whole Globe collection) under laminar flow hood in a sterile environment and then storage in MK or cornisol medium vial.
- Specular microscopy for endothelial cell count
- Microbiology (optional)—but always helpful

Storage (preservation) of the donor eye:
- **Short-term preservation (up to 96 hours)**
  - *Moist chamber method:* Whole globe at +4°C in a refrigerator for 24 hours.
  - *McCarey-Kaufman (M-K) medium:* C/S button at +4°C for up to 96 hours.
- **Intermediate-term preservation (up to 2 weeks):** Optisol-GS, Cornisol, Eusol-C and Life-4°C media.
- **Long-term preservation (months to years):**
  - *Viable:* Organ culture method, cryopreservation.
  - *Non-viable:* Glycerine preservation, lyophilization

Basic Ethics/Protocols of Eye Banking

- Eye tissue/cornea cannot be bought or sold
- Distribution of tissue irrespective of gender, race, creed, religion, etc.
- Distribution as per predefined priority; as per "waiting list" and as per "first come first basis" service
- Donor information cannot be shared with the recipient
- Donor/recipient identity cannot be disclosed to anyone/or any media, except for legal reason.
- No competition between the two eye banks

Counsel Patients and Family about Eye Donation *(OP 4.10)*

Two types of counseling: Post-death and pre-death (rarely)

Post-death counseling: In all cases pre-death counseling is not possible. Most of the time (or >95% of the cases)—it happens that counseling the relative has to be done only after the death of a patient.

The steps are:
1. **Approaching a donor family:** First to contact the ward nurse-in-charge of the deceased to identify the decision maker in the family.
2. **Wait:** Eye donation counselor (EDC) shall wait until the family members are found mentally relaxed.
3. **Introduce:** EDC introduces himself/herself by name and the eye bank he/she belongs to and begin counseling.
4. **Express sympathy and sharing the grief:** To understand the situation of grief—sudden death; young patient; head of the family; terminally ill
5. **Inform and talk about facts of eye donation:** Inform the family about the magnitude of the problem and the difference they can make by donating eyes.
   - Long waiting list for keratoplasty
   - Benefit to two corneally blind individuals
   - Explain the process of eye donation, and the functions of eye bank
   - Talk about *in-situ* C/S button excision and about 5 mL blood
   - Assure that there will be no disfigurement of face
   - Takes only 15–20 minutes

- Also assure that there will be no delay in funeral arrangements
- Confidentiality about the donor and recipient
- Assurance that eyes/corneas are not to be sold
- Certificate of Appreciation

6. **Give adequate time:** For the family members to discuss and decide about eye donation.
7. **Wait for positive reactions from the donor family:** Some examples:
   - Good listening from the side of donor family.
   - Good understanding the noble purpose and need for eye donation.
   - Calling other family members and involving them regarding eye donation.
   - Finally, accepting the fact and giving consent for eye donation.*
8. **Process involved in obtaining consent for eye donation**
   - Express gratitude to the family member for listening patiently
   - Get consent within the hospital
9. **Consent form:** To be filled and signed by one next of kin and two witnesses. Consent should be obtained before enucleation/*in-situ* excision.
10. **Express gratitude:** To the family member upon completing the eye donation procedure. Provide pamphlet and mobile number for further details/contact.

Negative reactions during counseling: Express gratitude to the family members of the deceased even in the absence of obtaining consent for eye donation.

Eye donation counselor shall never insist that the family donate eyes.

SCLERA (OP 5)

Episcleritis (OP 5.1)

Definition
It is a benign inflammatory process affecting the episcleral tissue that lies between the conjunctiva and the sclera. It is usually a mild and self-limiting disease, but recurrence is common.

Etiology
- Young adults, more in female.
- Two-third cases are idiopathic.
- But, in one-third of cases may have underlying systemic diseases:
  - *Collagen vascular diseases:* Rheumatoid arthritis, systemic lupus erythematosus, polyarteritis nodosa, seronegative spondyloarthropathies (ankylosing spondylitis, inflammatory bowel disease, psoriatic arthritis), Wegener granulomatosis, juvenile idiopathic arthritis
  - *Allergic reaction to endogenous toxins:* Streptococcal or tubercular.
  - *Infectious:* Herpes zoster, herpes simplex, syphilis, etc.
  - *Non-infectious conditions:* Behcet's disease, sarcoidosis, gout, acne rosacea

Pathologically, there is dense lymphocytic infiltrations in subconjunctival and episcleral tissue.

Symptoms
- Localized area of redness.
- Mild to moderate discomfort or irritation of the eye.
- Photophobia and watery discharge

Signs
Two clinical types: (1) Simple and (2) Nodular.
1. **Simple episcleritis:** More common type. Diffuse or sectorial redness with mild tenderness.
2. **Nodular episcleritis:** A small purple nodule with surrounding injection, is situated 2–3 mm away from the limbus (usually on the temporal side). The nodule is immobile and tender. Some patients with nodular episcleritis may have an associated systemic disease.

Complications
Normally, the condition is transient with spontaneous remission within a few days.

But sometimes, it may give rise to **following complications:**
- ❖ **Recurrent attacks:** When the attacks are fleeting but frequently repeated, it is called episcleritis periodica fugax
- ❖ Corneal dellen (adjacent to episcleral nodule)
- ❖ Deeper extension into the sclera, leading to scleritis
- ❖ Anterior and intermediate uveitis in some patients
- ❖ Adherence of conjunctiva with the sclera after repeated attacks.
- ❖ Cataract and secondary glaucoma due to overuse of steroid drops.

Indications for Referral
- ❖ More prolong course and multiple recurrences
- ❖ Nodular episcleritis with suspected/associated systemic disease
- ❖ Nodular episcleritis with dellen formation

Management
- ❖ Nonsteroidal anti-inflammatory drop, e.g., flurbiprofen, ketorolac or nepafenac eye drop—3 times daily.
- ❖ Oral anti-inflammatory agents—like ibuprofen, indomethacin or diclofenac.
- ❖ Weak corticosteroids drop (fluorometholone or loteprednol)—4 times daily, in selective cases
- ❖ Low dose oral aspirin or indomethacin for a prolonged period to prevent recurrence

Scleritis *(OP 5.2)*

Scleritis (inflammation of the sclera) is a more serious disease than episcleritis **(Table 3.9)**.

Etiology
- ❖ Usually bilateral and occurs most frequently in women.
- ❖ Associated systemic conditions:
  - ➢ *Connective tissue disorders:* In 50% of the cases:
    - ♦ Rheumatoid arthritis
    - ♦ Systemic lupus erythematosus
    - ♦ Polyarteritis nodosa
    - ♦ Seronegativespondyloarthropathies (ankylosing spondylitis, inflammatory bowel disease, psoriatic arthritis)
    - ♦ Wegener granulomatosis
    - ♦ Juvenile idiopathic arthritis
  - ➢ **Miscellaneous systemic conditions:** Tuberculosis, sarcoidosis, syphilis, leprosy, etc.
  - ➢ **Infectious local cause:** Herpes zoster or herpes simplex virus

Pathology
Deposition of immune-complex in the sclera leading to inflammation → marked infiltration of lymphocytes in the scleral lamellae with edema → breakdown of swollen lamellae with necrosis → scleral thinning → simultaneous inflammation of the uveal tract, causing uveitis.

TABLE 3.9: Differences between episcleritis and scleritis.

Features	Episcleritis	Scleritis
Definition	A superficial disease of episcleral tissue, a mild condition	A deep severe destructive disease of sclera; not a mild condition
Symptoms	Redness is the main presentation	Severe boring pain is the main presentation
Signs	Less tender. Bright red in color. Only superficial edema. No KPs, no feature of uveitis	More tender nodule. Purplish in color. Sclera appears thickened. Presence of keratic precipitates (KPs), feature of uveitis
Drug test with 10% phenylephrine	Quick blanching of blood vessels	No such blanching of blood vessels
Prognosis	Favorable, complications usually do not occur	Poor, complications like dimness of vision, scleral thinning, staphyloma and sometimes perforation may occur

Clinical Features

Symptoms

- Intense deep-seated pain with radiation towards the forehead.
- Redness and lacrimation.

Signs

- **Diffuse anterior scleritis:** The inflammation is more widespread involving either a segment of the globe, or the entire anterior sclera with intense deep-seated vascularization (brawny scleritis).
- **Nodular anterior scleritis:** An extremely tender, firm immobile nodule separated from the overlying congested episcleral tissue. Sclera is edematous over the nodule. Multiple nodules may extend around the limbus causing annular scleritis.
- **Anterior necrotizing scleritis with inflammation:** Avascular patches appearing in the episcleral tissue. Marked thinning of the sclera with increased visibility of underlying uvea. Associated anterior uveitis.
- **Anterior necrotizing scleritis without inflammation** (*scleromalacia perforans*): Typically occurs in female patients, with long-standing seropositive rheumatoid arthritis. The condition is painless and starts as a necrotic patch in the normal sclera. Eventually, extreme scleral thinning occurs, and the underlying uvea bulges through it. Spontaneous perforation is extremely rare.
- **Posterior scleritis:** It is usually not associated with specific systemic diseases. Inward extension (towards choroid) may give rise to *uveal effusion syndrome*—choroiditis, choroidal effusion, exudative retinal detachment, macular edema, etc. Outward extension onto the orbit may give rise to proptosis and extraocular muscles involvement.

Complications

- Nodular scleritis to multinodular scleritis to annular scleritis. Then scleral thinning ciliary staphyloma
- Anterior uveitis with its complications
- Sclero-keratitis, keratolysis, avascular necrotic scleral patch which may perforate
- Extreme scleral thinning with uveal tissue prolapses
- Uveal effusion syndrome in posterior scleritis
- Cataract and secondary glaucoma.

Indications for Referral

All patients with scleritis need referral to an advanced eye care facility and/or to a rheumatologist

- More prolong course and multiple recurrences
- Scleritis with suspected/associated systemic disease—to a rheumatologist for proper diagnosis and systemic management
- Scleritis with dellen formation—to a cornea specialist
- *Scleromalacia perforans*—to a cornea specialist
- Posterior scleritis with uveal effusion syndrome—to a retina specialist

Management

- **Investigations to find out the systemic cause:**
  - Total hemogram, serum uric acid
  - Collagen profiles for collagen vascular diseases, e.g., rheumatoid factor, antinuclear antibody, soluble immune-complex, lupus erythematosus (LE) cells, etc.
  - X-ray chest and sacroiliac joints
  - Mantoux test
  - VDRL and FTA-ABS for syphilis.
  - B-scan ultrasonography to detect posterior scleritis.
- **Treatment:**
  - *Tablet indomethacin*: 100 mg daily for 5 days, reducing to 75 mg daily until the inflammation resolves.
  - *Oral prednisolone*: 60–80 mg daily, then the dose can be tapered accordingly, as the inflammation subsides.

- Local corticosteroids are less effective, and subconjunctival injection is contraindicated for fear of perforation of the globe.
- *Immunosuppressive agents:* Oral methotrexate or azathioprine in severe and unresponsive cases.
- Biologicals for recalcitrant cases with the help of rheumatologist
- Atropine (1%) eye ointment—2 times daily for associated uveitis.

IRIS AND ANTERIOR CHAMBER (OP 6)

Iridocyclitis *(OP 6.1, 6,2 and 6,3)*

See page 55–57

Non-granulomatous Uveitis versus Granulomatous Uveitis *(OP 6.1)*

See page 58

Acute Iridocyclitis versus Chronic Iridocyclitis (Table 3.10) *(OP 6.2)*

According to standardization of uveitis nomenclature (SUN) working group: An acute iridocyclitis is defined as—"iridocyclitis of sudden onset and for limited duration."

The symptoms of are acute pain, redness, and photophobia that typically develop rapidly, over a few days.

These are resolved with appropriate anti-inflammatory therapy. If therapy can be tapered and inflammation does not recur for "at least 3 months off" of treatment, the disease is said to be of limited duration.

Chronic iridocyclitis: Defined as "persistent iridocyclitis for 6 weeks or longer, or with prompt relapse in less than 3 months, after discontinuation of treatment."

[**Recurrent iridocyclitis:** "Repeated episode of iridocyclitis separated by *periods of inactivity* without treatment for more than 3 months duration."]

Acute iridocyclitis: Such as HLA-B27-associated acute anterior uveitis

Chronic uveitis: Fuchs heterochromic cyclitis, JIA-associated uveitis, tuberculous uveitis.

TABLE 3.10: Acute iridocyclitis versus chronic iridocyclitis.

	Acute iridocyclitis	*Chronic iridocyclitis*
Onset and progression	Sudden onset with symptoms persisting for 6 weeks or less	Insidious onset, longer than 6 weeks
Symptoms	Redness, pain, diminution of vision, lacrimation, photophobia	Redness, diminution of vision, floaters
Signs	Ciliary congestion, fresh KPs/large mutton fat KPs, iris nodules, AC cells and flare, hypopyon	Stellate/old pigmented KPs, AC flare, ectropion uveae, PAS, secondary glaucoma
Pupil	Muddy iris, miosis, festooned pupil, *seclusio pupillae*	Iris atrophy, *occlusio pupillae*, iris bombe
Lens	Pigments on anerior lens capsule, posterior synechia	Total posterior synechia, complicated cataract
IOP	Initially low, then becomes raised	Low
Complications	Secondary glaucoma, pupillary block, macular edema	Band-shaped keratopathy (BSK), subluxated lens, hypotony—atrophic bulbi

Systemic Conditions that can Present as Iridocyclitis and their Ocular Manifestations (Table 3.11) *(OP 6.3)*

TABLE 3.11: Systemic conditions that can present as iridocyclitis and their ocular manifestations.

Acute anterior uveitis	Chronic anterior uveitis
• HLA-B27 positive (uveities only)	• Juvenile idiopathic arthritis (JIA)
• Ankylosing spondylitis	• Fuch's heterochromic iridocyclitis
• Reactive arthritis (Reiter's)	• Idiopathic
• Psoriatic arthropathy	• Sarcoidosis
• HLA-B27 negative (idiopathic)	• Syphilis
• Sarcoidosis	• Lupus
• Behcet's disease	• Herpes (zoster/simplex)
• Posner-Schiossmann syndrome	
• Crystaline lens-associated	
• Syphilis	
• Lupus	
• Trauma	

Ocular Manifestations of Systemic Conditions Causing Iridocyclitis *(OP 6.3)*

Juvenile Idiopathic Arthritis
- Silent (white uveitis)—painless, without photophobia and red eye.
- A/C—cells and flare along with anterior vitreous cells.
- Band-shaped keratopathy.
- Cataract.
- Glaucoma.
- Optic neuropathy and macular edema.
- Persistent hypotony from Cyclitic membrane formation may result in atrophic bulbi eventually.

Ankylosing Spondylitis
- Presentation with acute anterior uveitis (2–3%)
- HLA-B27 positivity.
- Sudden acute onset, severe iridocyclitis with fibrin in A/C.
- Pupillary membrane, pupillary block.

Reiters Syndrome
- Polyarthritis, urethritis, and conjunctivitis or uveitis,
- Non-granulomatous anterior uveitis is observed in 3–12% of patients.
- Nearly all patients with acute anterior uveitis and Reiter's syndrome are HLA-B27 positive.

Rheumatoid Arthritis
- **Corneal manifestations:** Keratoconjunctivitis sicca, filamentary keratitis, peripheral ulcerative keratitis, sclerosing keratitis, keratolysis, secondary Sjogren syndrome and dry eyes.
- **Episcleral manifestations:** Episcleritis (simple/nodular)
- **Scleral manifestations:** Anterior scleritis diffuse/nodular/necrotizing with inflammation), *scleromalacia perforans,* posterior scleritis
- **Other manifestations:** Venous stasis retinopathy, cranial nerve palsies, orbital apex syndrome, gold deposits (from treatment) in cornea and lens, HCQs related toxicity.

Behcet's Disease
- All eye structures can be affected by a non-granulomatous inflammation associated with necrotizing obliterative vasculitis.
- The classic finding is iridocyclitis with hypopyon.
- Vitreous cellular infiltration (vitritis) is always present during the acute phase.
- The classic fundus finding is necrotizing obliterative retinal vasculitis.
- Ophthalmoscopy shows Retinal edema is present in 10–20% of cases, especially in the macula.
- Severe vasculitis leads to thrombosis of vessels with secondary ischemic retinal changes.
- Bleeding from neovascularization into the vitreous cavity and subsequent fibrosis.

Sarcoidosis
- Granulomatous anterior uveitis,
- Anterior uveitis in 77–95% of cases, and a posterior uveitis in 14%.
- It also manifests acutely, and seventh-nerve palsy with other neurologic involvement, such as ophthalmoplegia is often present.

Tuberculosis
- Granulomatous anterior uveitis
- Posterior uveitis—choroidal tuberculoma
- Eales' disease with vitreous hemorrhage
- Multiple or recurrent phlyctens
- Tubercular scleral abscess
- Tubercular dacryoadenitis
- Antitubercular drug related (ethambutol) toxicity

Leprosy
- Granulomatous uveitis
- Madarosis
- Lagophthalmos
- Corneal exposure
- Interstitial keratitis
- Corneal ulceration and scarring
- Episcleritis and scleritis
- Iris pearl
- Conjunctival and scleral lepromas

Syphilis
- Both non-granulomatous and granulomatous uveitis
- Posterior uveitis
- Argyll Robertson pupil
- Keratouveitis
- Interstitial keratitis
- Cataract
- Retinal vasculitis
- Optic neuritis and optic atrophy

Hyphema and Hypopyon *(OP 6.4)*

Hyphema

Definition: Presence of blood in the anterior chamber of the eye.
Causes:
- **Blunt trauma** (most common) or open globe injury
- **During and after intraocular surgery,** e.g., cataract surgery, trabeculectomy, surgical PI, etc.
- **YAG laser peripheral iridotomy**
- **Uveitis-glaucoma-hyphema (UGH) syndrome:** Due to malpositioned IOL
- Spontaneous—as in rubeosis iridis, herpetic uveitis, intraocular neoplasm, etc.

Grading of hyphema:
Grade 0: No visible layer, but only RBCs within the A/C (micro-hyphema)
Grade I: Layered blood occupying <1/3rd of the A/C
Grade II: Blood filling 1/3rd to ½ of the A/C
Grade III: Layered blood filling ½ to < total of the A/C
Grade IV: Total filling of the A/C with blood, called total hyphema
'8' ball (black ball) hyphema: When the blood gets clotted, the hyphema appears as small blackball (like No. '8' ball in billiards game). This clotted blood causes secondary glaucoma more frequently.

Complications:
- Secondary glaucoma—due to blockage of angle by red blood cells, or breakdown products of the blood.
- Bloodstaining of the cornea.
- Secondary optic atrophy due to chronic glaucoma.
- Peripheral anterior synechia (PAS) or posterior synechia
- Rebleeding within first 5 days

Treatment:
- Complete bed rest with propped up position.
- Local corticosteroids to minimize traumatic uveitis.
- Secondary glaucoma—is treated with tablet acetazolamide and timolol (0.5%) eye drops.

Indications of anterior chamber paracentesis
- Blood does not get absorbed quickly by 5–7 days.
- Persistent high intraocular pressure (IOP) for 3–7 days depending upon the height of intraocular pressure.

- Early signs of bloodstaining of cornea.
- Limbal incision and removal of the clots may be urgently required in blackball hyphema.

Hypopyon

Definition: It is defined as milky white fluid level in the inferior part of the A/C, and usually accompanied by pain and red eye.

It occurs due to sedimentation of WBCs mixed with fibrin, secondary to inflammatory or infective process.

Causes:
- **Corneal ulcer:** It is sterile (sterile pus) in bacterial ulcer, but not sterile in fungal corneal ulcer.
- Acute severe iridocyclitis
- Endophthalmitis or panophthalmitis
- Herpetic anterior uveitis (hemorrhagic hypopyon)

Presence of hypopyon is always considered as serious sight threatening condition and needs immediate referral.

Inverse hypopyon: It is seen after a pars plana vitrectomy with silicone oil injection (in vitreoretinal surgery). With time, silicone oil emulsifies, and seeps into the anterior chamber and settles in the superior part (as it is lighter than aqueous humor, specific gravity: 0.97).

Pseudo-hypopyon: It refers to an accumulation of neoplastic cells in the anterior chamber. It is seen in, retinoblastoma, multiple myeloma, myeloblastic or acute lymphoblastic leukemia.

Angle of the Anterior Chamber and its Clinical Correlates *(OP 6.5)*

- The peripheral recess of the anterior chamber is known as the angle of the anterior chamber (also known as the "cockpit of glaucoma").
- It is bounded anteriorly by the corneo-sclera and posteriorly by the root of the iris and the ciliary body.
- At this part, in the inner layers of the sclera, there is a circular venous sinus (sometimes, broken up into more than one sinus) called the canal of Schlemm. It helps in the drainage of the aqueous. The Schlemm's canal is lined by endothelial cells.
- At extreme periphery, between the Schlemm's canal and the recess of anterior chamber—there lies a loose meshwork of tissues, known as trabecular meshwork.
- The trabecular meshwork is made up of circumferentially disposed flattened bands, and each is perforated by numerous oval openings. These tortuous openings communicate between the Schlemm's canal and the anterior chamber.

> **Circulation of Aqueous Humour**
> Aqueous is formed at the posterior chamber → via pupil into the anterior chamber → angle of anterior chamber → trabecular meshwork → canal of Schlemm → aqueous vein primarily, and also intrascleral plexus → finally drains into anterior ciliary veins.
> Some aqueous drains posteriorly into the uvea to suprachoroidal space (called **uveoscleral outflow**).

Clinical Correlations

Clinically, Van Herick slit-lamp grading system is used to estimate anterior chamber angle by comparing the depth of peripheral anterior chamber (PAC) to the peripheral corneal thickness (CT).

Grade 4: PAC >1 CT-wide open angle
Grade 3: PAC = ¼ – ½ CT—mild narrow angle
Grade 2: PAC = ¼ CT—moderately narrow angle
Grade 1: PAC < ¼ CT—extremely narrow angle

Angle of the anterior chamber is best visualized by a gonioscope. Normally, the angle is wide open, and is about 20–45°. If the angle is less than 10°, there will be every chance of developing angle-closure glaucoma.

Angle assessment is required:
- To get information both for glaucoma and non-glaucoma patient
- To diagnose glaucoma or glaucoma suspect
- To classify glaucoma: Primary open angle or angle-closure glaucoma
- To differentiate between open angle glaucoma from chronic angle closure glaucoma.

- **In case of angle-closure:** To identify subjects with 'occludable angle'
- To identify findings in other types of glaucoma—abnormal iris insertion, plateau iris syndrome, presence of goinio-synechia, pigmentation of trabecular meshwork, blood in Schlemm's canal, angle recession, angle neovascularization, evidence of anterior segment dysgenesis, etc.
- To see the patency of the ostium in trabeculectomy
- To treat the patients with minimally invasive glaucoma surgery (MIGS)

Common Clinical Conditions Affecting the Anterior Chamber (OP 6.6)

See page 15

GLAUCOMA (OP 6.7)

Definition: Glaucoma is a symptomatic condition of the eye, where the functional integrity of the eye is disturbed resulting in irreversible loss of visual field usually due to raised intraocular pressure.

Normal IOP

- **Schiotz:** 14 to 20 mm of Hg.
- **Applanation:** 16 mm ± 5 mm of Hg.

Classification of Glaucoma

A. **Congenital or developmental:**
- **Primary:** Due to primary developmental anomaly of the angle
- **Secondary:** Associated with ocular or systemic disorders

B. **Acquired:**
- **Primary:** Open angle glaucoma (POAG) and angle closure glaucoma (PACG)
- **Secondary:** Due to specific anomaly or eye disease, e.g., lens-induced glaucoma, glaucoma due to total hyphema, posterior synechiae, etc.

Buphthalmos

Definition: It is congenital or infantile glaucoma due to simple outflow obstruction as a result of failure in the development of tissues in the region of the angle of anterior chamber. It is generally bilateral and occurs more often in boys than in girls. It is mostly genetically transmitted.

Symptoms: Mother usually complains that the child is suffering from—watering, marked photophobia and blepharospasm. The child is irritable.

Signs:
- Eyeball gets enlarged, if the IOP is raised prior to 3-years of age. This enlargement looks like an ox eye, i.e., *buphthalmos*.
- Bluish sclera.
- Circumcorneal ciliary congestion.
- Cornea is enlarged, globular and steamy. Horizontal lines *(Haab's striae)* are seen due to rupture of Descemet's membrane. Corneal sensation is diminished.
- Deep anterior chamber.
- Tremulousness of the iris with patches of iris atrophy.
- Lens is flattened and displaced backwards, there may be subluxation.
- IOP is raised, but not marked.
- *Fundus*—cupping of the optic disc which may regress with treatment.

The patient is myopic (*but the amount of myopia is less than anticipated from axial length, owing to the flattening of the lens and its displacement backwards*).

Treatment:
- **Examination under anesthesia (EUA):** To check corneal diameter, anterior segment findings, IOP measurement and disc evaluation.
- **Timolol maleate (0.25%):** Twice daily, may be tried only for temporary period prior to surgery.
- **Surgical treatment:**
  - Trabeculotomy (goniotomy *ab-externo*, *gonio* means angle).
  - Goniotomy *(ab-interno)*.
  - Gonio-puncture.
  - Trabeculotomy with trabeculectomy may be more helpful.
- Penetrating keratoplasty may require if the cornea remains hazy.
- **Visual rehabilitation:** Amblyopia therapy is required after the surgery.

Primary Open-angle Glaucoma (POAG)

Mechanism: The increased intraocular pressure (IOP) is due to interference of aqueous outflow even though the angle is open.

Symptoms: POAG is usually asymptomatic (very silent disease) until it has caused a gross visual field loss. However, the patient may present with:
- Painless, progressive diminution of vision.
- Difficulty in near work and with frequent change of presbyopic glasses.

Signs: *Visual acuity may remain good till the late stage of POAG.*
- Cornea clear with normal anterior chamber depth
- Raised intraocular pressure (IOP)
- Cupping of the optic disc
- Gonioscopically, the angle of the anterior chamber is open.

The *classical triad* of POAG:
1. Raised intraocular pressure
2. Cupping of the optic disc
3. Field defects

Field defects in POAG: The field defects in POAG usually run parallel to the changes in the optic disc and nerve fiber bundles defect (NFBD). Central field is more important than peripheral field in early stage.

The defects are:
- One or more isolated small scotomatous area,
- A sickle-shaped defect extends from the blind spot above or below, or both—**Seidel's scotoma**.
- A larger area from blind spot in the form of an arc—**Bjerrum's scotoma**. This arcuate scotoma may pass above or below the fixation point and sometimes join to form an **annular scotoma**.
- Upper or sometimes, the lower nasal field tends to show sectorial defects which have a sharp horizontal edge—**Roenne's nasal step**.
- **In later stage:** Generalized constriction of peripheral field.
- Lastly, only a paracentral patch of temporal field persists, central vision being abolished.

Investigations of POAG:
- Gonioscopy
- Applanation tonometry
- Automated perimetry (Humphrey's, octopus, etc.).
- OCT of optic nerve head to study retinal nerve fiber layer (RNFL)

Treatment:
(1) Medical, (2) Surgical, (3) Laser, and (4) Combination therapy.

1. **Medical** (*see* also page 78)—*Topical preparations:* It may be given alone or in combination of two or three antiglaucoma medicines.
    - Timolol maleate (0.25% or 0.5%)—1 drop twice daily; Or betaxolol (0.5%) eye drop, a cardioselective, β-blocker—1 drop twice daily.
    - Brimonidine (0.2%) eye drop—twice daily.
    - Dorzolamide or brinzolamide eye drop (2%)—thrice daily.
    - Latanoprost (0.005%) eye drop or alternately, bimatoprost (0.03%) or travoprost (0.004%) eye drop—once daily at 9 PM.
    - Pilocarpine drop (2%)—1 drop 3 times daily.
2. **Surgical:** If medical treatment fails or there is non-compliance of the patient. Ideal choice is *trabeculectomy operation.*
3. **Laser:** One can also try *argon laser trabeculoplasty (ALT)*—a noninvasive OPD procedure, often helpful in early stage of the disease.
4. **Combined:** When surgery alone is not helpful, a drug may be added to control IOP effectively.

Normal tension glaucoma (NTG) or low-tension glaucoma (LTG): Few patients of POAG, develops characteristic field defects and cupping of the disc in spite of normal intraocular tension.

This type of POAG may be associated with cardiovascular abnormality (responsible for reduced optic nerve head perfusion).

Ocular hypertension: Patient is having bilateral high intraocular tension (i.e., above 21 mm of Hg) without any field defect and cupping of the disc.

These patients should be kept under observation as some of them may develop frank POAG in future.

Primary Angle-Closure Glaucoma (PACG)

PACG is an acute, subacute or chronic glaucoma due to obstruction of aqueous outflow, solely caused by closure of the angle by peripheral iris.

Etiological Factors

Age: 4th or 5th decade.
Sex: More common in female (4 times)

Type of eye predisposed for PACG:
- Small hypermetropic eye.
- Shallow anterior chamber.
- Narrow anterior chamber angle.
- Bigger size of the lens.
- Smaller cornea.

Laterality: Initially unilateral, later bilateral.
Personality: Emotional, nervous and anxious people

Mechanism of Angle Closure

- Pupillary block in mid-dilated position (in darkness or use of mydriatics).
- Forward ballooning of the peripheral iris resembling an 'iris bombe'.
- Crowding of iris root at the angle leading to peripheral anterior synechiae.
- Ultimately, it cuts off filtration channels of aqueous at the angle, leading to a sharp rise in IOP.

Stages of Angle Closure Glaucoma

It is divided into *four stages*:
1. Prodromal stage—characteristic symptom is coloured halos due to intermittent corneal edema
2. Acute congestive attack
3. Chronic congestive glaucoma
4. Stage of absolute glaucoma.

Colored halos: Colored halos are due to accumulation of fluid in the cornea. They are seen around the naked bulbs. The colors are distributed as in the spectrum of rainbow with red being the outermost and violet innermost. Similar colored halos may be seen in early cataract. Can be differentiated by *Fincham's stenopaeic slit test*. Here a stenopaeic slit is passed before the eye across the line of vision. As it passes, a glaucomatous halo remains intact but diminished in intensity, whereas a lenticular halo is broken up into segments which revolve as the slit is moved.

Clinical Picture of Angle-Closure Glaucoma in Acute Attack

Symptoms
- Acute intense pain radiating along the distribution of 5th cranial nerve.
- Headache with nausea and vomiting, often mistaken as acute abdomen.
- Marked dimness of vision.
- Redness, lacrimation, and sometimes photophobia.

Signs
- Vision reduced to hand movement to 'PL and PR'.
- Edema of the eyelids with narrowing of palpebral fissure.
- Tenderness of the globe.
- Both ciliary and conjunctival congestion with chemosis.
- Hazy, cloudy and insensitive cornea.
- Anterior chamber is very shallow.
- Pupil is moderately dilated and vertically oval. Reactions are absent.
- Iris pattern is lost and discolored. Iris bombe may present.
- *'Glaukomflecken'*—a type of anterior subcapsular cataract like 'spilled milk' caused due to ischemia of anterior lens capsule.
- Intraocular pressure is markedly raised.

- **Fundus:** Cannot be visualized due to corneal edema. But after instillation of glycerin drop (it clears the cornea temporarily), fundus may be visible with congested optic disc, small hemorrhages and spontaneous pulsation of retinal artery. But, there is no cupping.
- The fellow eye usually has a shallow anterior chamber and a narrow angle.

Termination of an Acute Attack
- Spontaneous improvement, due to lowering of tension.
- Recurrence of acute attacks—with marked loss of vision, permanent peripheral anterior synechia, irregular constriction of visual fields.
  Ultimately, all lead into chronic congestive stage.
- It may directly pass into chronic congestive stage.
- Rarely, may pass into absolute glaucoma with No PL vision.

Treatment of an acute attack: *It is an ocular emergency.*
- Press over the cornea with a sterile cotton bud or with gonioscope to open the pupillary block element.
- Tablet acetazolamide (Diamox 250 mg) 2 tablets stat and then 1 tablet 4 times daily along with potassium supplement.
- Injection mannitol (20%)—by IV infusion stat.
- Oral glycerol (50%)—1 oz (30 mL) of pure glycerol with equal amount of lemon juice stat, and then 3 times daily.
- Once the IOP reduces, then pilocarpine (2%) eye drop is instilled every 5 minutes till the pupil gets constricted. After that 3–4 times daily.
- Steroid-antibiotic eye drop to reduce congestions

After intensive medical treatment, the IOP may reduce to normal, or it may remain same.
- If eye becomes quiet with normal IOP, YAG laser peripheral iridotomy or surgical peripheral iridectomy is done on urgent basis.
- **If IOP remains same (i.e., medical treatment fails):** Trabeculectomy operation is to be considered.

  The second eye (i.e., fellow eye) is to be treated by laser peripheral iridotomy or surgical peripheral iridectomy (PI) as soon as possible.

Absolute Glaucoma

Definition

Absolute glaucoma is the end stage of any glaucoma whether congenital or acquired, primary or secondary, and is characterized by extremely high IOP with no perception of light.

Features
- **Vision:** Painful blind eye with no PL.
- **Conjunctiva:** Reddish-blue zone around the limbus, due to dilated anterior ciliary veins.
- **Cornea:** Edematous and insensitive. There may be bullous keratopathy.
- **Iris:** Patch of atrophy, neovascularization.
- **Pupil:** Dilated and grayish in appearance. No light reaction.
- **Optic disc:** Total and deep cupping with atrophy.
- **Tension:** Extremely high (stony hard).

Ultimately the sequalae may be:
- Scleral thinning → Staphyloma formation.
- Atrophic bulbi, due to atrophy of the ciliary body. There is decreased in aqueous production and shrinkage of the eyeball.
- Increased danger of scleral rupture

Treatment
- **Cyclo-cryotherapy:** A cryo-destructive procedure of ciliary processes, which reduces aqueous secretion and thereby reduction in lOP.
- **Cyclo-photocoagulation:** Another destructive procedure with laser.
- **Retrobulbar injection of alcohol (70%):** This is to destroy the ciliary ganglion.
- **Enucleation:** If the pain is still unbearable, and it is the last choice.

Secondary Glaucoma

Many of these may involve more than one mechanism of aqueous outflow obstruction for developing rise in IOP.

The Important Causes

- **Steroid induced glaucoma:** More with drops, prednisolone and dexamethasone are more important; least with loteprednol.
- **Lens-induced glaucomas:** Phacolytic glaucoma, phacomorphic glaucoma, lens particle glaucoma, with ectopia lentis (lens subluxation), etc.
- **Pseudoexfoliation glaucoma**
- **Pigmentary glaucoma**
- **Neovascular glaucoma:** With CRVO, diabetes, sickle cell retinopathy
- **Inflammatory glaucoma:** With iridocyclitis
- **Pupillary block glaucoma:** When air is kept in anterior chamber at the end of surgery, as in ICCE, endothelial keratoplasty, etc.
- **Traumatic glaucoma:** Due to hyphema or angle—recession
- **Glaucoma with intraocular tumors:** As in retinoblastoma
- **Malignant glaucoma:** Due to aqueous misdirection

INVESTIGATIONS OF A PATIENT WITH UVEITIS *(OP 6.8)*

Investigations in uveitis should be planned in a systematic tailored approach for each patient. Tests are ordered only if there is a strong clinical suspicion of a specific disease.

Proper investigations should start with:
- Detailed history taking (ocular and systemic)
- Complete ocular examination
- General physical examination
- Referral to medical specialists (for further evaluation)

General Investigations

- Complete blood count—CBC, ESR and C reactive protein
- Blood sugar and urine analysis (diabetes mellitus)
- Kidney and liver function tests if the patient need immunosuppressive drug or AT drugs.

Specific Investigations

I. Infectious Uveitis

A. **Bacterial diseases:**
- **Tuberculosis:** Chest X-Ray, Mantoux test, acid-fast stain of ocular fluid, quantiferon TB gold test
- **Syphilis:** VDRL, and FTA-ABS (fluorescent treponemal antibody absorption test)
- **Leptospirosis:** Microagglutination test, ELISA for leptospira antigens
- **Lyme disease:** *Borrelia burgdorferi* by ELISA and Western blot
- **Postsurgical/traumatic/endogenous endophthalmitis:** Gram's stain and cultures of aqueous and vitreous.

B. **Parasitic diseases:**
- **Toxoplasmosis:** ELISA for toxoplasmosis; skull X-ray for calcification.
- **Toxocariasis:** ELISA for serum anti-*Toxocara canis* IgG and IgM

C. **Viral diseases:**
- **Human immunodeficiency virus (HIV):** Western blot, ELISA, Tridot
- **HSV; herpes zoster virus and CMV;** aqueous and vitreous fluid for PCR (polymerase chain reaction),

II. Non-infectious Uveitis

- **Juvenile idiopathic arthritis (JIA):** ESR, ANA, X-ray
- **HLA-B27 related anterior uveitis:** HLA-B27 typing; X-ray sacroiliac joints
- **Sarcoidosis:** Angiotensin-converting enzyme; lysozyme, serum or urine calcium, chest radiography, gallium scan, biopsy for noncaseating granulomas, pulmonary function test, etc.

III. Collagen Vascular Diseases

- **Rheumatoid arthritis:** Anti-cyclic citrullinated peptide (anti-CCP); ANA (antinuclear antibody); CRP; ESR; rheumatoid factor; X ray of hand, wrist or knee joints

- ❖ **Systemic lupus erythematosus (SLE):** CBC (complete blood count); ANA; dsDNA; ssDNA (double- and single-stranded deoxyribonucleic acid)
- ❖ Progressive systemic sclerosis Hb; urinalysis for red blood cells; pulmonary function tests—restrictive lung disease; chest X-ray—fibrotic changes; elevated ESR and hypergammaglobulinemia
- ❖ **Relapsing polychondritis:** Biopsy showing granulomatous chondritis
- ❖ **Wegener's granulomatosis:** Chest radiography, sinus X-ray, cANCA (antinuclear cytoplasmic antibodies), urinalysis, tissue biopsy
- ❖ **Polyarteritis nodosa (PAN) group:** Serum eosinophils, pANCA, angiography; ESR

IV. Others

- ❖ **Behcet's syndrome:** Fundus fluorescein angiography (FFA); HLA-B51 and B52; FFA
- ❖ **Vogt-Koyanagi-Harada syndrome:** USG, (ultrasonogram); FFA
- ❖ **Sympathetic ophthalmia:** USG B scan; FFA; enucleation of the blind eye and histopathology
- ❖ **Retinochoroidal vasculitis:** ESR, VDRL/FTA-ABS, sarcoidosis tests, vitreous biopsy for lymphoma, viral PCR, toxoplasma and tuberculosis work up.

Antiglaucoma Medications *(OP 6.9)*

See page 78

Counsel a Patient with Anterior Uveitis *(OP 6.10)*

- ❖ Uvea is the middle layer among the three layers of eye ball.
- ❖ Inflammation of uvea is called uveitis.
- ❖ Uveitis is a disease of long duration and can be recurrent.
- ❖ The patient should be informed about the serious nature of anterior uveitis.
- ❖ Most cases of anterior uveitis respond favourably to early diagnosis and treatment.
- ❖ Some investigations are required time to time for early diagnosis

- ❖ Steroids (systemic, topical or local injection) are main mode of treatment; and sometimes, immunosuppressive drugs are required.
- ❖ Immunosuppressive drugs are very powerful and potent drugs. Dosage should be strictly followed.
- ❖ Patient should be informed about the possible side effects of side effects of long-term corticosteroid use (i.e., glaucoma and posterior subcapsular cataract) and immunosuppressants have some serious side effects on liver and kidney functions.
- ❖ Compliance with the therapeutic regimen and keeping all follow-up appointments are essential to achieve the therapeutic goals.
- ❖ It is important to keep well-documented medical record, and the patient should be reminded periodically throughout the course of treatment.
- ❖ Anterior uveitis may recur, especially when there is a systemic etiology. Therefore, both the clinician and patient must be alert for signs of recurrence and restart the therapy promptly.
- ❖ Patient should receive "strict report precautions" with alarming symptoms, such as—worsening pain, redness, photophobia. Blurring of vision, and floaters.

Counsel a Patient with Glaucoma *(OP 6.10)*

- ❖ Glaucoma is a disease that indicates—changes in optic nerve head and visual field changes associated with normal or increased eye pressure.
- ❖ Primary glaucoma based on the anatomy of the anterior chamber angle, is further divided into open angle and angle closure forms.
- ❖ Secondary glaucoma can be due to associated uveitis, disorders of lens, trauma, etc.

Open Angle Glaucoma

- ❖ Explains the nature of the disease—symptomless silent nature of disease with slow visual loss and field loss.

- Loss of vision or visual field in glaucoma cannot be recovered. It is permanent.
- This type of glaucoma are familial and hence close relatives are to be screened for the same.
- Eye drops are the first line of treatment that should be continued lifelong.
- Some eyedrops have side effects and at time they are serious.
- The importance of regular follow-up and use of medication to be explained to the patient seriously.
- Medicines only slow down the progress of the disease.
- The disease may progress despite regular use of medications. Change of medicine or addition of medicines are required.
- Surgery may be required at some point of the disease (when medical treatment fail) and has to be decided by the treating doctor.

Angle-closure Glaucoma

- Talk to a patient about pain, in certain angle-closure glaucoma suspect patient.
- Alert about rainbow halos around a naked light bulb.
- The condition is treatable and need to confirm the diagnosis by gonioscopy.
- Eye drop may be given temporarily to relieve their symptoms.
- Patient must be explained that the condition is recurrent, and preventive measures like a laser PI procedure has to be done in both eyes to stop future attacks.
- Surgery may have to be done at a later stage and will be decided by the doctor.

Congenital Glaucoma

- Parents should understand that their child is suffering from a serious eye condition that is present since birth or developing early in life.
- The child may require surgery under GA even when he/she is very young (weeks or months).
- Parents are made to realize that despite surgery and eye drops—the child may have poor vision, but that the treatment is essential to prevent further damage.
- Need for repeated follow up and long-term treatment, needs to be emphasized to the parents.
- Every time the child needs general anesthesia for proper evaluation of the eye condition

CRYSTALLINE LENS AND CATARACT *(OP 7)*

Surgical Anatomy of Crystalline Lens (Cataract) *(OP 7.1)*

- Lens is a transparent bi-convex body of crystalline structure.
- Diameter: 9–10 mm and thickness: 4–4.5 mm
- Lens is held in its position by suspensory ligament, called *zonules of Zinn*. They arise from the sides of the ciliary processes, and the valleys between them.
- The zonular fibers insert into the anterior and the posterior lens capsule near the equator and extend further over the anterior surface more than the posterior surface.

Surgically, the lens is divided into four zones:
1. Capsule and capsular bag
2. Superficial cortex
3. Epinucleus
4. Hard nucleus.

- **Capsule:** It completely envelops the lens, and the cells of origin are completely contained in it. The thickness at the posterior pole is 2.8–4 µm and at anterior pole is 15.5 µm.
  In cataract surgery: An opening (capsulorrhexis) is made in the anterior capsule of the lens as a first step. At the end of the procedure—*capsular bag* is created for 'in-the-bag' PC IOL implantation.
- **Cortex:** Is a soft, thin layer present immediately beneath the capsule and envelopes the epinucleus. It is aspirated out of the capsular bag with ease.
- **Epinucleus:** Is a layer of semi-soft lens matter around the nucleus. It can

be aspirated better by a phaco-probe ("epinucleus mode") during phacoemulsification.
- ❖ **Nucleus:** Is the hard lens substance forming the greatest portion of the lens substance. The hardness varies with the grading of nuclear cataract. The cataractous lens nucleus is fragmented in multiple pieces and then emulsified before aspiration. *Preoperative nucleus grading (after dilatation) gives us valuable input towards the surgical plan.*
- ❖ **Zonules:** Zonular attachments and morphology are also important for surgical planning, e.g., subluxation or dislocation of the lens, overall zonular weakness in myopic eye, and pseudoexfoliation; zonular dehiscence during surgery, etc.

Metabolism of Crystalline Lens *(OP 7.1)*

The lens fibers are composed entirely of soluble and insoluble proteins.

Water-soluble proteins (85%): Are α-crystalline, β-heavy and β-light crystalline, and γ-crystalline; and they are found mainly in the lens cortex.

Water-insoluble protein (15%): Albuminoid fraction and found mainly in the lens nucleus. With age insoluble protein increases.

The lens epithelium generates energy from carbohydrate metabolism:
- ❖ Anerobic glycolysis by Embden-Meyerhof pathway—85%
- ❖ Hexose-monophosphate shunt
- ❖ Kreb's cycle
- ❖ Sorbitol pathway

The lens epithelium maintains low concentration of sodium and water within the lens by active Na-K-ATPase pump system.

Pump mechanism of the lens-fiber membranes, maintain relative dehydration of the lens.

Glycolysis provides the necessary ATP energy.

Auto-oxidation: High concentration of reduced glutathione in the lens, maintains the lens protein in a reduced state and ensures the integrity of the cell-membrane pump.

Transparency of Crystalline Lens

It transmits almost 80% of light energy. Its transparency is due to:
- ❖ Sparsity of cells
- ❖ Single layer of epithelial cells, which is not thick.
- ❖ Close alignment of individual cells (the lens extracellular space is less than 5% of its total volume, so the zone of discontinuity is very small compared to the wavelength of light).
- ❖ Semipermeable character of the lens capsule.
- ❖ Avascularity
- ❖ It's index of refraction ranges from about 1.406 at the center (nucleus) to about 1.386 in outer cortical layers, making it a gradient index lens.

ETIOPATHOGENESIS, STAGE OF MATURATION AND COMPLICATIONS OF CATARACT *(OP 7.2)*

Etiopathogenesis of Cataract (Table 3.12)

Age related is the most common type and the pathogenesis is multifactorial and not fully understood. It includes the following factors:
- ❖ Compactness and stiffening of central lens substance (nuclear sclerosis) as new layers of outer cortical fibers continue to proliferate with age
- ❖ Structural and chemical changes in lens proteins (crystallins) resulting in loss of transparency
- ❖ Pigmentation of lens proteins (yellow to brown)
- ❖ Changes in the ionic components of the lens fibers

Stage of Maturation of Cataract

"Maturity" terminology is only for the senile cortical cataract.

Senile Cortical Cataract

- ❖ **Stage of lamellar separation:** Only appreciated by slit lamp examination

TABLE 3.12: Etiopathogenesis of cataract.

Cataract type	Causes	Vulnerable people
Senile	Aging, systemic disease, oxidative stress, smoking, lack of essential dietary factors	Elderly person above 50 years of age
Congenital or developmental	Hereditary, maternal—malnutrition, infection, drugs; fetal hypoxia, birth trauma, idopathic	
Traumatic	Blunt trauma, open globe injury, foreign body, damage to the capsule	People working in factory, glass furnace, sport injuries
Complicated	Complications of some chronic inflammatory or degenerative eye diseases	Patients with skin diseases, allergy, uveitis, asthma, etc.
Metabolic	Diabetes mellitus, galactosemia, myotonic dystrophy, etc.	Patient deficient with some hormones or enzymes
Toxic	Some drugs or toxins, e.g., steroids	Patient on steroid therapy or toxic drugs
Electrical or radiational	Infrared rays, UV rays, powerful electric current	Patients with exposure to UV rays, excessive sunlight, radiation, high-voltage current

- **Stage of incipient cataract:** Few flakes of grayish white opacity from periphery towards center in a spoke-like or saucer-shaped pattern of the posterior capsule (posterior subcapsular cataract)
- **Stage of immature senile cataract (ISC):** Further progresses bit with some clear cortex
- **Stage of mature senile cataract (MSC):** Complete opacification and whole cortex is involved
- **Stage of hypermature senile cataract (HMSC):**
  - *Morgagnian type:* Liquefaction of cortical contents with bag of milky fluid. Brownish nucleus sinks at the bottom.
  - *Sclerotic type:* Cortex becomes integrated, and nucleus shrunken.

Senile Nuclear Cataract

Advancement (maturity) depends on color of nucleus and hardness.
Nuclear sclerosis 1: Gray appearance nucleus—**softer**
Nuclear sclerosis 2: Yellowish nucleus—**soft**
Nuclear sclerosis 3: Amber color nucleus—**medium**
Nuclear sclerosis 4: Brown nucleus (*cataracta brunescens*)—**hard**
Nuclear sclerosis 5: Black nucleus (*cataracta nigra*)—**suprahard**

Lens Opacities Classification System III (LOCS III)

- The most popular grading/staging system of cataract.
- LOCS III uses a reference set of standard photographs that defines the extent of opacities in cortical and subcapsular zones and the color/grade of the nuclear opacity.
- Using LOCS III, the cataract can be classified as: Nuclear color/opalescence = NC/NO: 1-6, cortical opacities = C: 1–5 and posterior subcapsular opacities = P: 1–5.

Complications of Cataract

- Cataracts can become "hypermature" which may cause:
  - Phacolytic glaucoma
  - Phacomorphic glaucoma
  - Phacogenic/phacoanaphylactic uveitis
  - Subluxation, or even dislocation of cataractous lens
  - If neglected more—can lead to optic atrophy and permanent blindness
- Cataracts left untreated can impair vision so much that accidental other injuries (e.g., patient may fall with hip or femur

fracture, or head injury; car accidents, etc.) can occur.
- Nucleus becomes so dense/hard that surgical removal becomes risky and consequently more complications
- **In congenital or developmental cataract**—unilateral or bilateral amblyopia if not treated earlier within first year of life.

Technique of Ocular Examination in a Patient with Cataract *(OP 7.3)*

See page 22–24

Types of Cataract Surgery: Steps, Intra- and Postoperative Complications of Extracapsular Cataract Extraction Surgery *(OP 7.4)*

See page 177–181

Participate in the Team for Cataract Surgery *(OP 7.5)*

- The purpose of a team is to work together towards a common goal.
- Surgical team must ensure that an informed patient, who is relaxed and mentally prepared for the cataract surgery and back home again.
- **The student must participate at all levels.**

Preoperative

- Diagnosis and possible type of cataract surgery.
- To observe—cataract surgery so that they can inform patients about the procedure and about the hospital policy
- To counsel the patient about cataract surgery
- To check all reports and investigations including biometry
- Help for medical reimbursement or cashless medicare policy

Just Before Surgery

- **To check about systemic conditions of the patient:** BP, blood sugar, ECG report or any other significant comorbidity, e.g., deafness, parkinsonism, asthma, cardiac problem, allergy, etc.
- **Help to check patient preparation:**
  - Confirm the eye to be operated and mark it
  - Pupillary dilatation
  - Confirm about cataract surgery under LA or topical anesthesia
  - Checking biometry and confirm IOL selection

After Operation on Day of Surgery

- Check for operated eye condition
- Check for the vitals before discharge
- Explain about postoperative medications in the discharge paper
- Explain about Dos and Don'ts in the postoperative period
- Help to get medical certificate for medical leave

Follow-up Visit

- A cataract patient must come back to the hospital/community for follow-up visits, including detection of complications and referral back to the surgi-center if needed.
- Informing patients about postoperative complications—what to look out for and what they should do (including where they should report)

Final Visit for Refraction

- The patient's journey is completed only when the patient has been followed up for final refraction, and is satisfied with the outcome.
- A system for recording patient satisfaction, taking any needed action, and giving feedback to staff.

Informed Consent for Cataract Surgery *(OP 7.6)*

Before cataract surgery, we must use an informed consent process:
- To educate our patients
- Explain to them the likely outcome of the surgery
- Describe potential risks

- Help them make an appropriate decision.

It helps a patient understand the risks, alternatives, benefits, and indications for cataract surgery.

It involves several aspects such as:
- The discussion with the patient
- The explanation of the procedure
- The signing of a written consent form.

From the patient's perspective, there may be some fear or anxiety factors, e.g., will cataract surgery painful? Will it be under injection? What if I blink during surgery? What if I move during surgery? Need to change the lens implant? Will there be stitches placed in the eye? Will I be able to see right away? What are the risks? How long an IOL last? Will I still need spectacles after surgery? And so on...

Concurrent Ocular Conditions and Comorbidities

Patients must understand that pre-existing ocular conditions may limit their vision and cataract surgery may only partially address their visual needs.

Cataract surgery can correct pre-existing corneal astigmatism and that is to be addressed. But other *comorbidities* are typically not correctable simply by performing cataract surgery.

Glaucoma, retinal disease, such as diabetic retinopathy or AMD, will limit the post-operative visual outcomes from cataract surgery and some retinal conditions may even worsen after cataract surgery.

Patients should be explained—even in otherwise normal eye, a man-made IOL will not have the same optical performance as a natural crystalline lens.

Some patients may have *additional comorbidities that increase the risks of cataract surgery* and these, too, should be explained to the patient:
- Patient with pseudoexfoliation may be prone for zonular dehiscence during surgery which could result in IOL decentration or
- A posterior polar cataract may be complicated by posterior capsule rent and requiring anterior vitrectomy and a multi-piece IOL.
- Patient with prior refractive surgery has a higher risk of wrong IOL power calculation.
- Patient with Fuchs' endothelial dystrophy is at a higher risk for corneal decompensation following cataract surgery.

Audiovisual recording during consent process is becoming popular in recent times—because of medicolegal reasons.

Preoperative Counseling of Cataract Patient *(OP 7.6)*

- Preoperative counseling a prospective patient both for risks and benefits is important for medicolegal, moral, and ethical reasons.
- It respects patient's autonomy and right to make decisions regarding treatment plan.
- However, surgeon is also expected to provide guidance and expert advice on: benefits of surgery versus risks.
- Proper preoperative counseling helps to prepare patients for surgery and increase their satisfaction with the entire process.

Topics Covered During Counseling

Certain essential information must be provided to the cataract patient prior to surgery on individual basis. Patients should know about:
- Preoperative assessment and IOL selection
- Type of anesthesia
- Intraoperative procedures
- Postoperative recovery

Preoperative assessment: Biometric assessment and IOL selection, macular function tests, systemic examination to determine anesthetic risk, and expectations on the day of surgery.

IOL options and selection: With the ever-increasing range of available IOLs, the choice of lenses—monofocal, trifocal, multifocal, aspheric, and toric—should be discussed with the patient.

The surgeon must guide the patient so as to what type of IOL will be most suitable for the individual. A thorough discussion of the patient's lifestyle and priorities are essential before the doctor and patient can jointly reach a decision on whether a given IOL is suitable. The option of astigmatic correction with toric IOLs or limbal relaxing incisions should also be covered.

Surgical procedure: Major steps of cataract surgery should be explained, preferably with the aid of short video-film or animations. Choice of anesthesia (topical or injectable) and use of intraoperative sedation to be discussed with the patient.

Complications: There are many possible intra-operative and postoperative complications, which are usually listed on an informational sheet available to the patient prior to surgery. However, the surgeon should give emphasis on some risk factors, such as posterior polar cataract, suprahard cataract, high myopia or hypermetropia, compromised cornea as in Fuchs' dystrophy, etc., and discuss about possible problems on those.

Postoperative care: Patient should be informed about the follow-up visits and duration of postoperative restrictions, visual recovery time, and need for postoperative eye drops.

Allow the patient to ask question: Finally, a patient should have the opportunity to ask questions and clarify with the surgeon in case of any doubt. Some anxious patient requires 'extra' counseling by the team—surgeon, anesthetist, nurse, trained counsellor to reduce the fear factors during surgery.

RETINA AND OPTIC NERVE (OP 8)

Retinal Vascular Occlusions (OP 8.1)

There are **two types** of retinal vascular occlusion. The type depends on which blood vessel is affected:
1. **Retinal artery occlusion:**
   - Central retinal artery occlusion (CRAO)
   - Branch retinal artery occlusion (BRAO)
2. **Retinal vein occlusion:**
   - Central retinal vein occlusion (CRVO)
   - Branch retinal vein occlusion (BRVO)

Etiology
- Above 60 years of age
- Atherosclerosis of the arteries
- Embolism from elsewhere to the eye: Hollenhorst plaques (cholesterol emboli) often responsible, calcium and platelet-fibrin emboli
- Blockage or narrowing of carotid arteries
- Heart problems, arrhythmia or valve issues
- Diabetes, high blood pressure
- Hyperlipidemia
- Coagulopathies
- Obesity, pregnancy, oral contraceptives
- Intravenous (IV) drug abuse
- Open angle glaucoma
- Smoking
- Inflammatory disorders, e.g., giant cell arteritis

Pathology
- Retinal vascular lumen is obstructed by an embolus, thrombus or inflammatory/traumatic vessel wall damage or spasm. Giant cell arteritis may be associated with this condition.
- **Occlusion of the retinal arteries** results in ischemia of the inner retina. When the inner retina is damaged, it is very edematous. Over time, the edema resolves and the inner retina atrophies. Thus, the vision loss is often permanent, may be with only mild visual recovery.
- **In branch retinal artery** occlusion, only part of the retina is involved. The area affected by the occluded vessels is associated with the area and degree of visual loss.
- **The pathogenesis of CRVO:** Follows the principle of Virchow's triad for thrombogenesis—involving endothelial damage, venous stasis and hypercoagulability. Central retinal vein and artery share a common sheath at a crossing posterior to the lamina cribrosa and atherosclerotic changes of the artery compress the vein, and precipitate CRVO. So, the pathogenesis of CRVO is critically related to the changes in central retinal artery.

- RVO is essentially an obstruction of venous circulation that drains blood from the retina. With blockage, pressure builds up within capillaries, leading to hemorrhage and leakage of fluid. This leads to macular edema if the leakage is near the macula.
- Macular ischemia occurs with nonperfusion of these capillaries and without oxygen supply. Neovascularization (abnormal new blood vessels) then occurs, which can lead to neovascular glaucoma, vitreous hemorrhage, and in late cases, tractional retinal detachment.

Clinical Features

Retinal Artery Occlusion

Symptom: Painless, unilateral sudden loss of vision.
Signs: Vison is only PL to no PL; RAPD,
Fundus: Larger arteries are thread-like, and the smaller arterioles are invisible. A **cherry red spot** at the fovea appears within few hours and seen against cloudy-white retinal edema. In branch retinal artery occlusion: cattle-tract or box cart appearance, cloudy white edematous retina corresponding to the area of ischemia. An atheromatous embolus may be visible as a pale refractile body within the artery (Hollenhorst plaque),

Retinal Venous Occlusion

Symptoms: Painless moderate to severe visual loss.
Signs: May be with RAPD, ophthalmoscopically, mild tortuosity and dilatation of all branches of the central retinal vein; dot and blot; and flame-shaped hemorrhages are seen throughout the fundus. Cotton-wool exudates may be present. Mild to moderate swelling of the optic disc. Macular edema may or may not be present. The appearance is sometimes called **'blood and thunder'** fundus.

Management

For CRAO: Urgent management in OPD: Adoption of a supine posture, ocular massage, anterior chamber paracentesis, sublingual isosorbide dinitrate to induce vasodilation, 'rebreathing' into a paper bag or breathing 'CARBOGEN',
Short admission: Hyperosmotic agents—mannitol or glycerol or intravenous acetazolamide 500 mg to achieve sustained lowering of intraocular pressure.
Transluminal Nd:YAG laser lysis of the embolus.

Further management of retinal artery occlusions involves a multidisciplinary approach including neurologists with stroke expertise.

Treatment of retinal vein occlusions is provided by ophthalmologists:
- General systemic investigations to find out the cause
- Fundus fluorescein angiography (FFA)
- Treatment of macular edema—by NSAID drops and anti-VGEF injections
- Laser photocoagulation—panretinal or scatter photocoagulation for CRAO and sectorial or focal laser for BRVO
- Treatment of neovascularization
- Follow-up care for prevention of neovascular glaucoma

INDICATIONS OF LASER THERAPY IN RETINAL DISEASES (OP 8.2)

Since the introduction of intravitreal injections (anti-VGEFs or triamcinolone), role of laser therapy is reduced in treatment of some retinal diseases. However, retinal laser therapy is still considered a standard of care in the management of a number of retinal diseases.

Indications for Retinal Lasers

- **Diabetic retinopathy:**
  - *Proliferative diabetic retinopathy (PDR):* Treatment of PDR remains the most common indication for laser photocoagulation till today. Panretinal photocoagulation (PRP) reduces the hypoxic load and promotes inner retinal oxygenation.
  - *Diabetic macular edema (DME):* In addition to anti-VEGF injection, focal retinal laser is useful for treatment of

extrafoveal edema. Focal laser requires for leaking microaneurysms or grid laser for areas of diffuse leakage on the retina.

- **Retinal vascular occlusions:**
  - Grid laser is effective in macular edema secondary to branch retinal vein occlusion (BRVO)
  - Scatter photocoagulation in the management of neovascularization in central retinal vein occlusion (CRVO) for prevention of glaucoma.

  Macular or peripheral laser to ischemic areas in recalcitrant cases.
- **Central serous choroidoretinopathy (CSCR):** Lasers have long been used for management of focal leaks in the treatment of persistent cases of non-resolving CSCR.
- **Retinal breaks:** Laser retinopexy around retinal breaks (retinal hole or tear) is required to achieve chorioretinal adhesion and sealing the area of break. This is important in prevention of retinal detachment.
- **Exudative retinal vascular disorders:** In case of coats' disease, retinal microaneurysm or capillary hemangioma—laser photocoagulation may be used directly to close the leaking vessels by promoting thrombosis.
- **Retinochoroidal neovascular diseases:** Retinochoroidal neovascular diseases, can be treated with laser photocoagulation efficiently.
- **Peripheral retinal ischemic retinopathies:** In vasculitis and retinopathy of prematurity (ROP), laser can help to reduce the hypoxic load on the retina and prevent devastating complications.
- **Tumors:** For vasoproliferative retinal tumors, angiomas, etc., laser photocoagulation can promote closure.
- **Foveoschisis secondary to optic disc pit:** Can be addressed by laser prior to considering surgery.
- **Hyaloidotomy:** To disrupt the hyaloid interface in eyes with subhyaloid hemorrhages.
- **Transpupillary thermotherapy (TTT):** A more intense, destructive modality of laser used for the treatment of choroidal melanomas, retinoblastoma, subfoveal CNVMs and other ocular tumors.
- **Photodynamic therapy (PDT)** A scatter laser photocoagulation, is used to shrink abnormal new blood vessels.
- **Micropulse laser:** Subthreshold micropulse laser is thought to limit damage to adjacent tissue. This has been most extensively explored in the treatment of DME.
- **Nanopulse laser:** Subthreshold laser—a new modality to treat RPE without much damage as compared with conventional laser.
- **Targeted retinal photocoagulation (TRP):** Is to block a specific target, e.g., feeder vessel photocoagulation in CNMV, focal photocoagulation in DME, or selective laser to areas of nonperfusion.

Fundus Examination *(OP 8.3)*

See page 19

Enumerate and Discuss Treatment Modalities in Retinal Diseases *(OP 8.4)*

What are the common retinal diseases?

Retinal diseases can present in many different forms:

- **Retinal tear:** With aging, vitreous tends to separate from the retina, creating a posterior vitreous detachment (PVD). In most cases, a PVD does not cause any complications. But in some eyes, it pulls the retina with enough force to cause the retinal tissue to tear.

  Rarely, a retinal tear may occur as a result of ocular injury.
- **Retinal detachment (RD):** RD generally occurs when fluid travels through a retinal tear and causes the retina to detach from the rest.

  Symptoms depend on the extent of RD, and vary from no symptoms at all, to seeing floaters, flashing lights, and a shadow that blocks the peripheral vision and sometimes central vision as well.

Three main types of RD:
1. *Rhegmatogenous:* Most common, occurs as a result of a retinal tear. May be caused by aging, or after trauma or surgery and myopia
2. *Tractional:* Typically occurs in proliferative diabetic retinopathy
3. *Exudative:* Occurs as a result of choroidal tumor

❖ **Diabetic retinopathy (DR):** It is a serious sight-threatening complication of diabetes that can lead to blindness.
DR affects 1 in 3 people with diabetes. 95% of people with DR can avoid severe vision loss with early treatment.
Diabetes damages the small blood vessels throughout the body, including the fine capillaries in the retina.
Eventually, these fine blood vessels leak blood and other fluids into the eye, and cause the macular edema, resulting in cloudy or blurred vision.
As these blood vessels are damaged, new abnormal blood vessels are produced. These new vessels are fragile and are even more susceptible to leaking and bleeding fluid into the eye.

Different types of DR:
1. *Non-proliferative diabetic retinopathy (NPDR):* It is the earliest stage of the disease. In this stage, microaneurysms develop, which eventually rupture and bleed, giving rise to "dot-and-blot" hemorrhages. There are also soft and hard exudates formation. This is further sub-divided as mild, moderate and severe.
2. *Proliferative diabetic retinopathy (PDR):* It is the more severe form of the disease. In this stage, abnormal vessels begin to grow in the retina (neovascularization). These new vessels eventually break, causing bleeding into the vitreous (vitreous hemorrhage). Associated fibrovascular scarring causes tractional RD with severe visual loss and even blindness.
3. *Diabetic macular edema (DME):* It is a complication of diabetic retinopathy. DME occurs when damaged blood vessels leak fluid into the macula. It may cause blurry or wavy vision with central visual loss.

❖ **Retinal vascular occlusions:** Retinal artery occlusion and vein occlusions (*see* page 128)

❖ **Age-related macular degeneration (AMD):** There are two types of macular degeneration: wet macular degeneration (wet-AMD) and dry macular degeneration (dry-AMD)

❖ **Epiretinal membrane (ERM):** Also known as cellophane maculopathy, or macular puckers. ERM are semi-translucent, fibrocellular, and avascular membrane with few or no blood vessels. It forms on the inner retinal surface, and if it affects the macula, then causes visual distortions.

❖ **Macular hole:** Development of a small hole or defect in the macular area due to abnormal traction between the retina and vitreous; or following an injury to the eye.

❖ **Retinopathy of prematurity (ROP):** History of prematurity and low birth weight (<1,500 g) are present; history of prolonged exposure to oxygen for first 10 days; bilateral in 100% of cases; first noted in neonatal period; presence of tractional retinal detachment. Intraocular pressure is normal.

❖ **Retinitis pigmentosa (RP):** RP is a rare, genetic, ocular disease that causes retinal receptor damage and vision loss.
In initial stage—patients present with night blindness (nyctalopia), mid-peripheral visual field loss and difficulty of vision in low light. Progression of RP continues to destroy cells in the central visual field—resulting in tunnel vision, reduced visual acuity, and loss of color vision.

Treatment Modalities

The main goals of treatment are to stop or slow disease progression and preserve, improve or restore patient's vision.

It is important to make correct diagnosis. **Some investigations** may be done to determine the location and extent of the disease:
- **Amsler grid test:** Test to see the clarity of central vision. If the lines of the grid seem faded, broken or distorted to understand better about the extent of macular damage. In AMD, the patient is asked to use this grid test at home for self-monitoring the condition.
- **Ultra-wide field fundus photography:** To capture the image of the extreme peripheral retina. It is important for patient counseling and to show the pre-treatment and post-treatment images of diseased area at the periphery.
- **Optical coherence tomography (OCT):** An excellent technique for capturing precise images of the central retina to diagnose epiretinal membranes, macular holes and macular edema, to monitor the extent of wet AMD, and to monitor responses to treatment.
- **Fundus autofluorescence (FAF):** FAF may be used to determine the advancement of retinal diseases, including macular degeneration.
- **Fundus fluorescein angiography (FFA):** Fluorescein dye is used to see retinal blood vessels under a special spectrum of light. This helps to identify blocked blood vessels, leaking blood vessels, abnormal new blood vessels and subtle changes in the retina.
- **Optical coherence tomography angiography (OCTA):** A noninvasive method to examine retinal vasculature
- **Indocyanine green angiography (ICGA):** Indocyanine green dye that lights up when exposed to infrared light. The resulting images show retinal vessels and the deeper, choroidal blood vessels which are important in choroidal vascular diseases.
- **Ultrasound B scan:** This test uses ultrasound wave which helps to view the vitreoretinal structures in the eye. It can also identify some eye tumors.
- **CT and MRI:** In rare instances, these imaging methods may be used to help evaluate eye injuries or tumors.

Treatment

Treatment of retinal diseases may be complex, multipronged and sometimes urgent based on the retinal disease and its characteristics.

Options include:
1. **Conservative treatment:** Medications: is helpful in some retinal diseases, e.g., anti-inflammatory injections, antibiotics, antivirals, NSAID drops, or corticosteroids, etc.). The main goal of conservative treatment is to alleviate inflammation and infections.
2. **Laser photocoagulation:** As discussed in *see* page 129
3. **Retino-cryopexy:** May be used alternately to treat a retinal tear. Intense cold freezes the retina and the treated area will later scar and secure the retina.
4. **Posterior sub-Tenon injections:** Triamcinolone in macular edema or retinochoroiditis
5. **Intravitreal injections:** Anti-VGEFs, triamcinolone, dexamethasone implants and specific anti-infective agents. *See* page 74
6. **Surgical treatment (vitreoretinal surgeries):** VR interventions are often complex and based on the retinal disease and its presentation.
    - *Pneumatic retinopexy:* Air or gas is injected into the eye to repair retinal detachment. May be with cryopexy or laser photocoagulation
    - *Scleral buckling:* Used to repair a retinal detachment. A small piece of silicone sponge/band is stitched to the sclera to indent the sclera and reduce the force of the vitreous on the retina, for reattachment of retinal.
    - *Vitrectomy:* Vitreous is removed with a cutter and air, gas (C_3F_8 or SF_6) or silicon oil is injected in to the space for internal tamponade. It may also be performed in vitreous hemorrhage.

It is performed in a macular hole, diabetic retinopathy, epiretinal membrane, endophthalmitis, eye injury or a retinal detachment.
- *Silicon oil removal:* Injected silicon oil needs to be removed after 3–6 months to prevent silicon oil emulsification.
- *Perfluorocarbon liquids (PFCL) injection:* Used to facilitate VR surgery in some conditions, e.g., giant retinal tears, drainage of suprachoroidal hemorrhages, dislocated crystalline or intraocular lenses, etc.
- *Retinal prosthesis:* Implantation of a small electrode chip in the retina. It relays visual information and then process the inputs to a video camera attached with eyeglasses. This is for severe vision loss or blindness caused by retinal disease.
- *Macular translocation:* Involves moving of macula to a healthier section of the retina.
- *Telescopic IOL implantation:* Is surgically placed inside one eye to provide central vision in that eye and the other eye provides peripheral vision for end-stage AMD patients

7. **Low vision aids (LVA):** It is useful in some retinal diseases with low vision and when all treatments fail. The aim is to magnify existing central vision to widen the field of view and eliminate glare.

DISEASES OF OPTIC NERVE AND VISUAL PATHWAYS *(OP 8.5)*

Correlated Anatomy

The visual signals (electrical impulses) originate at the *end-organ:* neural epithelium of the rods and cones; and connecting ultimately to visual cortex. (*See* page 147)
- **The first-order neuron:** It is the bipolar cell with its axons in the inner layers of the retina.
- **The second-order neuron:** It is the ganglion cell of the retina. Its axon passes into the nerve fiber layer optic nerve contains approximately 1 million nerve fibers, which are axons of the retinal ganglion cells of and along the optic nerve to the lateral geniculate body.
- **The third-order neuron:** Originates in the cells of lateral geniculate body, then travels by way of the optic radiations to the occipital cortex (visual center).

The visual pathways thus consist of:
- Two optic nerves
- An optic chiasma
- Two optic tracts
- Two lateral geniculate bodies
- Two optic radiations and
- Visual cortex on each side

In the visual system of human eye, the visual information processed by retinal photoreceptor cells travel in the following way:

Retina → Optic nerve → Optic chiasma (here the nasal visual fibers of both eyes cross over to the opposite side) → Optic tract → Lateral geniculate body → Optic radiation → Visual cortex (primary and secondary).

It follows that a lesion of the optic radiation, optic tract, or occipital lobe will cause blindness of the temporal half of the retina of the same side and nasal half of the opposite side.

Projecting this outward, such lesion will cause loss of vision in the opposite half of visual field a condition known as *hemianopia.*

Optic Nerve and Visual Pathways Diseases *(OP 8.5)*

Common Diseases with Etiologies

1. **Papilledema:** Intracranial space occupying lesions, malignant hypertension, idiopathic intracranial hypertension
2. **Optic neuritis:** Inflammation of the optic nerve. Causes include viral infections and multiple sclerosis.
3. **Anterior ischemic optic neuropathy (AION):** Atherosclerosis, giant cell arteritis, collagen diseases, smoking, anemia, etc.
4. **Optic atrophy:** Atrophy of the optic nerve. Causes are—congenital, multiple sclerosis, tabes dorsalis, trauma and secondary to

optic nerve disease or retinal diseases (retinitis pigmentosa, CRAO, etc.)
5. **Toxic optic neuropathies (toxic amblyopia):** Ethambutol, quinine, tobacco—alcohol amblyopia and methyl alcohol toxicity (poisoning)
6. **Visual pathway diseases are mainly due to intracranial causes:** Space occupying lesions, infarcts, thrombosis, hemorrhage, etc.

Common Symptoms

- **Loss of vision:** The main symptom.
- **Visual field loss**
- Disturbances in color vision.
- Severe headache
- Nausea and vomiting
- Pain is conspicuously absent, except it may be a prominent symptom in retrobulbar neuritis.

Common Signs

- Reduced visual acuity
- Diminished contrast sensitivity
- Relative afferent pupillary defect (RAPD)
- **Ophthalmoscopy:** Attention is directed to the margins of the optic disc, its surface and color, pulsation of the central retinal vein, and the size of the physiological cup.
  - *Papilledema:* Bilateral disc hyperemia, edema, blurred margin
  - *Optic neuritis:* Unilateral disc edema, hyperemia, blurred margin
  - *AION:* Sectorial disc edema with splinter hemorrhage
  - *Optic atrophy:* Pale, white disc with clear margin; in glaucomatous optic atrophy-associated with total cupping

Differences between Papilledema and Optic Neuritis (Table 3.13)

Diagnostic Tests

- Blood pressure—to rule out malignant hypertension
- Systemic neurological examination (physician referral)
- Color vision test
- *Swinging flash light test:* To see relative afferent pupillary defect (RAPD)
- Confrontation visual field test

TABLE 3.13: Difference between papilledema and optic neuritis.

Features	Papilledema	Optic neuritis
History	Headache and vomiting, initially no visual symptom	Sudden loss of vision: History of fever or upper respiratory tract infection
Laterality placement	Usually bilateral	Usually unilateral
Visual acuity	Remains normal until late stage	Severely reduced (6/60 or less)
Pain or tenderness of the eyeball	Absent	May be present
Pupil	Normally reacting	Relative afferent pupillary defect (Marcus-Gunn's pupil)
Disc swelling	More than +3D (1 mm) elevation in the established case	Usually +2D to +3D elevation
Hemorrhage and exudates	More in established case	Relatively less
Visual fields	Enlargement of blind-spot and later gradual constriction Colored field not much affected	Central or centrocecal scotoma More with colored objects
CT scan or MRI	Intracranial space occupying lesion may be detected	Demyelinating disorder may be seen
Recovery of vision	May not be complete even after treatment	Usually complete with adequate treatment

(CT: computed tomography; MRI: magnetic resonance imaging)

- Perimetry—by Humphrey field analyser (HFA)
- Electroretinogram (ERG)—assess the function of the rod and cone photoreceptors in secondary optic atrophy
- **Visual evoked potential (VEP):** Optic neuritis delays the latency of visual evoked potentials. Helpful in diagnosis of optic atrophy in children
- Lumbar puncture—cerebrospinal fluid (CSF) examination
- Blood tests—routine and for collagen vascular disorders

Imaging
- OCT imaging—for retinal nerve fiber layer (RFNL) thickness
- Fundus fluorescein angiography (FFA)—to study the optic nerve head
- X-ray skull—for pituitary tumor
- CT scan—for space occupying lesions in papilledema
- Magnetic resonance imaging (MRI)—to rule out multiple sclerosis in optic neuritis or intracranial lesion in papilledema

Management

Treatment depends on type of disorder. Some optic nerve disorders, patient may get vision back. With others, there is no treatment, or treatment may only prevent further vision loss.

Treatments may include:
- Control of blood pressure, diabetes, weight, and other risk factors
- Avoidance of smoking and alcohol
- Withdrawal of drug, e.g., ethambutol
- Corticosteroids—intravenous (methyl prednisolone in optic neuritis), oral steroids in some cases of AION
- Antibiotics to control infection
- Neuro-vitamin supplements—*injection hydroxycobalamine* (in the form of B_1, B_6 and B_{12} injection) may be added
- Surgical decompression of the optic nerve
- Low vision aids, including magnifiers, large-print devices, and talking watches
- Neurological/rheumatology consultation
- Periodic follow up and co-management with physician

MISCELLANEOUS *(OP 9)*

Demonstrate the Correct Technique *(OP 9.1)*

Examination of Extraocular Movements (Uniocular and Binocular)

See page 10

Fundus Examination Techniques

See page 19

Ocular Examination of a Patient with Cataract

See page 22-24

Counsel Patients and Family about Eye Donation

See page 109

Elicit Appropriate History in a Patient Presenting with Red Eye

See page 94

Demonstrate, Document and Present the Correct Method of Examination of Red Eye

See page 94

Demonstrate the Symptoms and Clinical Signs of Different Lid Disorder

See page 86

Steps in Performing Visual Acuity Assessment for Distance Vision, Near Vision, Color Vision and Pin-hole Test

See page 7-9

Bell's Phenomenon (Palpebral Oculogyric Reflex) *(OP 9.1)*

It is a sign that allows clinician to notice an upward and outward movement of the eye when the eyelids are forcibly closed.

It is important in facial palsy or ptosis evaluation. This specific type of ocular movement is present 80% of the normal population, and is a defensive mechanism (e.g., when an attempt is made to touch a patient's cornea).

How to Elicit Bell's Phenomenon?

- **In case of facial palsy:** It is elicited by simply asking the patient to close the lids. It becomes obviously noticeable.
- **In normal patient or in patient with ptosis:** Ask the patient to close the eyelids tightly. The examiner then tries to prevent eyelid closure by thumbs and notes the position of the eyeball. Normally, the eye will elevate and move outwards.

Regurgitation Test of Lacrimal Sac (OP 9.1)

Also called ROPLAS (Regurgitation on Pressure over the Lacrimal Sac) Test

See page 61

Massage Technique in Congenital Nasolacrimal Duct Obstruction (NLDO)/ Congenital Dacryocystitis

See page 89

Demonstrate and Describe the Technique of Removal of Foreign Body from Eye

See page 101

STRABISMUS (SQUINT) AND INDICATIONS FOR REFERRAL (OP 9.2)

Definition: It is defined as misalignment of the visual axes of the two eyes, when they are directed towards a fixation object.

Normally, the visual axes of two eyes are essentially parallel in all directions of ocular movements, except in convergence and divergence.

Pseudo-strabismus: Here, the visual axes are in fact parallel, but the eyes seem to have squint.

Causes: Prominent epicanthic folds or hypertelorism.

Classification of Strabismus (Squint) (Flowchart 3.1)

Types: Mainly two types:
1. **Concomitant:** (i) Latent (*heterophoria*) and (ii) Manifest (*heterotropia*)
2. **Noncomitant or paralytic.**
   i. **Latent squint or heterophoria (phoria):** Here, eyeball tends to deviate but this

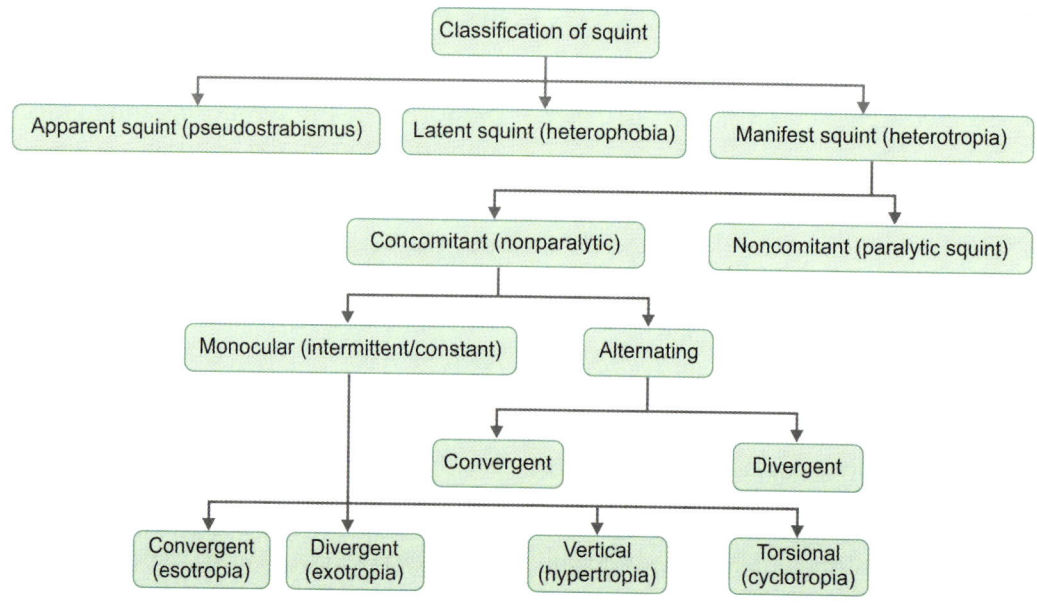

Flowchart 3.1: Classification of strabismus (squint).

deviation can be prevented by the effort of fusion between two eyes for the interest of binocular vision.

Types:
1. **Exophoria:** Tends to deviate outwards.
2. **Esophoria:** Tends to deviate inwards.
3. **Hyperphoria:** Tends to deviate upwards.
4. **Hypophoria:** Tends to deviate downwards
5. **Cyclophoria:** Tendency of torsional deviation.

Methods of diagnosis

Cover test: One eye is covered, and the other eye is made to fix on an object. In presence of heterophoria, the eye undercover, deviates. When the cover is removed, the covered eye corrects the deviation, and regains its normal position quickly.

Other tests are *Maddox rod, Maddox wing* and *Synoptophore* evaluation to know range of fusion.

ii. **Manifest squint or heterotropia:** Deviation persists in spite of effort of fusion by both the eyes.

Types: (i) *Concomitant* and (ii) *Paralytic*
- *Exotropia:* Outwards deviation
- *Esotropia:* Inwards deviation
- *Hypertropia:* Upwards deviation
- *Cyclotropia:* Torsional deviation

(Exo = Divergent; Eso = Convergent)

Diagnosis of Heterotropia

- **Visual acuity testing:** By Snellen's chart, 'illiterate E', etc.
- **Refraction under atropine:** To find out any refractive error.
- **Ocular motility:** To find out any limitations of ocular movement.
- **Cover test:** To find out the squint is uniocular or alternating.
- **Fixation behavior:** To find out foveal (centric) fixation or eccentric fixation.
- **Anterior segment and fundus:** To rule out any organic lesion which may be the cause of squint.
- **Measurement of the angle of squint:**
  - *Corneal reflection test (Hirschberg):* Estimating the distance of corneal light reflex (Purkinje's first image) from pupillary center. 1 mm decentration of reflex corresponds to about 7° of ocular deviation. This test is also useful to differentiate it from pseudo-strabismus.
  - *Prism reflex test (Krimsky):* Prisms are placed in front of the deviating eye until the corneal light reflexes become symmetrical.
  - *Prism-bar-cover test (PBCT):* The prism power required to negate the ocular movements, equals to the angle of deviation, and it is measured in prism diopter (Δ). Roughly, 10 of ocular deviation equals to 2 prism diopter (2Δ) deviation. It is the most accurate method of measuring the angle of deviation.
- **State of binocular vision:** All three grades of binocular vision (SMP, fusion and stereopsis) are determined by synoptophore.
- **Worth's 'four-dot' test:** To diagnose the presence of suppression and abnormal retinal correspondence in a manifest squint.
- **Diplopia charting:** It is done in a dark room, with red glass placed in front of right eye and green glass in front of left, to dissociate the images. Position of two images is recorded on a chart with nine squares (representing nine positions of gaze) marked on it.
- **Hess screen (chart):** The eyes are dissociated similarly with red and green goggles and note the patient's response to the dissimilar images formed by each eye while viewing a different target (dot and line) on Hess screen.
- **Forced duction test (FDT):** This test is used to differentiate defective ocular movements due to physical restriction, from a muscle paralysis.

Differences between Concomitant and Paralytic Squint (Table 3.14)

Principle of Treatment

A. **For concomitant squint:** Remember four 'O's:
1. "O" for Optical correction (refraction).
2. "O" for Occlusion (for amblyopia).

TABLE 3.14: Difference between concomitant and paralytic squint.

Concomitant squint	Paralytic squint
Mostly developmental, usually not associated with trauma/disease	Mostly acquired, usually associated with trauma/disease
Occurs in infants and children	Usually in adults
Diplopia absent	Diplopia present
No abnormal head posture	Abnormal head posture to avoid diplopia
Absence of false projection (i.e., false localization of object)	False projection is present
Angle of squint is usually constant in all directions of gaze	Angle of squint is variable in different directions of gaze
Ocular movements are normal and there is no restriction	Ocular movement is restricted in the direction of action of paralyzed muscle
Secondary angle of deviation is always equal to primary deviation	Secondary deviation is greater than primary deviation
Amblyopia is present	No amblyopia
Surgical result is usually good	Surgical result is not satisfactory, and at times, surgery may be contraindicated

3. "O" for Orthoptic exercises.
4. "O" for Operative correction.

Main idea of the treatment is to give binocular single vision as well as alignment of the visual axes between the two eyes.

B. For paralytic squint:
❖ Investigations to find out the cause (e.g., neurological consultation, X-ray skull, CT scan and MRI of brain, blood sugar, thyroid profile, etc.)
❖ Observation for at least 6 months for maximum recovery.
❖ Treatment of diplopia:
  ➢ Occlusion of the worse eye.
  ➢ Prism correction
❖ Neuro-vitamin injection, e.g., vitamin-B_1, B_6 and B_{12} for few weeks.
❖ **Surgical correction**—as a last measure and usually performed after 6 months.

Indications for Referral in a Patient with Strabismus

❖ All children with strabismus
❖ Strabismus with amblyopia
❖ Strabismus with diplopia
❖ Acute onset strabismus at any age
❖ Paralytic strabismus of recent onset with double vision—to exclude nerve palsy—need urgent referral to a neurologist
❖ Strabismus due to thyroid ophthalmopathy or myasthenia gravis—needs referral to a physician

Headache in Ophthalmic Practice and Referral *(OP 9.3)*

Headache as a primary symptom to an ophthalmologist often presents a diagnostic challenge.

In all cases of headache, the ophthalmologist's basic responsibility is to detect the serious cause of headache early. *It may be an intracranial neoplasm by detecting the papilledema.*

There by, he can refer the patient as early as possible.

Causes of headache in ophthalmic practice:
❖ **Associated with refractive errors and ocular-muscle imbalance:**
  ➢ Astigmatism and hypermetropia
  ➢ Presbyopia
  ➢ Heterophoria or latent squint
  ➢ Convergence insufficiency
  Management
  ➢ These headaches are relieved by proper cycloplegic refraction and spectacle correction.

- Untreated hypermetropia can result in persistent attempts for accommodation, leading to ciliary muscle spasm and headache. Thus, relaxing accommodation with proper convex-power spectacles may lessen the eye spasm and headache.
- Phorias or convergence insufficiency can be corrected by orthoptic exercises.

❖ **Secondary to organic eye diseases:**
- Acute attack of angle closure glaucoma
- Acute iridocyclitis
- Acute keratitis, contact lens over—wear or photokeratitis
- Scleritis
- Secondary glaucoma of acute onset

Treatment of these headaches is directed towards the cause.

❖ **Secondary to ENT pathology:** Mainly due to sinusitis (frontal or others), need early referral to an ENT specialist.

❖ **Related to systemic diseases: Indications for quick referral**
- Papilledema as in *raised intracranial tension* (urgent referral to a neurologist) or in *malignant hypertension* (urgent referral to a physician)
- Temporal arteritis (referral to a physician)
- Migraine (referral to a physician)
- Psychogenic (anxiety or tension headache)—need psychiatrist's help.

AVOIDABLE BLINDNESS, NPCBVI AND VISION 2020 *(OP 9.4)*

Avoidable Blindness *(OP 9.4)*

Uniform Definition of Blindness (WHO)

"Best corrected visual acuity (BCVA) in the better eye is less than 3/60 (Snellen's) or its equivalent" or *in the absence of visual acuity chart*—"Inability to count fingers in daylight at a distance of 3 meters" (to indicate less than 3/60 or its equivalent).

Avoidable blindness: This includes both preventable blindness and/or curable blindness. 80–85% of the blindness is estimated to be avoidable. According to WHO estimate 45 million people are blind in the World as of 2000.

Curable blindness: The type of blindness where the visual loss is reversible by prompt management. It is almost synonymous with cataract blindness. Others are—uncorrected refractive errors, glaucoma, inflammation of ocular tissues, etc.

Preventable blindness: The loss of vision that could have been completely prevented by timely effective preventive or prophylactic measures:

❖ Corneal blindness (infectious keratitis, vitamin A deficiency, injuries, chemical burns, etc.)
❖ Industrial blindness (by improving occupational safety conditions)
❖ Retinopathy of prematurity (ROP)
❖ Diabetic retinopathy, etc.

Rapid Assessment of Avoidable Blindness (RAAB) Study by NPCBVI (2015–2019)

Major causes of blindness in population aged ≥50 years (percentage-wise):

Cataract	66.2
Corneal blindness	7.4
Cataract surgical complications (including PCO)	7.2
Posterior segment disease (excluding DR & ARMD)	5.9
Glaucoma	5.5
Diabetic retinopathy (DR)	1.2
Age-related macular degeneration (AMD)	0.7

Major causes of visual impairment (VI)* in population aged ≥50 years (percentage-wise):

Cataract	71.2
Refractive error	13.4
Cataract surgical complications (including PCO)	5.9

*Visual impairment (VI): *Presenting visual acuity is <6/18 in better eye with available correction.*

National Program for Control of Blindness *(OP 9.4)*

National Programs for Control of Blindness (NPCB) is renamed as **"National Programme** for Control of Blindness and Visual Impairment (NPCBVI)" in the year 2019.

NPCBVI was launched in the year 1976 as a 100% centrally sponsored scheme with the goal to reduce the prevalence of blindness from 1.4% to 0.3%. As per survey in 2001–2002, prevalence of blindness was 1.1%. Various initiatives undertaken during the five year plans under NPCBVI are targeted towards achieving the goal of reducing the prevalence of blindness to 0.3% by the year 2020.

RAAB study conducted between 2015 and 2019 showed prevalence of blindness in all age groups = 0.36%.

Goals and Objectives of NPCBVI in the XII Plan

- To reduce the backlog of blindness through identification and treatment of blind at primary, secondary and tertiary levels based on assessment of the overall burden of visual impairment in the country.
- Develop and strengthen the strategy of NPCBVI for "eye health" and prevention of visual impairment; through provision of comprehensive eye care services and quality service delivery.
- Strengthening and upgradation of RIOs to become center of excellence in various subspecialties of ophthalmology.
- Strengthening the existing and developing additional human resources and infrastructure facilities for providing high quality comprehensive eye care in all districts of the country.
- To enhance community awareness on eye care and lay stress on preventive measures.
- Increase and expand research for prevention of blindness and visual impairment
- To secure participation of voluntary organizations/private practitioners in eye care

Methods of Intervention

Primary (peripheral) level: *By community health worker* and *ophthalmic assistant*—at Primary Health Center (PHC), Block Primary Health Center (BPHC) and rural hospitals.

Service: *Primary eye-health care*
- Treatment of common eye aliments, e.g., conjunctivitis, superficial foreign body, trachoma, etc.
- Correction of refractive errors
- Screening for cataract
- Treatment of xerophthalmia
- Vitamin A prophylaxis
- Tele-ophthalmology services via vision centers
- Appropriate and timely referral to secondary or tertiary centers

Secondary (intermediate) level: By ophthalmologist and paramedical ophthalmic assistant (PMOA) at sub-divisional hospitals and district hospitals.

Service: *Secondary eye-health care* (in addition to primary eye care).
- Treatment of common blinding conditions. e.g., cataract, glaucoma, trichiasis, entropion, ocular trauma, etc.
- Screening of diabetic retinopathy
- Cataract surgery eye camp via outreach program
- Appropriate and timely referral to tertiary centres

Central (tertiary) level: By ophthalmologist and paramedical ophthalmic assistant (PMOA), postgraduate students, nurses and other trainees at:
- Medical colleges
- State eye hospitals/institutes
- Regional institutes of ophthalmology (RIOs)
- National (apex) eye institute.

Service: *Tertiary eye-health care* (in addition to secondary eye care).
- Sophisticated eye care, e.g., retinal detachment, corneal grafting, oculoplasty and other complex surgeries.
- To provide eye bank services.
- To provide specialized training programs for all staff
- To train postgraduate ophthalmology students for 2–3 years
- To arrange CME program for the ophthalmologists

- To undertake and promote research activities in ophthalmology

Apex center (National Eye Institute) is to function as a center of excellence to provide overall leadership, supervision and guidance in technical matters in planning and implementation of the program.

Dr Rajendra Prasad Center for Ophthalmic Sciences, AIIMS, New Delhi, is identified for this purpose.

Vision 2020: The Right to Sight *(OP 9.4)*

It is the global initiative for the elimination of avoidable blindness, a joint program of the World Health Organization (WHO) and the International Agency for the Prevention of Blindness (IAPB).

It was launched in 1999. Vision 2020 India was launched in 2004.

Five conditions have identified as immediate priorities within the framework of Vision 2020 program.
1. Cataract
2. Trachoma
3. Onchocerciasis
4. Childhood blindness and
5. Refractive errors and low vision

Target seven diseases identified under '**Vision 2020' India:**
1. Cataract
2. Childhood blindness
3. Refractive errors and low vision
4. Corneal blindness
5. Diabetic retinopathy
6. Glaucoma
7. Trachoma (focal geographical areas)

Cataract

To improve the quantity and quality of cataract surgery. Targets and strategies include:
- To increase the cataract surgery rate 6000 by 2020.
- IOL surgery for >80% by the year 2005 and for all by the year 2010.
- YAG capsulotomy services at all district hospitals by 2010

Childhood Blindness

Prevalence: 0.8/1000 children.

Common causes are vitamin A deficiency, measles, conjunctivitis, ophthalmia neonatorum, injuries, congenital cataract, retinopathy of prematurity (ROP) childhood glaucoma.

To identify areas where childhood blindness from preventable disease is common and to encourage preventive measures, for example:
- Measles immunization
- Vitamin A supplementation
- Nutrition education
- Avoidance of harmful traditional practices
- Monitoring of use of oxygen in newborn

To provide specialist training and services for the management of surgically remediable visual loss in children from:
- Congenital cataract
- Congenital glaucoma
- Corneal scar
- Retinopathy of prematurity

Refractive errors and low vision:
- Refraction services to be available in all PHC/BPHC by 2010.
- Availability of low—cost, good quality spectacles for children
- Low vision services are to be established at 150 tertiary level eye care institutions.

Corneal Blindness

Major Causes

Corneal ulcers due to infections, trachoma, ocular injuries and keratomalacia due to vitamin A deficiencies.

Actions to be Taken
- Vitamin A supplementation
- Measles vaccination
- Better water supply and sanitation for reduction in trachoma and other infections.
- Eye banking support

Glaucoma

- Glaucoma screening at eye care institutions for all persons above the age of 35 years, those with diabetes mellitus, and with family history of glaucoma.

- Community based referral by multi-purpose workers of all persons with diminution of vision, colored haloes, rapid change of glasses, ocular pain and family history of glaucoma.
- Glaucoma screening at eye camps in all patients above the age of 35 years.

Diabetic Retinopathy

Awareness generation by health workers:
- All known diabetics to be examined and referred to eye surgeon by the ophthalmic assistant.
- To provide laser treatment to all those requiring it at tertiary level

Trachoma

Implementation of **SAFE** strategy (*See* page 99):
- **S**—**S**urgery to correct trichiasis and/or entropion
- **A**—**A**ntibiotics
- **F**—**F**acial hygiene
- **E**—**E**nvironmental hygiene

Five Basic Strategies

To combat blindness are:
1. Disease control and prevention
2. Training of personnel
3. Strengthening the existing eye care infrastructure
4. Use of appropriate and affordable technology
5. Mobilization of resources

EVALUATION, INITIAL MANAGEMENT AND REFERRAL IN PATIENT WITH OCULAR INJURY (OP 9.5)

Types of ocular injury are:
1. Blunt injury (closed globe injury)
2. Penetrating injury (open globe injury)
3. Chemical injury.

Evaluation and referral depends upon the type and severity of the Injury.
1. **In blunt injury the effects are:**
    - *Eyelids:* Ecchymosis (black eye) 'Panda Bear sign', lid laceration, emphysema (crepitation due to paranasal sinus injury).
    - *Conjunctiva:* Subconjunctival hemorrhage, chemosis, conjunctival laceration.
    - *Cornea:* Abrasions, Descemet's tear, edema, blood staining of the cornea, rupture cornea.
    - *Sclera:* Scleral rupture (mostly near the limbus).
    - *Anterior chamber:* Hyphaema, clotted blood in A/C.
    - *Iris:* Iridodialysis, traumatic aniridia, traumatic iritis
    - *Pupil:* Miosis, mydriasis, irregular pupil with sphincteric tear, D-shaped pupil (due to iridodialysis), reaction—impaired.
    - *Ciliary body:* Angle recession glaucoma (separation of circular and radial muscle fibres of the ciliary body from longitudinal fibers).
    - *Lens:* Vossius' ring (imprint of miosed pupil on the anterior surface of the lens), traumatic cataract (rosette cataract), subluxation of the lens, dislocation of the lens.
    - *Vitreous:* Vitreous hemorrhage.
    - *Choroid:* Choroidal rupture, detachment of the choroid.
    - *Retina:* Macular edema (Berlin's edema), hemorrhage, tear or hole, retinal detachment.
    - *Optic nerve:* Avulsion of the optic nerve, Optic atrophy.
    - *Tension:* Hypotony, secondary glaucoma.
    - *Lacrimal apparatus:* Subluxation of the lacrimal gland; injury to the medial canthus and lacrimal canaliculi.
    - *Orbit:* Orbital or retrobulbar hemorrhage, orbital fracture and, blow-out fracture.

In blunt Injury the primary physician can manage—ecchymosis of lids, subconjunctival hemorrhage, corneal abrasion, small hyphema, etc.

The cases where urgent referral is required in blunt injury:
- With moderate to severe visual loss, e.g., vitreous hemorrhage, retinal detachment or traumatic optic neuropathy
- Large conjunctival laceration, cornea or scleral rupture
- Moderate to severe hyphema
- Subluxation/dislocation of lens
- Diplopia—due to orbital blow-out fracture

2. **In penetrating (or open globe) injury:**
   - The primary physician examines the eye to assess the severity of injury.
   - It may be small cornea tear to severe globe rupture and with or without retained intraocular foreign body.
   - Close the lids properly after antibiotic drop/ointment and sterile pad and bandage. Then refer the patient to a tertiary eye care center.
   - It is always an emergency. Urgent referral is required in all cases.
   - The primary goal—is to address closure of the wound to prevent infection (endophthalmitis).

3. **Chemical injury:**
   It is a true emergency situation. So, the treatment should be started immediately even before testing vision, unless an associated open globe injury is suspected.
   Role of primary physician: *First emergency treatment, then referral*
   - Anesthetic drop and eye lid speculum
   - Copious but gentle wash of the eye(s) using normal saline or Ringer's lactate solution for 30 minutes or more
   - Tap water can be used in absence of these solutions
   - Upper and lower fornices must be everted and irrigated thoroughly
   - Conjunctival fornices are to be swept with moistened cotton buds
   - If any lime particle seen, it has to be removed gently
   - If necessary, double eversion (Desmarres' retractor) of upper lid is important in removing particles from the deep fornix
   - *Wait for 5–10 minutes:* Assess the severity of the chemical burn
   - *If it is mild grade* (grade 1 or 2 without limbal ischemia)—treat the patient with antibiotic drops, steroid drops, tears substitutes and tablet vitamin C, etc., and observe for 48 hours. If not respond to treatment—then refer to a secondary/tertiary eye care center.
   - *If it is of moderate severe grades* (grade 3 or 4 with limbal ischemia): After initial management, refer the patient to a tertiary eye care center as early as possible.

OCULAR MANIFESTATIONS AND ASSOCIATIONS OF COVID-19

The eyes are important clinically in COVID-19. The spike proteins of virus SARS-CoV-2 binds to the angiotensin converting enzyme which is present in various ocular structures.

The eyes are thought to be an independent route of entry apart from naso- and oropharynx.

COVID-19 causes ocular symptoms directly and indirectly.
- **Direct manifestation:** COVID conjunctivitis (behaves like any viral conjunctivitis)
- **Rarer manifestations:** Episcleritis, panuveitis and optic neuritis.

Indirect manifestation due to CNS involvement, hypercoagulable state and drug side effects:
- Retinal artery and venous occlusion
- Cranial nerve palsy
- Orbital apex syndrome
- Rhino-orbital-cerebro mucormycosis
- Optic neuritis and papilledema
- Post-COVID dry eye worsening
- Contraindication for eye donation

EXPLAIN EFFECT OF PITUITARY TUMORS ON VISUAL PATHWAY (AN 30.5)

Effect of pituitary tumors on visual pathway and corresponding visual field defects are caused by tumor compression on the optic nerve or chiasm leading to axonal damage. Depending on the size and location of the tumor, as well as the anatomical relationship of the chiasm to the pituitary stalk, the severity and symmetry of the visual field defect may vary.

Monocular Visual Field Deficits

Asymmetric tumors may preferentially involve one side of the chiasm or an optic nerve, and most commonly presents as a superotemporal quadrantanopia.

The patient may have a unilateral or bilateral optic neuropathy or develop an optic neuropathy in one eye and a contralateral superotemporal defect in the fellow eye, (i.e., the junctional scotoma).

Chiasmal Field Deficits

Classically, lesions at the level of the optic chiasm produce a bitemporal hemianopia. Pituitary adenomas, which grow upward from the pituitary stalk, compress the chiasm from below, which preferentially involves the inferior, nasal, and macular nerve fibres. This corresponds to superior, bitemporal, and central vision loss. While these field defects typically respect the vertical midline, pituitary adenomas large enough to cause compression of optic nerve and also reduce visual acuity with diffuse central depression of visual field. In case of tumors that preferentially grow posteriorly, selective compression of macular fibers may cause a bitemporal hemianopsia involving the central visual field while sparing the peripheral field.

Optic Tract

Rarely, pituitary adenomas can compress the optic tract and produce a homonymous hemianopia.

Optic Atrophy

Chronic tumor compression can lead to optic atrophy. Some atrophy is reported to be present in approximately 50% of pituitary lesions with visual field defects. If only the fibers nasal to the macula are damaged, only the nasal and temporal optic disc may be atrophic, often described as "bow-tie"

or "band-shaped" pattern in both eyes in a bitemporal hemianopsia and only in the eye with the temporal visual field loss (nasal fiber loss) in a homonymous hemianopsia from an optic tract lesion.

DESCRIBE ANATOMICAL BASIS OF HORNER'S SYNDROME (AN 31.3)

Horner syndrome (or oculo-sympathetic paresis) results from interruption of the sympathetic nerve supply to the eye. It is characterized by the *classic triad* of 'miosis', 'partial ptosis', and 'hemifacial anhidrosis', as well as apparent enophthalmos.

Horner syndrome may develop from lesions at any point along the cervical sympathetic pathway.

It inactivates the dilator muscle and thereby produces miosis. It inactivates the Muller's muscle in superior tarsus which produces ptosis. Depending on the level of the lesion, impaired flushing and sweating may be found ipsilaterally. With central first-order neuron lesions, anhidrosis affects the ipsilateral side of the body. Lesions affecting second-order neurons may cause anhidrosis of the ipsilateral face.

The pupils react normally to light and accommodation. Heterochromia of iris (affected eye being hypopigmented) is seen in congenital Horner syndrome.

EXPLAIN THE ANATOMICAL BASIS OF OCULOMOTOR, TROCHLEAR AND ABDUCENT NERVE PALSIES ALONG WITH STRABISMUS (AN 31.5)

Oculomotor (3rd) Nerve Palsy

Ptosis due to weakness of levator. Eyeball rotates outward (divergent) and slightly downward due to unopposed action of the lateral rectus (N VI) and superior oblique (N IV) muscles. Intorsion of the eyeball on attempted down gaze, due to action of superior oblique muscle. Ocular movements are restricted in all direction, except outward (due to lateral rectus). Pupil is dilated and does not constrict to light or convergence. In pupil-sparing 3rd nerve palsy (e.g., in diabetes mellitus), pupil reacts normally.

Trochlear (4th) Nerve Palsy

Trauma is the most common cause of isolated fourth nerve palsy, which may be bilateral. It causes paralysis of the superior oblique muscle. *The clinical features are as follows:* Abnormal head posture—chin depression, head tilt and slight face turn to the opposite (normal) side. Diplopia is most troublesome, as it occurs more in downgaze. Eyeball deviated upward and inward (ipsilateral hypertropia). Extorsion of the globe (excyclotropia). Restriction of the ocular movements on downward and inward.

Abducens (6th) Nerve Palsy

This is the most common type, and commonly occurs in raised intracranial tension. The long intracranial course, and its angulation over the petrous tip of the sphenoid bone, make it vulnerable in raised intracranial tension. In this situation, the sixth nerve palsy is a false localizing sign. *Signs:* They are due to paralysis of lateral rectus. The eyeball is rotated inward (convergent squint). Defective abduction of the eye, partially or completely. Face turn toward the field of action of paralyzed muscle (e.g., a patient with right sixth nerve palsy will turn his face to the right).

DESCRIBE AND DEMONSTRATE PARTS AND LAYERS OF EYEBALL *(AN 41.1)*

See page 68

Describe the Anatomical Aspects of Cataract, Glaucoma and Central Retinal Artery Occlusion *(AN 41.2)*

Anatomical aspect of cataract: *See* page 123

Anatomical aspect of glaucoma: *See* page 116

Anatomical aspect of central retinal artery occlusion (CRAO)

The central retinal artery is the first branch of ophthalmic artery. It supplies nerve fibers in the optic nerve as well as the inner layers of the retina. After entering the eye, the central retinal artery divides into superior and inferior branches.

In addition, the cilio-retinal artery may be present in 30–40% of the individual. It is a branch of the short posterior ciliary artery, which is a separate branch of the ophthalmic artery. When present, it supplies the papillo-macular bundle, which contains the most photoreceptors cells which are essential for central vision. In these patients, the macula may still be perfused in acute CRAO. This means, these patients still maintain good central vision.

The exact location of blockage in CRAO is debated. Anatomically, the narrowest part of central retinal artery lumen is where it pierces the dural sheath of the optic nerve and not at the lamina cribrosa. This is the most common location where blockage occurs.

The blood-flow through any of these vessels may be disrupted during a retinal artery occlusion. CRA occlusion may be caused by emboli, vasculitis, or spasms.

DESCRIBE THE POSITION, NERVE SUPPLY AND ACTIONS OF INTRA-OCULAR MUSCLES *(AN 41.3)*

See page 73

DESCRIBE AND DISCUSS FUNCTIONAL ANATOMY OF EYE, PHYSIOLOGY OF IMAGE FORMATION, PHYSIOLOGY OF VISION INCLUDING COLOR VISION, REFRACTIVE ERRORS, COLOR BLINDNESS, PHYSIOLOGY OF PUPIL AND LIGHT REFLEX *(PY 10.17)*

The pupillary reflexes: Three reflexes are of clinical importance:

1. **Light reflex:** If light enters an eye, the pupil of this eye constricts (direct light reflex),

and there is an equal constriction of the pupil of the other eye (consensual light reflex).
2. **Near reflex:** A constriction of pupil occurs on looking at a near object, a reflex largely determined by the reaction to convergence.
3. **Psychosensory reflex:** A dilatation of the pupil occurs on psychic or sensory stimuli.

Light Reflex (Fig. 3.2)

Rods and cones → optic nerve → optic chiasma (partially decussate) → optic tract → pretectal nucleus (instead of running to the lateral geniculate body) → partial decussation in the midbrain → Edinger-Westphal nucleus on each side → third nerve → inferior division → branch to inferior oblique → short root of ciliary ganglion → ciliary ganglion → short ciliary nerves → sphincter pupillae muscle

This decussation is important to explain the mechanism of consensual reaction, as well as direct reaction to light, and for several pathological reactions.

Near Reflex

It initiates mainly by the fibers from the medial rectus muscle, which contracts on convergence.

Medial rectus muscle → via third nerve → mesencephalic nucleus of fifth nerve → a presumptive center for convergence at pons → Edinger-Westphal nucleus → along the third nerve → accessory ciliary ganglion → sphincter pupillae muscle of the iris.

DESCRIBE AND DISCUSS THE PHYSIOLOGICAL BASIS OF LESION IN VISUAL PATHWAY (PY 10.18)

The end-organ: It is the neural epithelium of the rods and cones.
The first-order neuron: It is the bipolar cell with its axons in the inner layers of the retina.
The second-order neuron: It is the ganglion cell of the retina. Its axon passes into the nerve-fiber layer and along the optic nerve to the lateral geniculate body.
The third-order neuron: It originates in the cells of lateral geniculate body, then travels by way of the optic radiations to the occipital cortex (visual center).

The visual pathways thus consist of:
❖ Two optic nerves
❖ An optic chiasma
❖ Two optic tracts
❖ Two lateral geniculate bodies
❖ Two optic radiations
❖ Visual cortex on each side.

In general, the fibers from the peripheral retina enter the periphery of the optic nerve, and the fibers near the optic disc enter the central part of the nerve. The fibers from the macular area form the papillomacular bundles, which have a separate course. Partial decussation occurs where the nasal fibers cross at the chiasma. The fibers of the peripheral retina have two distinct groups, corresponding to the nasal and temporal halves of the retina.

The fibers of the temporal half enter the chiasma and pass to the optic tract of same side, and then to the lateral geniculate body. The fibers from the nasal half enter the chiasma, decussate, and then pass to the optic tract of opposite side, then to the lateral geniculate body.

The third-order neurons pass by the optic radiation into the corresponding occipital lobe. It follows that a lesion of the optic radiation,

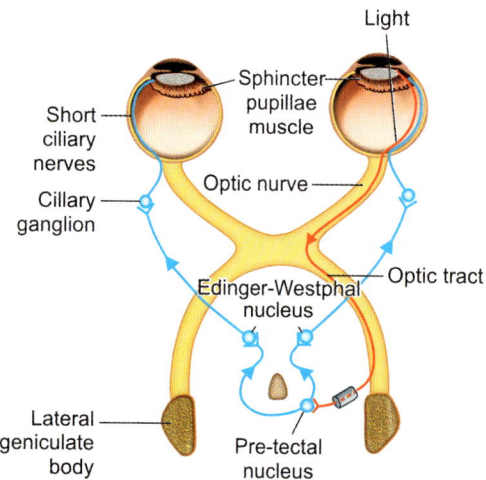

Fig. 3.2: Pathway of the light reflex.

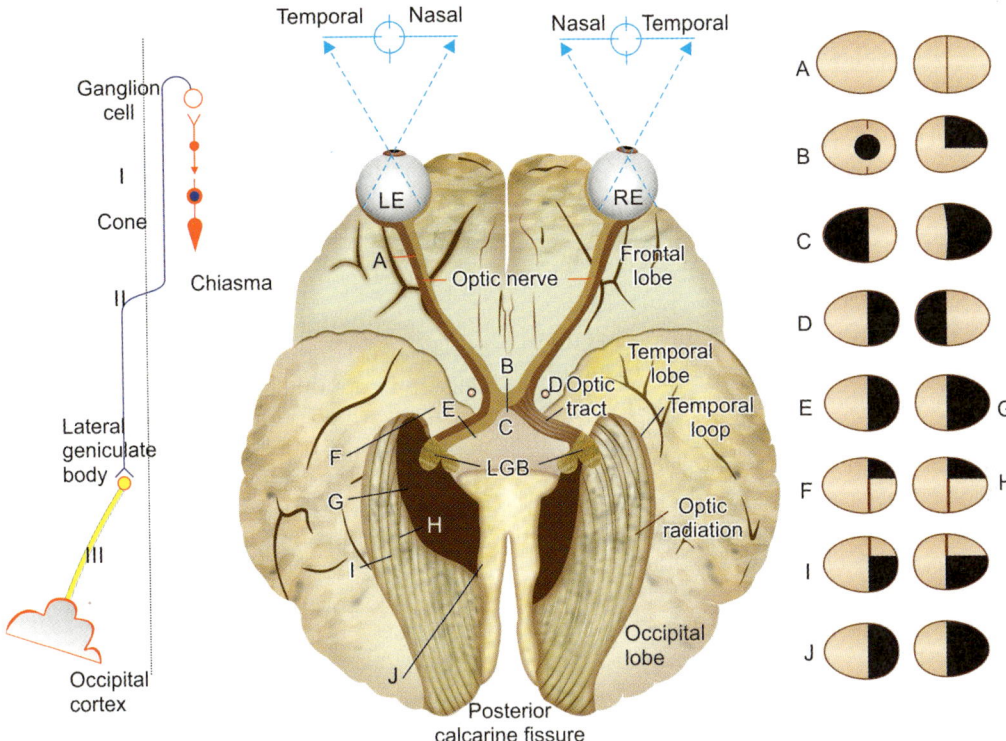

Fig. 3.3: Optic (visual) pathways—all the right and left nasal fibers decussate at the chiasma.

The sites of lesions and corresponding visual field defect are: (A) Through optic nerve—ipsilateral blindness; (B) At the proximal part of optic nerve at chiasmal junction—ipsilateral blindness with contralateral superior quadrantopia (Traquair's junctional scotoma); (C) Middle of chiasma—bitemporal hemianopia; (D) From lateral sides of chiasma—binasal hemianopia; (E) Of optic tract—contralateral homonymous hemianopia; (F) Of temporal lobe—contralateral quadrantic homonymous defects; (G) Whole optic radiation—contralateral homonymous hemianopia; (H) Anterior part of the optic radiations—contralateral inferior homonymous quadrantic defects; (I) Posterior part of the optic radiations—contralateral superior homonymous quadrantic defects; (J) Occipital cortex—contralateral homonymous hemianopia with macular sparing.

optic tract, or occipital lobe will cause blindness of the temporal half of the retina of the same side and nasal half of the opposite side. Projecting this outward, such lesion will cause loss of vision in the opposite half of visual field a condition known as hemianopia. **Figure 3.3** describes the anatomical sites of lesions and the corresponding visual field defects in classical cases.

Describe and Discuss Visual Evoke Potentials *(PY 10.19)*

See page 79

Demonstrate Testing of Visual Acuity, Color and Field of Vision in Volunteer/ Simulated Environment *(PY 10.20)*

See page 7–9

DESCRIBE THE ETIOLOGY, GENETICS, PATHOGENESIS, PATHOLOGY, PRESENTATION, SEQUELAE AND COMPLICATIONS OF RETINOBLASTOMA *(PA 36.1)*

Etiology

Incidence: 1 in 20,000 live births.
Laterality: 25–30% of cases are bilateral.
Age: The neoplasm is probably congenital, but the average age of diagnosis is 18 months. Most cases become clinically apparent before the age of 3 years.
Inheritance: A positive family history is present only in 6% of cases (mostly in bilateral cases). Mode of inheritance is autosomal dominant. Remaining 94% of cases are sporadic.
Chromosomal abnormalities: In 5% of cases, it is associated with deletion of the long arm of chromosome-13 and with trisomy-21.

Clinical Presentation

Leukocoria or amaurotic cat's eye reflex: The most common mode of presentation (60% of cases) and is due to reflection of light from the yellowish-white mass in the retrolental area.
Squinting of the eye: The second most common mode of presentation (20%).
Secondary glaucoma which may be associated with buphthalmos.
Proptosis (due to orbital involvement).
Endophthalmitis or anterior uveitis may also be a presenting feature.
Visual difficulties: Noticed by the parents.
Nystagmus in bilateral cases if it occurs within 6 months.

Histopathology

Gross examination: A chalky-white, friable tumor with dense foci of calcification.
Microscopic: Retinoblastoma consists of small, round, densely packed cells with large basophilic nuclei. It may be well differentiated or poorly differentiated. Well-differentiated retinoblastoma is characterized by presence of rosettes and fleurettes.
Flexner-Wintersteiner rosette: Cells arrange in a single layer around a central clear lumen. This is true rosette and highly characteristic.
Homer–Wright rosette: It is a radial arrangement of cells around a central triangle of neural fibers (rather than clear lumen) and is mainly found in neuroblastoma or medulloblastoma.
Pseudorosette: In necrotic retinoblastoma, several layers of cells may be seen around a blood vessel, within the areas of extensive necrosis with the formation of pseudorosette.
Flurette: It is composed of group of tumor cells and contains pear-shaped eosinophilic processes which project through a fenestrated membrane.
Histology of metastatic lesions outside the retina shows a change of character of the cells. They resemble sarcomatous cells and rosettes are in rarity.

Sequelae

- ❖ Retinoblastoma is a highly malignant tumor. If left untreated, retinoblastoma can be fatal. It will continue growing and can invade the entire eyeball with subsequent metastasis.
- ❖ It remains within the eyeball and curable within 3–6 months of its first presentation (if the child presents with leukocoria). Delay in the diagnosis will decrease the survival rate.
- ❖ Death may occur within one year of metastasis.
- ❖ Metastasis may occur via the following possible routes:
  - ➢ Direct invasion of the CNS via the optic nerve. Sometimes, or it may extend into the orbit as a fungating mass.
  - ➢ Through the subarachnoid space to the contralateral optic nerve
  - ➢ Through the cerebrospinal fluid to the CNS
  - ➢ Via the hematogenous route to the lungs, bone, and brain
  - ➢ Via the lymphatics if the tumor invades anteriorly into the conjunctivae, eyelids, or extraocular tissue.
  - ➢ Spontaneous regression of the tumor is a rare occurrence but may occur in a small number of cases.

Complications
- Retinal detachment
- Retinal necrosis
- Massive choroidal invasion
- Tumor invasion into the anterior chamber
- Neovascularization of the iris
- Glaucoma
- Recurrence of tumor
- Trilateral retinoblastoma
- Elevated intracranial pressure (ICP)
- Subsequent metastasis
- Complications related to retinoblastoma treatment and these include:
  - The formation of a cataract, can occur as a result of radiation therapy
  - Surgical infection or bleeding
  - Temporal bone hypoplasia
  - Chemotherapy reactions, e.g., nausea, diarrhea, bleeding, and tiredness
  - Spread of the retinoblastoma
  - Loss of vision
  - Secondary neoplasm arising from elsewhere

Prognosis: The overall mortalities from retinoblastoma are between 15 and 20%. Mortality rate is higher with optic nerve involvement, large size tumor, poorly differentiated tumor and when there is choroidal invasion.

If retinoblastoma is left untreated patient is likely to develop the following complications:
- Orbital invasion
- Optic nerve invasion
- Blindness
- Intracranial extension
- Secondary neoplasms
- Metastasis
- Tumor recurrence
- Temporal bone hypoplasia
- Cataract
- Radiation neuropathy
- Radiation retinopathy

DESCRIBE DRUGS USED IN OCULAR DISORDERS *(PH 1.58)*

See page 74

VISUAL LOSS IN THE ELDERLY *(IM 24.15)*

Vision loss is very common in the elderly people. The prevalence of vision loss is increasing as the population ages. When people start to lose their sight they often report difficulty reading small print, cooking, mobility, taking medication and recognising faces. Visual acuity, contrast sensitivity and visual field - all may be affected.

International Classification of Diseases (ICD) 11 (2018) classifies vision loss into **two groups**—visual loss for distance and for the near.

Distance vision impairment:
- Mild—visual acuity worse than 6/12 to 6/18
- Moderate—visual acuity worse than 6/18 to 6/60
- Severe—visual acuity worse than 6/60 to 3/60
- Blindness—visual acuity worse than 3/60

Near vision impairment: Near visual acuity worse than N6 at 40 cm.

Globally, at least 2.2 billion people have a near or distance vision impairment. In at least 1 billion or almost half of these cases, vision impairment could have been prevented or has yet to be addressed.

Globally, the leading causes of visual loss in elderly are:
- Uncorrected refractive errors
- Cataract
- Age-related macular degeneration
- Glaucoma
- Diabetic retinopathy
- Corneal opacity
- Trachoma

Clinical presentation and diagnosis of all these conditions require comprehensive eye heath check-up in elderly people. There are some diseases which are silent, e.g., glaucoma, diabetic retinopathy, ARMD, etc., need routine screening by the eye care professionals at a regular interval.

Sudden onset loss of vision is an ocular emergency and need to be evaluated at a secondary or tertiary eye care centre.

Each eye condition requires a different, timely response. There are effective interventions covering promotion, prevention, treatment and rehabilitation which address the needs associated with eye conditions and vision impairment; some are among the most cost-effective and feasible of all healthcare interventions to implement. For example, uncorrected refractive error can be corrected with spectacles or surgery while cataract surgery can restore vision.

Rehabilitation

Vision impairment severely impacts quality of life among adult populations. Adults with vision impairment often have lower rates of workforce participation and productivity and higher rates of depression and anxiety. In the case of older adults, vision impairment can contribute to social isolation, difficulty walking, a higher risk of falls and fractures, and a greater likelihood of early entry into nursing or care homes.

Vision rehabilitation is very effective in improving functioning for people with an irreversible vision impairment that can be caused by eye conditions such as diabetic retinopathy, glaucoma, consequences of trauma and age-related macular degeneration.

Low-vision Devices

A typical example of low-vision devices is ergonomic, optical, electrical devices, smartphones, tablets, etc. Post-clinical and functional assessment, the low-vision team will comment on whether magnification, minification, voice-over devices can be used to improve vision. Following are of low-vision and speech-output device:

- ❖ Optical/electronic device
- ❖ Stand or handheld magnifiers
- ❖ Closed-circuit television system
- ❖ Handheld monoculars or binoculars
- ❖ Non-optical devices: Large print books, reading stands, lamps, Handwriting implements

Prevention

Ultraviolet light exposure and smoking are associated with accelerated cataract formation. It is reasonable to counsel older patients to reduce their exposure to ultraviolet light when feasible and to stop smoking. Smoking is also linked to an increased risk of vision loss associated with age-related macular degeneration.

CHAPTER 4

Common Eye Instruments

EYE SPECULUMS (FIGS. 4.1A TO C)

The types are — (1) universal eye speculum, (2) guarded eye speculum, and (3) wire speculum.

Universal Eye Speculum (Fig. 4.1A)

Identification: It has a spring and two limbs, and a screw to adjust the limbs. It is called universal because it can be used on either side.

Method: It is fixed to the eyelids in such a way that screw should face outward and forward.

Uses: It is used to separate both eyelids for good exposure of the eyeball mainly during extraocular operations, for example:
- Pterygium excision
- Squint operation
- Evisceration or enucleation
- Debridement and scraping of corneal ulcer
- To give subconjunctival or sub-Tenon's injection
- Removal of corneal foreign body
- Removal of conjunctival cyst or mass
- During suture removal

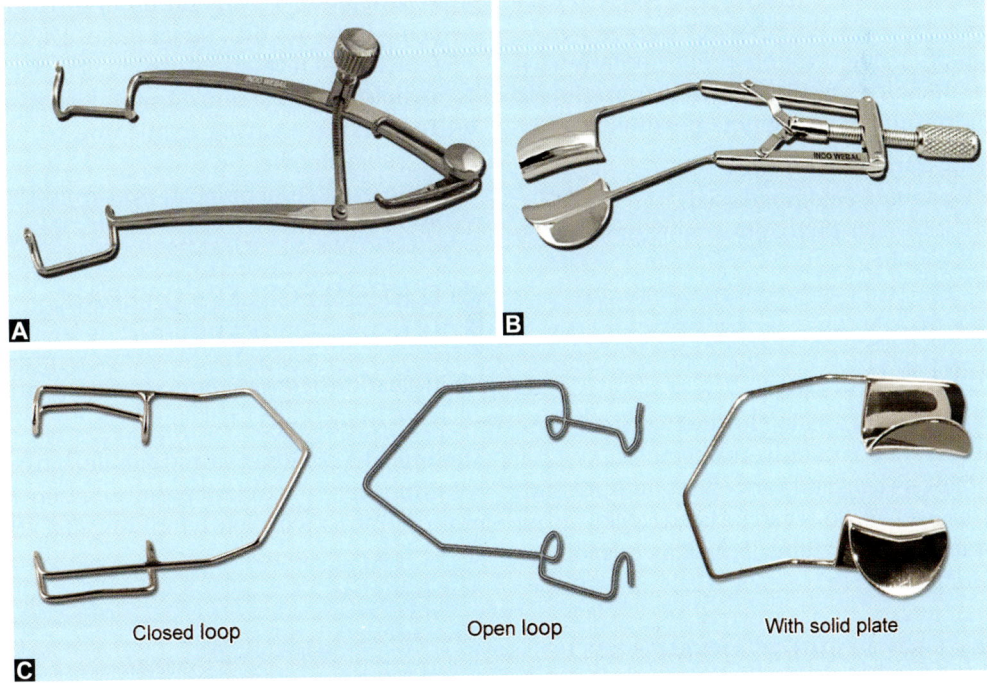

Figs. 4.1A to C: (A) Universal eye speculum; (B) Guarded eye speculum; (C) Wire speculum.

It is not used routinely in intraocular operations as it gives pressure over the globe. This causes rise in intraocular pressure (IOP) during surgery. One can put a cotton pellet or assistant can lift the instrument during intraocular operation to avoid rise in IOP.

Disadvantages
- Since it has no guard, eyelashes of upper lid (larger) come in the field of operation.
- Not used in intraocular operation because of more vitreous-upthrust and risk of vitreous loss by direct pressure on the globe.

The speculum should not be confused with Muller's retractor, which has got two or three right-angle sharp pointed pins (teeth) underneath to engage the skin flap.

Guarded Eye Speculum (Fig. 4.1B)

Identification: The upper limb of the speculum is having a guard plate which keeps the eyelashes of the upper lid away from the field of operation. So, two instruments are required, one for the right eye and the other for the left eye.

Uses: Same as universal eye speculum. It is especially useful in squint operation in children and in pterygium operation.

Disadvantages:
- Operating field is reduced.
- It is heavier, hence gives more pressure on the globe.

BARRAQUER'S WIRE SPECULUM (FIG. 4.1C)

It is made up of a stainless-steel wire and there is no screw. It is of universal type.

It is very light and hence gives little pressure on the eyeball. So, it can be used safely during intraocular operations as well as extraocular operation.

ARTERY FORCEPS (HEMOSTAT) (FIG. 4.2)

Identification: This is a medium-sized, fully serrated forceps with catch. It may be straight

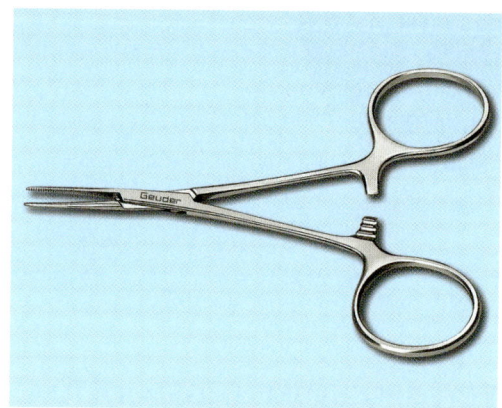

Fig. 4.2: Artery forceps (hemostat).

or curved. The curved forceps are used more frequently.

Uses:
- Used as needle holder for passing superior rectus bridal suture
- To crush lateral canthus in lateral canthotomy.
- For hemostasis during DCR or DCT, especially if the angular vein is damaged.
- Fasanella-Servat operation of ptosis (to clamp conjunctiva, tarsal plate, Muller's muscle and levator muscle).
- To hold muscle stump during enucleation.
- To make irrigating cystitome from a 26-gauge needle.
- To hold whole lacrimal sac prior to excision of sac in DCT.

FIXATION FORCEPS (EYEBALL FIXATION FORCEPS) (FIG. 4.3)

Identification: It is a medium size forceps with 2:3 teeth (may be 3:4) at its tip.

Method: The conjunctiva and episcleral tissue are firmly held at 6 o'clock position within 3–4 mm of limbus with left hand. Because, the

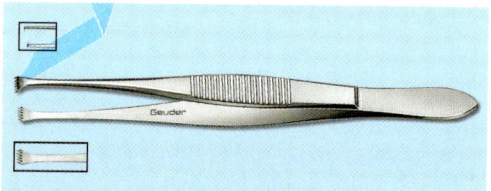

Fig. 4.3: Fixation forceps.

conjunctiva is firmly adhere to episcleral tissue and sclera around the limbus, and it is 4–5 layers thick. It may be used at other part around the limbus (e.g., 3 o'clock, 9 o'clock, etc.).

Uses:
- To fix the eyeball during operative procedures, like:
  - Cataract surgery
  - Paracentesis
  - Pterygium surgery,
  - Needling, etc.
- To catch superior rectus muscle to pass bridle suture.
- To catch other tissues, e.g., skin, Tenon's capsule, etc.
- To lift bulbar conjunctiva during sub-conjunctival or sub-Tenon injection.
- Used in forced duction test (FDT) in case of squint to know any mechanical restriction is present or not.
- To hold the sponge piece, gauze piece or cotton ball for swabbing.

SCALPEL HANDLE (BARD PARKER HANDLE) (FIG. 4.4)

Identification: It is a flat handle with a short, grooved neck. Handle No. 3 is used in ophthalmic surgeries. The blades are fitted with the neck is No. 11 or No. 15 (No. 11 is triangular blade and No. 15 has curved elliptical tip).

Method: In cataract operation. The knife is held in pen holding position. Eyeball is fixed with fixation forceps. A groove (partial thickness) is made at the limbus with the knife (preferable with No. 15 blade). A puncture is made at 11–12 o'clock position to enter into the anterior chamber (preferably with 'No. 11' blade). Posterior or scleral lip is depressed to drain aqueous very slowly. Then the section is enlarged with the corneal scissors.

Uses:
- Ab externo corneoscleral section for cataract surgery.
- Trabeculectomy operation for making scleral flap.

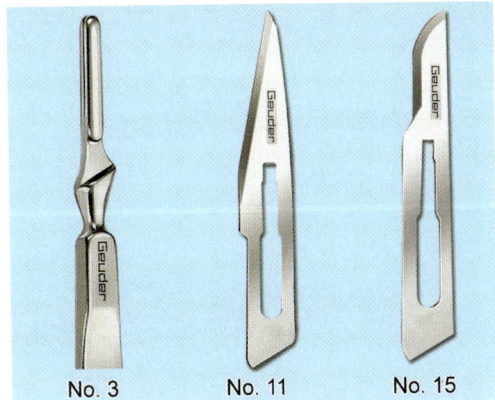

Fig. 4.4: Scalpel handle and blades.

- Skin incision as in DCR, ptosis or other lid surgeries.
- To dissect the pterygium head from the cornea.
- To give incision in chalazion operation.
- For suture removal after cataract operation or keratoplasty.
- Advantages in cataract operation
- It is a 'guarded' section. As there is slow release of aqueous, the chance of quick decompression of the globe is almost nil.
- It is 'stepped', i.e., biplaner or triplaner incision—so wound security is better.
- Easier for the beginners.

Disadvantages:
- Conjunctival flap is usually necessary before giving section.
- It is time consuming.

BLADE BREAKER (FIGS. 4.5A TO C)

Identification: It is an instrument to break the razor blade (must be a carbon-steel blade, e.g., 'Bharat' blade). It is of medium size, with two jaw-like plates at its tip to catch the razor blade firmly. The other end of the instrument is having catch for better grip of the blade. At least eight blade-fragments can be made from a single razor blade.

Advantages:
- It is cheaper than any other knife-blade.
- It is sharper than No. '11' or No. '15' blade.

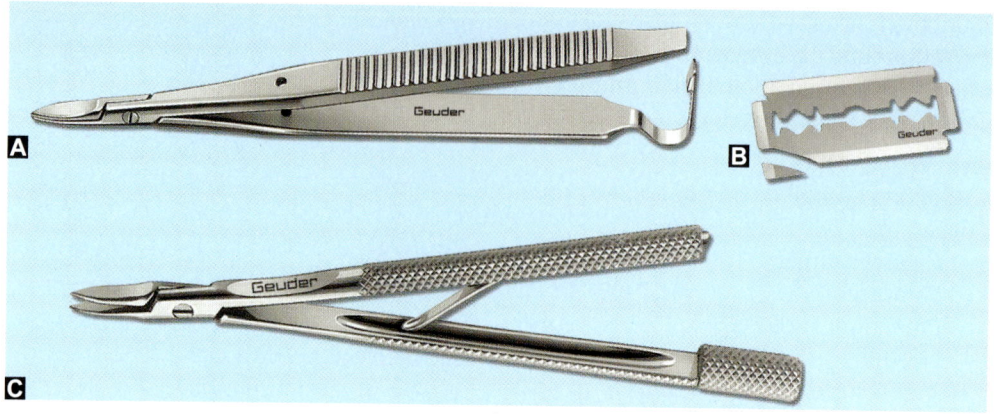

Figs. 4.5A to C: (A and B) Carbon-steel blade; (C) Blade breaker.

Disadvantages: As only the breakable carbon-steel razor blade is used—rust formation is a problem.

Uses: Blade breaker with razor blade-fragments is having the same uses as Bard Parker handle with knife.

(Instruments used for corneoscleral section are: (a) Bard Parker knife, (b) Blade breaker with razor blade, (c) Disposable keratome, (d) Sapphire or diamond knife and (e) Femtosecond laser.

THERMOCAUTERY (HEAT CAUTERY) (FIG. 4.6)

Identification: It is a metallic ball with pointed tip, attached to the end of a handle. The ball is made up of steel or brass (*brass retains heat for a longer time*).

Method: The metallic ball is heated over the flame of a spirit lamp before cauterization. When it is sufficiently hot, the pointed tip is applied to the bleeding points for hemostasis.

Uses: To cauterize any superficial bleeding points during operation on the eyeball (e.g., in cataract operation and glaucoma operation after making the conjunctival flap).

- To cauterize the bare scleral area in pterygium surgery.
- To cauterize the margin of a progressive corneal ulcer.
- To cauterize small iris prolapse.
- Temporary punctal occlusion.

Advantages: It is cheap and easily available.

Disadvantages:
- As the application of heat is not uniform—there may be more tissue charring at the beginning of cautery.
- More tissue charring may excite more tissue reaction.

The best method of hemostasis is by **wet field cautery** (*Hemostatic eraser*) or diathermy where the hemostasis is uniform; and tissue charring and reaction are minimal.

CORNEAL SPRING SCISSORS (UNIVERSAL) (FIGS. 4.7A AND B)

Identification: It is a small, curved spring scissors with sharp small blade It is called universal, as it is used to cut both right and left half of the section.

ote

Right sided corneal scissors mean to cut right half of the section and left sided for left half of the section. In case of universal scissors to cut the right half of the section, surgeon must use his left hand and to cut the left half, use right hand. But those who are no proficient with the left hand—they use right and left corneal scissors, and both are operated by right hand.

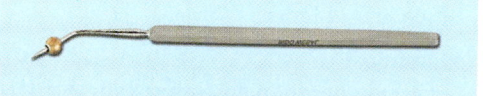

Fig. 4.6: Thermocautery.

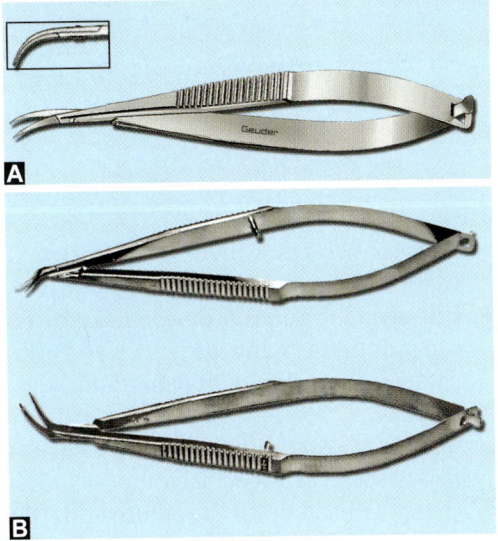

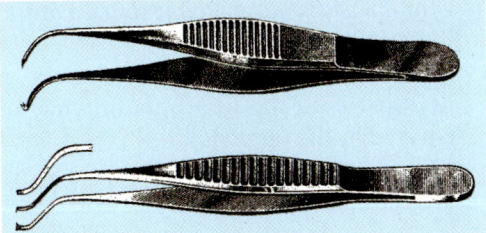

Fig. 4.8: Iris forceps.

Figs. 4.7A and B: (A) Corneal spring scissors (universal); (B) Corneal scissors—right and left sided.

Method: In case of cataract surgery, after making corneoscleral groove and entering into AC, one blade of the scissors is introduced into the anterior chamber, the other blade is being outside. Scissors are held in pen holding position, and with small snips, the section is enlarged on either side for 120–160°. Left hand is used for making right half of the section.

Uses:
- To extend 'ab-externo' section in cataract operation.
- To cut the corneal button from the donor and recipient eyes in case of keratoplasty.
- It may be used to cut the 8-0 suture ends.
- It may be used to cut the iris for iridectomy.
- To make conjunctival flap in cataract or trabeculectomy surgery.

IRIS FORCEPS (FIG. 4.8)

Identification: It is a small light-weight forceps with 1:2 teeth on the inner side of its tips. The shape of the forceps may be straight, curved or angular.

Method of iridectomy:
- Enter into the AC with close tips and touch the peripheral iris.
- Open the forceps a little to catch a pinch of iris tissue and take out as a triangular fold of iris outside the section.
- Cut a small triangular piece of iris tissue radially with de-Wecker's scissors or Vannas scissors.
- Always check the severed iris tissue by rubbing it over the drape.
  This is to see the pigmented layer has cut or not, i.e., if there is release of pigment—it means iridectomy has done in full thickness.

Uses: To grasp the iris—tissue in various types of iridectomies.

There is usually *no bleeding during iridectomy* as iris vessels are highly contractile. Iridectomy is avoided in case of diabetic cataract and rubeosis iridis as there may be chance of bleeding.

Types of iridectomy with indications:
1. Peripheral iridectomy (at 11 or 1 o'clock position)—indications are:
   - Angle closure glaucoma.
   - As a part of trabeculectomy operation and
   - Sometimes, in penetrating keratoplasty operation.
   - In intracapsular cataract extraction with anterior chamber IOL.
   - At *6 o'clock position*—in vitreoretinal surgery and endothelial keratoplasty (DMEK or DSEK)

   Peripheral iridectomy is done to prevent pupillary block glaucoma. It is not mandatory in extracapsular cataract extraction (ECCE, manual SICS or phacoemulsification).
2. **Optical iridectomy:** In case of central corneal opacity where the facility for

keratoplasty is not available or it is contraindicated.
3. It is done in the lower part of the iris, as in upper part, the new opening may be covered by the upper lid.
4. **Broad or complete iridectomy:** To facilitate the extraction of lens (when pupil is small and rigid, or if there is extensive synechiae, and may be in presence of pseudoexfoliation.
5. **Iridectomy for prolapsed iris.**
6. **Iridectomy to remove tumor or cyst of the iris.**

Iridotomy: Puncture of the iris without abscission of any portion.

YAG laser-peripheral iridotomy (YAG-PI): Is better to prevent acute angle-closure glaucoma as it is noninvasive (so, no chance of infection) OPD procedure. It is also less expensive for the patient.

Others:
- To create an artificial pupil when the true pupil is closed or severely up drawn.
- '4-point iridotomy' is done by a von Graefe's cataract knife to treat secondary glaucoma in iris bombe'.

DE-WECKER'S IRIS SCISSORS (FIG. 4.9)

Identification: It is a butterfly-shaped spring scissors with the cutting blades bent at an angle of 60° with the handle. On the handle, there are two wings for index finger and thumb. Its one blade has pointed tip and the other blade has rounded tip.

Method: Scissors is held in such a way that the plane of blade lies at the same plane as of iris, whereas the handle is almost vertical.

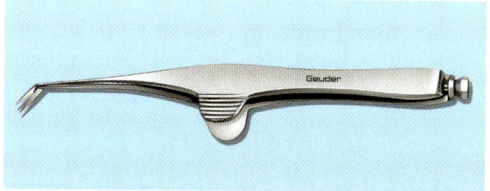

Fig. 4.9: De-Wecker's iris scissors.

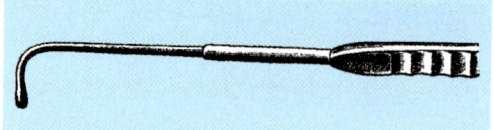

Fig. 4.10: Lens expressor (hook).

Uses:
- It is used to cut a piece of iris tissue in iridectomy.
- It is used for anterior or open-sky vitrectomy, if there is any vitreous loss during cataract extraction or in penetrating keratoplasty.
- It is used to cut the trabecular tissue with a part of sclera in trabeculectomy operation.
- It may be used to cut the suture ends (8-0 or 10-0 sutures) during corneoscleral suturing.

LENS EXPRESSOR (LENS HOOK) (FIG. 4.10)

Identification: It has a flat corrugated handle with a curved, olive-pointed blunt tip. The plane of the flatness of the handle is perpendicular to the plane of curvature of the limb.

Uses:
- In case of extracapsular cataract operation—to deliver the nucleus.
- It may be used to hook the extraocular muscles.
- It may also be used as a tissue retractor, particularly in DCR operation to retract the sac during punching or breaking the bone.
- Rarely for intracapsular extraction of the lens, either by intracapsular forceps or by Smith-Indian technique.

IRIS REPOSITOR (FIG. 4.11)

Identification: It is an elongated 'S' or 'Z'-shaped instrument with a stout handle and two long narrow flattened extremities. Both the edges and tips are blunt. Its one end may be curved, and another end may be angulated.

Method: A few strokes over the peripheral iris on its upper part is required to reposit the iris.

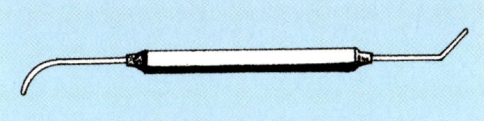

Fig. 4.11: Iris repositor.

When the iris properly repositioned, the pupil becomes perfectly circular and central.

Uses:
- To reposit the iris after the delivery of lens nucleus in ECCE.
- To reposit the iris after iridectomy.
- To bring air from posterior chamber to anterior chamber.
- To break the adhesions in synechiae (synechiolysis).
- To bring back the folded conjunctiva to cover the wound.
- Lamellar dissection of the cornea in lamellar keratoplasty.

Precaution: Iridectomy site should be avoided during repositioning of the iris. If reposition is not done properly there may be:
- Iris incarceration at the wound
- Prolapse of the iris
- Chance of infection
- Gaping of the wound
- Non-reformation of the anterior chamber.

NEEDLE HOLDER (BARRAQUER'S AND CASTROVIEJO'S) (FIGS. 4.12A AND B)

Identification: It is a medium-sized spring needle holder with two narrow and fine curved jaws. It may be available with or without a catch.

Uses:
Barraquer's—used to hold fine needles (of 8-0 to 10-0 sutures) for:
- Corneoscleral suturing after cataract operation.
- Scleral suturing in squint, detachment and trabeculectomy operation
- Corneal suturing in keratoplasty and open globe injuries.
- Suturing the mucosal flaps in DCR operation.
- Sometimes in conjunctival suturing.

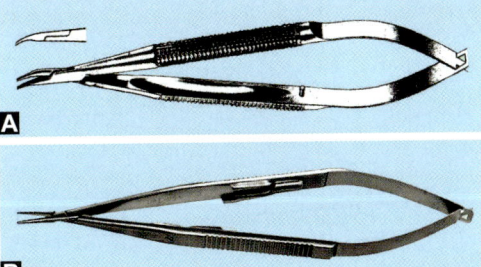

Figs. 4.12A and B: Needle holder. (A) Barraquer's; (B) Castreveijo's.

Castroviejo's—is required to hold slightly larges needles (of 4-0 to 6-0 sutures) for conjunctival suturing as in squint, glaucoma, pterygium or retinal detachment.

COLIBRI FORCEPS (FIG. 4.13A)

Identification: It is a curved or angular forceps with fine limbs, having 1:2 teeth at its tip. It is thicker and stout.

ST. MARTIN'S FORCEPS (FIG. 4.13B)

Identification: It is a straight small but stout forceps with 1:2 teeth at its' fine tip.

LIM'S SCLEROCORNEAL FORCEPS (FIG. 4.13C)

Identification: It is small, lightweight forceps, with 1:2 teeth at the end of curved tip and serrated thumb rest.

Uses: All three instruments have similar uses:
- To hold limbal tissue/sclera for fixing the globe
- To hold corneal or scleral lip during suturing as in cataract surgery, corneal tear repair, in keratoplasty, etc.
- To hold the scleral lip for dissection and scleral suturing (as in trabeculectomy).
- To catch the iris tissue for iridectomy.

SUPERIOR RECTUS HOLDING FORCEPS (FIG. 4.14)

Identification: It is a stout forceps with double curvature (S-shaped) at its ends. It has 1:2 teeth

Chapter 4: Common Eye Instruments

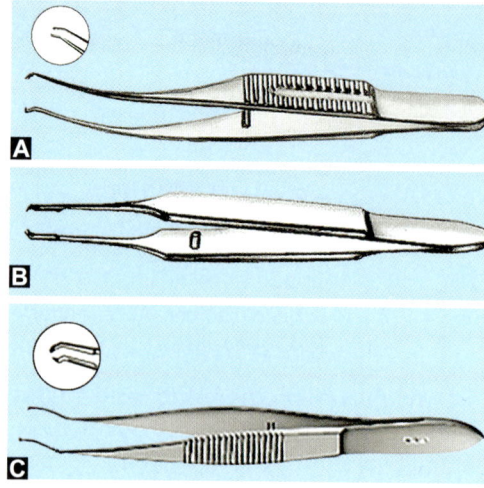

Figs. 4.13A to C: (A) Colibri forceps; (B) St. Martin's forceps; (C) Lim's forceps.

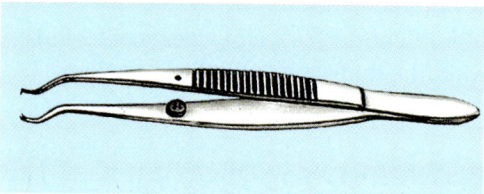

Fig. 4.14: Superior rectus holding forceps.

at its tip. Its curvature at the tip is to fit with the curvature of the globe.

Uses: It is used to catch the superior rectus muscle belly for passing stay (bridle) suture, so that the eyeball can be rotated and fixed downwards in cataract, glaucoma or other surgery.

SUTURE TYING FORCEPS (FIG. 4.15)

Identification: It is a small straight or curved forceps with long fine limbs. It does not have any tooth at its tip. The tips are made stout by extra thick platform.

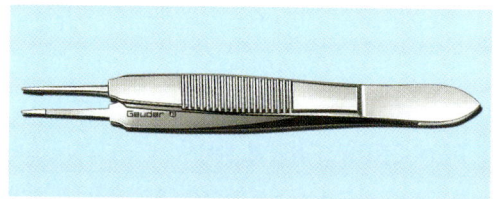

Fig. 4.15: Suture tying forceps.

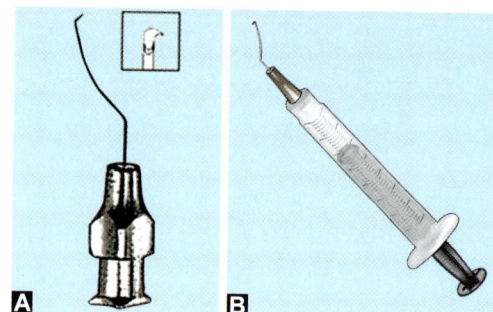

Figs. 4.16A and B: (A) 26-G cystitome; (B) BSS filled 2 mL syringe with needle cystitome.

Uses:
- To hold the suture ends during tying the sutures.
- To hold the cut ends of the suture during its removal.
- To remove caterpillar hair.

CYSTITOME OR CAPSULOTOME (FIGS. 4.16A AND B)

It is made from disposable 26-G needle. The tip is bent 60–90° with a needle holder opposite to the beveled side. The body of the needle is also bent about 45° at the junction of shaft.

Uses: The bent-tipped 26 gauze needle is fitted with a 2 mL syringe. The syringe is filled with balanced salt solution (BSS) or Ringer's lactate to keep the anterior chamber well formed during needle manipulation. The capsule is cut with the bent tip of the needle in a continuous curvilinear capsulorhexis (CCC), or by interrupted multiple punctures for 'Can-opener' capsulotomy.

CAPSULORHEXIS FORCEPS (UTARATA FORCEPS) (FIG. 4.17)

Identification: It is a fine long forceps with curved sharp tip without any tooth.

Uses:
- To perform continuous curvilinear capsulorhexis (CCC) in manual SICS or in phacoemulsification.

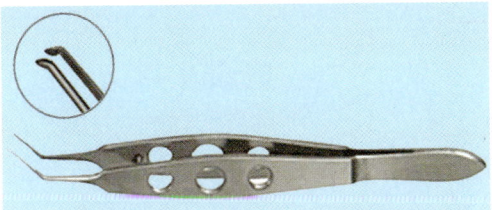

Fig. 4.17: Capsulorhexis forceps (Utrata).

- The initiation of rhexis is started with cystitome, and then completed with the rhexis forceps, or it may be with the rhexis forceps alone.
- It may be used to remove small capsular tag.

IRRIGATING VECTIS (FIG. 4.18)

Identification: It is a hollow vectis fitted with a needle base. Its tip has 3–5 small openings for free passage of irrigating solution. The maximum horizontal diameter of the vectis is 5.0–5.5 mm.

Use: The vectis is connected with the tubing system of a Ringer's lactate or BSS bottle, or it may be fitted with a Ringer's lactate or BSS filled 2 mL syringe during nucleus delivery.

The irrigating fluid creates hydrostatic pressure and at the same time mechanical pull by the vectis is to deliver the nucleus out. Posterior scleral lip depression and simultaneous counter balancing force by S/R bridle suture are the important steps during nucleus delivery.

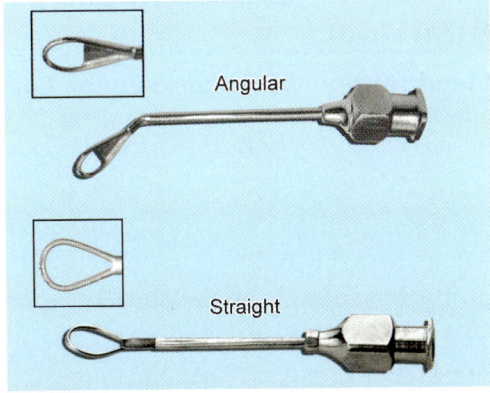

Fig. 4.18: Irrigating vectis.

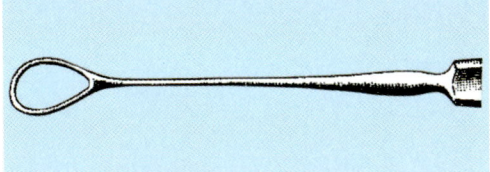

Fig. 4.19: Wire vectis.

VECTIS (WIRE VECTIS) (FIG. 4.19)

Identification: It is a ring of wire (round or oval) at the end of a narrow limb, attached to a handle (like a large platinum loop). It may be little curved like a spoon.

Methods: Pupil must be fully dilated. The lens edge should be visible. Carefully pass the vectis behind the lens. Lift the lens and then take the lens out. Vitreous loss is inevitable in vectis delivery in case of ICCE.

Uses:
- To remove a subluxated or dislocated lens.
- To deliver the lens nucleus in ECCE (better with irrigating vectis).

IRRIGATION-ASPIRATION CANNULA (SIMCOE) (FIG. 4.20)

Identification: It is a two-way cannula, one end of which is attached to a blunt needle via a silicone tube. Normally, this end is fitted with an irrigation or infusion system and the two-way cannula itself is fitted with a 2 mL or 5 mL syringe for aspiration.

Method: After delivery of the nucleus in ECCE, the cannula in introduced into the anterior chamber. The infusion is slowly started either from a hanging Ringer's lactate or BSS bottle. As the anterior chamber is formed, the surgeon starts aspirating cortical material slowly till the posterior capsule is cleaned (as appreciated by brilliant fundal glow under coaxial illumination of the operative microscope).

Uses:
- For simultaneous irrigation and aspiration of cortical materials in case of ECCE or ECCE with PCIOL.

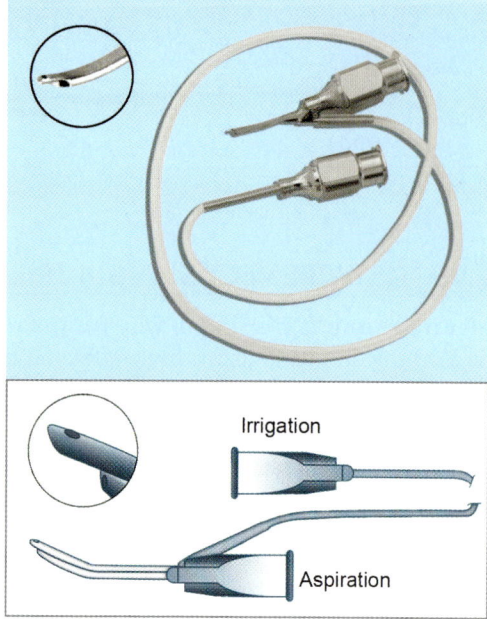

Fig. 4.20: Irrigation-aspiration two-way cannula (Simcoe cannula).

- To remove viscoelastic material after insertion of IOL.
- May be used to remove blood in hyphema or pus in hypopyon.

McPHERSON'S FORCEPS (FIG. 4.21)

Identification: It is a fine medium size toothless forceps with an angulation at about 7–8 mm from its tip.

Uses:
- It is used to hold the IOL during its placement in the capsular bag or sulcus or in the anterior chamber.
- It is used to catch and remove the loose anterior capsule after completion of capsulotomy.

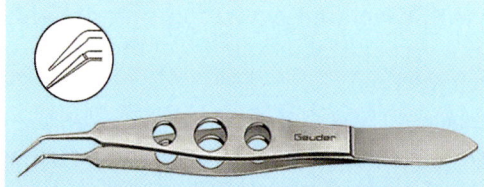

Fig. 4.21: McPherson's forceps.

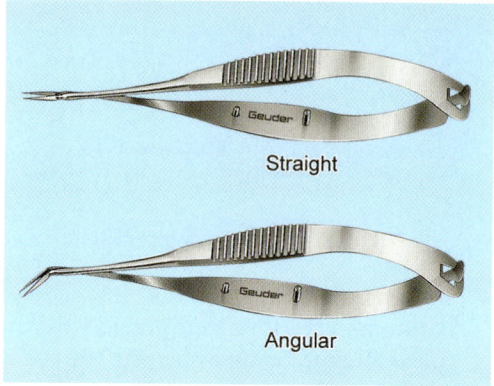

Fig. 4.22: Vannas' scissors.

- It may be used as a suture tier during suturing with 10-0 nylon.

VANNAS' SCISSORS (FIG. 4.22)

Identification: It is much smaller scissors with spring action. It may be straight, curved or angular.

Uses:
- To cut 10-0 sutures in cataract or keratoplasty operation.
- To prepare fine conjunctival graft as in pterygium autograft.
- To cut trabecular flap in trabeculectomy.
- To cut anterior capsular tags in ECCE.
- To cut vitreous in open-sky vitrectomy, as in vitreous loss during ICCE or ECCE and keratoplasty.
- To cut iris in different types of iridectomy.

IOL DIALER (SINSKY'S HOOK) (FIG. 4.23)

Identification: It is an angular fine hook attached to a long round solid handle.

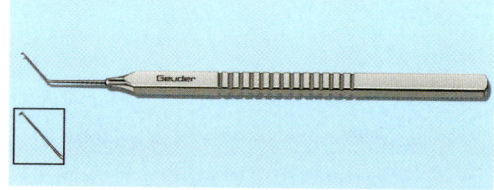

Fig. 4.23: IOL dialler (Sinsky's hook).

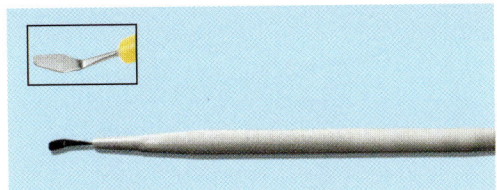

Fig. 4.24: Crescent knife.

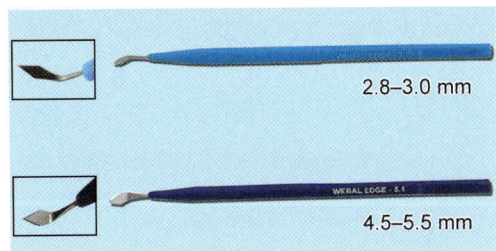

Fig. 4.25: Angular keratome.

Methods and uses:
- To dial the IOL for proper placement in-the-bag or in sulcus and for centration. The hook is positioned in the dialing holes of the PMMA IOL optic, and then to rotate in a clockwise manner.
- Used as a left-hand instrument during phacoemulsification in softer cataract:
  - For nucleus rotation
  - For breaking the lens nucleus after trenching
  - As a chopper
- May be used to break the posterior synechiae in cataract surgery

CRESCENT KNIFE (SCLERO-CORNEAL SPLITTER) (FIG. 4.24)

Identification: It has a thin crescentic blade, at the end of a neck and attached to a polycarbonate handle. The cutting-edge of the blade may be beveled-up or beveled-down. The blade has a forward angulation of 45° for better and parallel movement during dissection.

It is available as a disposable blade in pre-sterile pack. It may be reused for 3–4 times after ETO sterilization.

Uses:
- To make sclerocorneal tunnel in manual SICS
- For lamellar dissection of the cornea in lamellar keratoplasty.
- For partial thickness scleral flap or for fine limbal dissection

ANGULAR KERATOME (FIG. 4.25)

Identification: It has a thin triangular blade, at the end of neck and attached to a polycarbonate handle. The cutting-edge of the blade may be beveled-up or beveled-down. The blade has a forward angulation of 45° for better and parallel movement during dissection. The width of the blade may be 1.8–3.0 mm diameter (for phacoemulsification) or 4.5–5.5 mm for manual SICS.

It is also available as a disposable blade in pre-sterile pack.

Uses:
- Used for making corneal/limbal section in phacoemulsification.
- Used to enter into the anterior chamber after making sclerocorneal tunnel in manual SICS or phacoemulsification.
- 4.5–5.5 mm diameter keratome is used to enlarge SICS tunnel.

SIDE-PORT BLADE (FIG. 4.26)

Identification: It has a thin, long straight blade (15° angle), at the end of a neck and attached to a polycarbonate handle. The maximum width of the blade is to pass a 20 G needle.

It is available as a disposable blade in pre-sterile pack.

Uses: To make the side port (to enter into the anterior chamber from the sides of main incision) in cataract surgery.

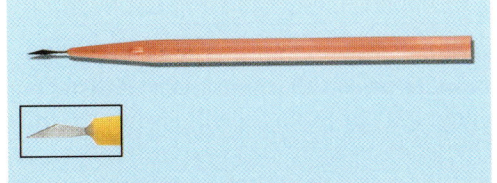

Fig. 4.26: Side-port blade.

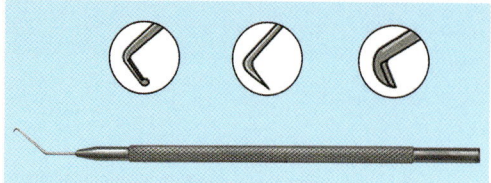

Fig. 4.27: Phaco chopper.

- Indication of side-port in cataract surgey:
  - To inject viscoelastic substance.
  - To inject trypan blue dye.
  - To clean sub-incisional lens cortex by IA cannula.
  - To manipulate second instrument. (Sometimes, two side-ports are given on either side for bimanual irrigation and aspiration.
  - To insert the anterior chamber maintainer.
- To inject/titrate BSS and air for donor manipulation in endothelial keratoplasty.
- For paracentesis to drain blood in hyphema.
- To remove small intracameral foreign body.

PHACO CHOPPER (FIG. 4.27)

Identification: Solid round handle fixed to long fine limb with an angulation at the distal part. The tip is bet at 90° and the inner edge of the tip has sharp cutting edge (*sharp chopper*). Inner edge may be blunt (called *blunt chopper*).

Uses: It acts as a second instrument to manipulate the nucleus during phacoemulsification. It is mainly used to split or crack the nucleus into multiple small fragments.

PHACO HANDPIECE WITH CONNECTING CORD (FIG. 4.28)

Identification: Cylindrical metal body (like a fountain pen) with a short neck at distal end where the phaco tip (needle) is fitted tightly. The proximal end has two ports—one for irrigation and the other for aspiration. The electric cord at the proximal end connects the hand piece with the phaco machine (console).

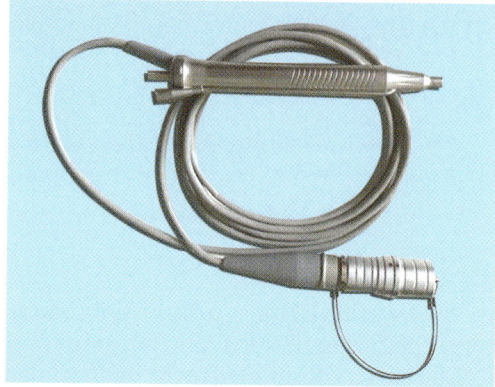

Fig. 4.28: Phaco handpiece with connecting cord.

Irrigation and aspiration system are also connected to the machine.

Uses: Nucleus emulsification and aspiration of nucleus material during phaco procedure. It also emulsifies and aspirate epi-nucleus after that.

EPILATION FORCEPS (CILIA FORCEPS) (FIGS. 4.29A AND B)

Identification: It is a small stout forceps with blunt flat ends. The inner surfaces of the tip are reinforced by extra thick platform which may be rhomboidal or elliptical.

Uses:
- To remove the offending, misdirected eyelashes in trichiasis.
- To remove the involved eyelash in stye.
  Topical anesthesia may be required for epilation. It is not a permanent and ideal procedure. As the root is not destroyed, eyelash grows again within 6–8 weeks and causes same problem.

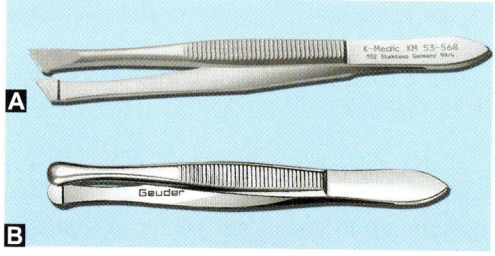

Figs. 4.29A and B: (A) Rhomboidal tip; (B) Elliptical tip.

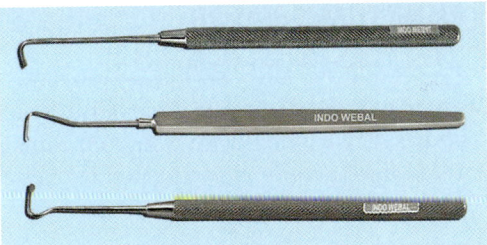

Fig. 4.30: Strabismus hooks.

Ideal method should be permanent where the hair-root is destroyed.

Ideal methods are:
- **Electrolysis:** Anesthesia is required. A fine needle (the negative pole) is introduced into the hair follicle and a current of 2 mAmp is passed. End point is noted by appearance of foam.
- **Electro-diathermy:** A current of 30 mAmp is applied for 10 seconds.
- **Cryosurgery:** Pigmentation is a problem.
- If more than 1/3rd lid margin is involved—partial entropion correction operation is a better choice.

STRABISMUS HOOK (MUSCLE OR SQUINT HOOK) (FIG. 4.30)

Identification: It has a solid handle with a long narrow limb with 90° bent at its tip. The tip may be sharp or knobbed. The handle is not corrugated and the plane of curvature of the limb is same as the plane of handle.

Uses:
- It is used to hook the extraocular muscles during:
  - Squint operation
  - Retinal detachment (buckle) operation
  - Enucleation operation
- It may be used as a tissue retractor

LID RETRACTOR (DESMARRE'S) (FIG. 4.31)

Identification: It is a saddle-shaped folded instrument at the end of a metallic handle. It is of varying size depending upon the size of the palpebral aperture. It is not self-retaining.

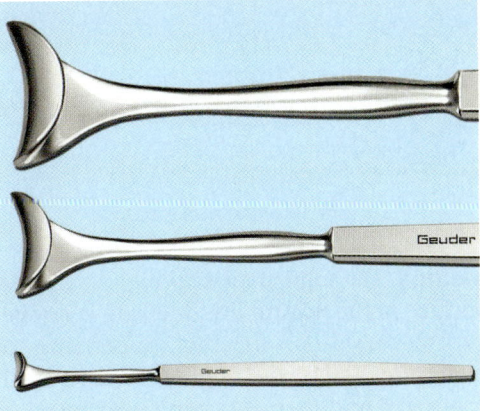

Fig. 4.31: Desmarre's lid retractor.

Method (for children):
- Patient is made to lie on the table and an assistant must fix his head.
- Anesthetic eye drop is instilled.
- Lid retractor is applied from the temporal side sliding against the eyeball.
- Upper lid is retracted, and the eye is examined.
- As the lower lid can be easily retracted by finger, lower lid retractor is not necessary. In children and in severe blepharospasm, two retractors are needed.

Uses:
- Used for examination of conjunctiva and anterior segment:
  - In children and non-cooperative patient
  - In case of severe blepharospasm and photophobia
  - In case of lid edema
- To examine upper fornix by double eversion of the lid.
- It may be used as a tissue retractor (e.g., to retract conjunctiva and Tenon's capsule in squint and retinal detachment operation).

CHALAZION FORCEPS (CLAMP) (FIG. 4.32)

Identification: It is a forceps with a large screw for fixing and tightening the limbs like a clamp. One limb has a solid disc-shaped plate, and the other limb has a ring at its end. It is hemostatic and self-retaining.

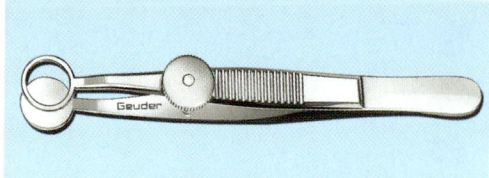

Fig. 4.32: Chalazion forceps.

Method: The solid plate is applied on the skin surface of the lid and the ring side is applied on the tarsal conjunctiva, encircling the chalazion. The screw is tightened, and the lid is everted and then chalazion is exposed for incision.

Uses:
- To fix the chalazion for surgery and also to ensure hemostasis.
- To give intralesional steroids injection in chalazion
- Excision of a small granuloma or papilloma of the lid.

CHALAZION SCOOP (CURETTE) (FIG. 4.33)

Identification: It is a small scoop with sharp edge, attached to a handle. The size of the scoop may vary. Two different sized scoops may be attached to ends of same handle.

Uses: To scoop out the granulation tissue after giving incision on chalazion. Scooping of the chalazion must be complete, otherwise there may be chance of recurrence.

After removal of the chalazion forceps, the bleeding is controlled by pressure over the lid, against the incised area. A pressure bandage is applied for few hours with antibiotic ointment.

PUNCTUM DILATOR (NETTLESHIP'S) (FIG. 4.34)

Identification: It is a long narrow solid cylindrical instrument with a smooth conical pointed tip. Its body is corrugated for better gripping with thumb and index finger.

Uses:
- To dilate the punctum and part of the canaliculus before introducing lacrimal cannula for syringing.
- To dilate the punctum for probing in case of congenital dacryocystitis.
- To dilate the punctum and then probing to identify lacrimal sac during DCR operation.
- For dilatation of the punctum in congenital or acquired punctal stenosis.
- Before dacryocystography (DCG).

Method of syringing:
- Anesthetize the eye with 4% lignocaine or 1% proparacaine drop.
- Pull the lower lid and identify the lower punctum in bright light.
- Hold the punctum dilator vertically by right index and thumb and place it on the punctal opening.
- Twist it with light pressure and introduce into the punctum.
- Then hold the punctum dilator horizontally and push it medially by rotatory movement—following the course of the canaliculus (first vertically then horizontally). Then withdraw it.
- Take the lacrimal cannula, fitted in a syringe, filled with distilled water and introduce it in the same direction.
- Push the piston of the syringe to inject water into the canaliculus and ask the

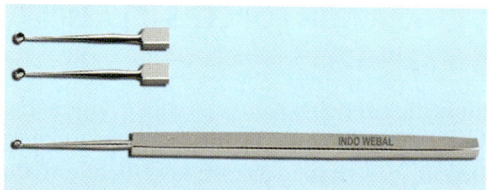

Fig. 4.33: Chalazion scoop.

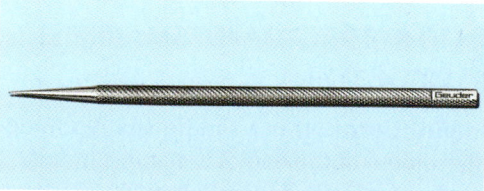

Fig. 4.34: Punctum dilator.

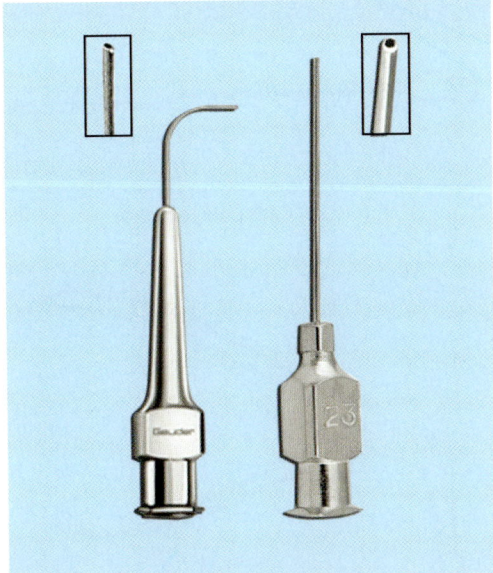

Fig. 4.35: Lacrimal cannula.

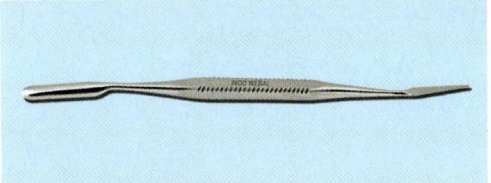

Fig. 4.36: Lacrimal dissector with scoop.

patient about water has reached the throat or not. Alternatively, note the swallowing movement of the neck.
* In case of obstruction, note fluid regurgitation from same or the upper punctum.

LACRIMAL CANNULA (FIG. 4.35)

Identification: It is a small straight angulated or curved cannula with blunt tip. It can be fitted to any syringe.

Method: Same as punctum dilator.

Uses:
* Syringing or patency test of the lacrimal passage.
* For dacryocystography (DCG).
* During probing and syringing in congenital dacryocystoitis.
* Postoperatively, it is used to check the patency after DCR operation.

LACRIMAL DISSECTOR WITH SCOOP (LANG'S) (FIG. 4.36)

Identification: It is a narrow long instrument with a stout pointed dissector at one end, and the other end is having an elongated scoop.

Uses:
* **Dissector end:**
  ▹ It is used for blunt dissection of lacrimal sac after giving skin incision (both in DCT and DCR operation).
  ▹ It is used to clean the bone pieces from the punch, while punching or cutting the bone of DCR.
* **Scoop end:** To scoop out the tissue remnants by scraping from the upper end of bony NLD after excision of the lacrimal sac (only in DCT).

ROUGINE (FIG. 4.37)

Identification: It is rectangular blade attached hy a narrow neck to a corrugated handle. The blade is sharp at its distal end, which is beveled on one surface, the other surface being plane. Basically, it is a small periosteal elevator.

Uses:
* To dissect and disinsert the medial palpebral ligament to find out cleavage between lacrimal sac and the lacrimal fossa.
* Dissection of the lacrimal sac from the medial wall and the floor of the lacrimal fossa, by separating the periosteal tissue surrounding the sac.
  It is used both in DCT and DCR operation.

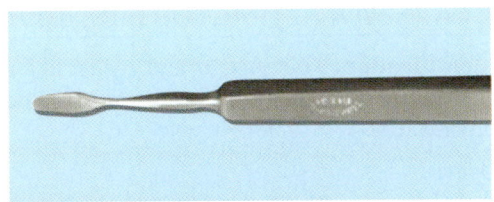

Fig. 4.37: Rougine.

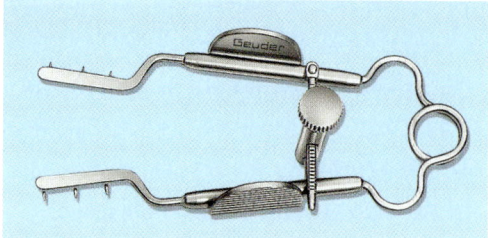

Fig. 4.38: Muller's retractor.

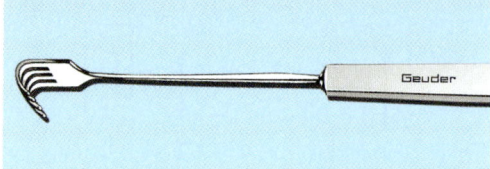

Fig. 4.39: Cat's paw retractor.

MULLER'S RETRACTOR (FIG. 4.38)

Identification: It is made up of two limbs with a screw to fix the limbs in a retracted position. Each limb has got two or three right-angled curved pointed hooks (pins) for engaging the incised edges of the skin and deeper tissues.

Uses: To retract the incised edges of the skin and deeper tissues during DCT and DCR operations.

Its hemostatic effect is due to angled hooks causing compression of the blood vessels by the spring action of the retractor.

This instrument has disadvantage of reducing field of operation. Instead, one can pass 3 deep stay sutures on each skin-edge of incision to achieve retraction and hemostasis.

The complications may occur during giving incision to the skin are:
- Injury to the angular vein
- Cutting the medial palpebral ligament
- Injury to the lacrimal sac inadvertently.

The structures cut to reach the lacrimal sac proper are:
- Skin
- Subcutaneous tissue
- Few fibers of orbicularis oculi
- Medial palpebral ligament
- Anterior lacrimal fascia.

CAT'S PAW RETRACTOR (FIG. 4.39)

Identification: This instrument is just like a small dinner fork. The ends of the fork are bend downwards.

Uses:
- It is used to retract the skin, subcutaneous tissues and ligament during lacrimal sac surgery.

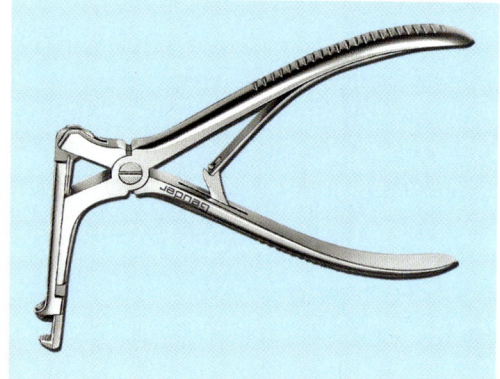

Fig. 4.40: Bone punch.

- It may also be used in other plastic operations of the eye lid.

BONE PUNCH (FIG. 4.40)

Identification: It is a large instrument, which consists of a spring handle and two long blades. The upper blade has a hole with sharp cutting edge and the lower blade has a cup like depression with sharp edge.

Use: It is used to punch or break the bones (lacrimal bone, adjacent nasal bone and frontal process of the maxilla) in DCR operation to create a bony ostium. Ideally, two different sized bone punches are required to make a round bony opening of about 10 mm diameter.

HAMMER, CHISEL AND BONE GOUGE (FIGS. 4.41A TO C)

These stout and heavy instruments are not routinely used during DCR operation. But when the bones of the lacrimal fossa are seemed to be hard, these instruments are then used for making a bony ostium (osteotomy) in DCR surgery.

Chapter 4: Common Eye Instruments

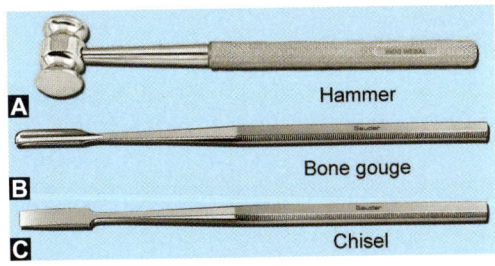

Figs. 4.41A to C: (A) Hammer; (B) Bone gouge; (C) Chisel.

Sometimes used in various orbitotomy procedures.
[*Usually, first the lacrimal bone is broken with a lens hook or blunt dissector, then the bony window is made with help of a bone punch*].

EVISCERATION SCOOP OR SPOON (FIG. 4.42)

Identification: It has a large rectangular or oval shallow spoon attached to a handle. Its shape is almost like a spade.

Uses: It is used to scoop out the intraocular contents during evisceration. Evisceration is the removal of the contents of the globe with inner two coats while leaving the sclera and the optic nerve intact.

The structures scooped out are:
- Lens
- Vitreous
- Whole uvea
- Whole retina.

Indications of evisceration:
- Panophthalmitis
- In case of expulsive hemorrhage—to assist auto-evisceration if the process is incomplete—rarely performed.
- Painful blind eye

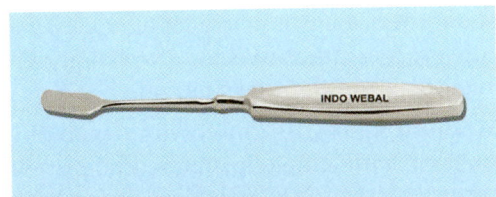

Fig. 4.42: Evisceration scoop.

- Cosmetic procedure for disfigured eyes/phthisical eyes—combined with a scleral implant and prosthetic shell.

Method: Steps of operation (*See* page 184).

ENUCLEATION SCISSORS AND SPOON (FIGS. 4.43A AND B)

Identification: It is a broad, stout scissors having uniformly curved blades with blunt tips. It is curved to fit the curvature of the globe.

Use: It is used to cut the optic nerve with its sheaths during enucleation surgery.

Enucleation is the surgical removal of the eyeball and a portion of optic nerve from the orbit.

Enucleation Spoon

Use: After severing all the recti muscles, it is passed from the lateral side deep inside the orbit to get hold the optic nerve.

Then the scissors are used to cut the optic nerve.

Indications of enucleation:
a. **Absolute indications:** When there is risk of life, or risk to the other eye due to the disease.
   - Malignant melanoma in adult.
   - Retinoblastoma in children.
   - Non-repairable severe open globe injury to prevent sympathetic ophthalmia in the other eye.

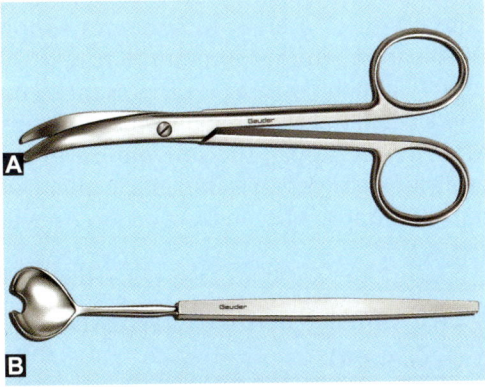

Figs. 4.43A and B: (A) Enucleation scissors; (B) Enucleation spoon.

b. **Relative indications:** Enucleation may be done in case of:
   - Painful blind eye due to absolute glaucoma, chronic iridocyclitis, intraocular hemorrhage, etc.
   - Phthisis bulbi with calcification.
   - Disfigured eye, e.g., anterior staphyloma, ciliary staphyloma, etc.
   - Sympathetic ophthalmia.
c. **To collect whole globe from the cadaver in eye banking:** *In general, this is the most common indication of enucleation.*

Method: Steps of operation (*See* page 183).

The structures cut by enucleation scissors are:
- Optic nerve with its meningeal sheaths.
- Central retinal artery and vein.
- Two long posterior ciliary arteries.
- Two long ciliary veins.
- Short posterior ciliary vessels and nerves.
- Lastly, two oblique muscles.

In case of malignant tumors: At least more than 10 mm optic nerve stump is to be cut behind the globe. This is because the central retinal artery enters the optic nerve at this distance. So, when the extraocular vascular spread occurs—it may be detected by histopathology of the optic nerve. Thereby, subsequent treatment by radiation or exenteration may be considered.

In panophthalmitis: Enucleation is contraindicated because infection may spread via the meningeal sheaths or their spaces into the brain leading to meningitis or encephalitis.

Cosmetic appearance of artificial eye is better with evisceration than with simple enucleation without implant. Because the muscle attachments are still present to the scleral shell (later form a ball like structure) after evisceration, the movement of the artificial eye is possible. But enucleation with an orbital implant has always a better cosmetic result.

LACRIMAL PROBE (BOWMAN'S) (FIG. 4.44)

Identification: It is a thin, long probe with round lip. It is made up of stainless steel or silver.

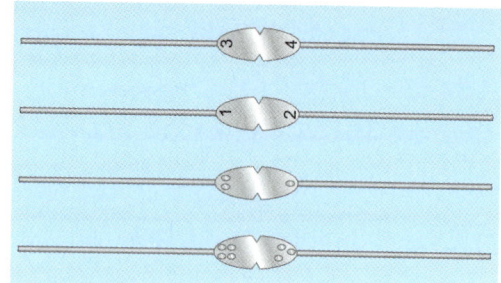

Fig. 4.44: Lacrimal probe (Bowman's).

They are of different diameters (size 00 to 08). Each instrument has two different size probes attached centrally with a flat handle.

Uses: To probe nasolacrimal passage in:
- Congenital punctal stenosis.
- Congenital dacryocystitis. If probing fails to achieve the patency of nasolacrimal passage, then DCR may be considered.
- During DCR to identify the exact position of lacrimal sac for giving incision on the sac wall.

Uses: *Method (probing and syringing)*
- Under general anesthesia.
- Probing is usually done through the upper punctum.
- Start with a smaller size probe and gradually increase the size.
- Always follow the direction of nasolacrimal passage during probing.
- Syringing is done 2–3 minutes after the probing.

Complications of probing:
- False passage.
- Nasal bleeding.
- Orbital cellulitis.

LID SPATULA (PLATE) (FIG. 4.45)

Identification: It is a flat solid instrument of about 10 cm long. Its both ends are round and convex. It is little curved or grooved at right angle to its long axis, near its end.

Method: Before its application, eyeball is smeared with antibiotic ointment to prevent corneal abrasion. It is introduced under the lid to provide a solid support during lid surgery.

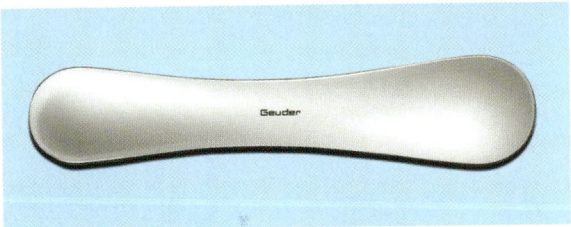

Fig. 4.45: Lid plate (spatula).

Three stay sutures are usually passed along the lid margins so that the assistant can hold the sutures together along with lid plate for better support during dissection.

Use: It is used in various lid surgeries, e.g., ptosis, entropion, etc. It gives more exposure of operative field than a clamp, but it does not help in hemostasis.

ENTROPION FORCEPS (FIG. 4.46A)

Identification: It is just like chalazion forceps except its shape is horizontally oval, and it is bigger in size. It is used for both sides.

ENTROPION CLAMP (FIG. 4.46B)

Identification: It is a stout clamp with two limbs, and one screw for fixation. One limb has got a solid semilunar plate and the other limb has U-shaped curved rim corresponding to the semilunar plate. Right and left sided clamps are different.

Method (Same for both instruments): Eye is smeared with antibiotic ointment before its application to prevent corneal abrasion. Its solid plate is applied on the tarsal conjunctival side and the fenestrated or rim-side is on the skin surface (in reverse order of chalazion forceps). The screw is tightened for fixation.

Use (Same for both): It is used to fix the lid during entropion operation. By tightening the screw, it helps in hemostasis during operation. But it reduces the area of operative field.

CALIPER (CASTROVEIJO'S) (FIG. 4.47)

Identification: It is a measuring caliper in which the measurement (in mm) is adjusted by spring action of a screw. The measuring ends are pointed like a compass, and the scale is fixed to the opposite end.

Methods: The exact measurement is taken by adjusting the spring action of the screw which is indicated by the pointed end on the scale.

Uses:
- ❖ To measure the size of the cornea, as in buphthalmos, megalocornea, microcornea, etc.
- ❖ To use in various surgeries:
  - ➢ *Phacoemulsification or SICS:* Length of incision.
  - ➢ *Trabeculectomy:* Length of scleral flap.
  - ➢ *Squint operation:* Amount of resection or recession of muscle.
  - ➢ *Keratoplasty:* To determine the size of the donor and recipient corneal button.

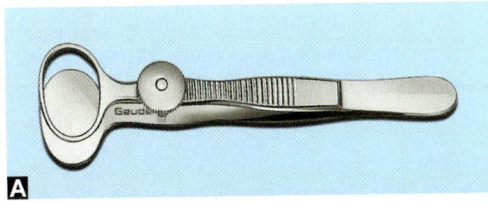
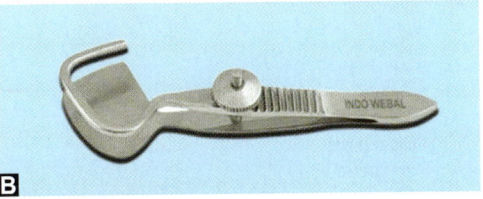

Figs. 4.46A and B: (A) Entropion forceps; (B) Entropion clamp.

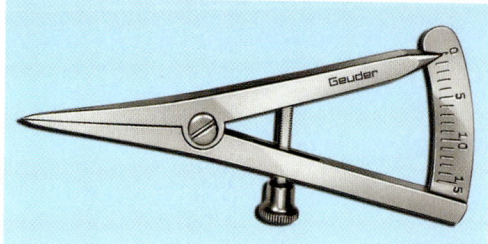

Fig. 4.47: Caliper.

- *Retinal detachment surgery:* To measure the distance for passing encircling band or to make port at pars plana.
- *Ptosis surgery:* To measure the amount of LPS to be resected.
- To measure the length for any purpose.

CORNEAL TREPHINE (CASTROVEIJO'S) (FIG. 4.48)

Identification: It is a cylindrical instrument which has three parts:
- A circular blade.
- An adjustable inner core or 'obturator'
- A cover to protect the sharpness of the blade.

It is available in different diameters (like 6.0, 6.5, 7.0, 7.5 ... 10, 10.5, etc. in mm).

The obturator has a scale (marking 0, 2, 4, 6, etc., in 1/10th of mm) which helps the surgeon to select exact depth of the cornea to be cut. This is important in lamellar keratoplasty.

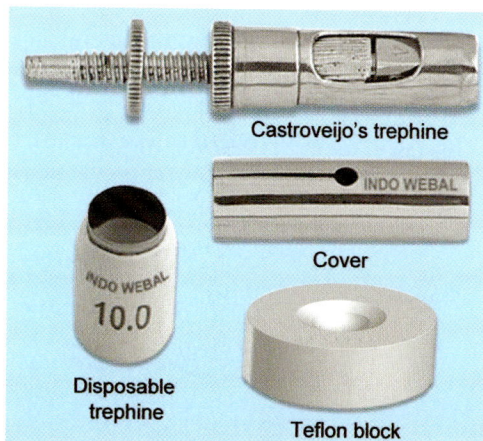

Fig. 4.48: Corneal trephine.

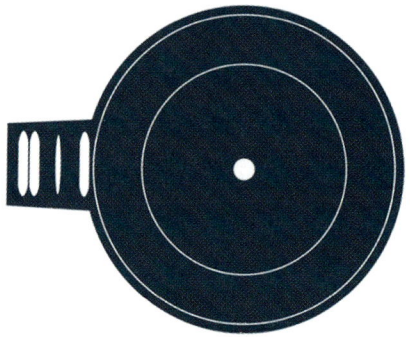

Fig. 4.49: Pin-hole.

Uses: To cut the 'donor' and 'recipient' corneal button in penetrating and lamellar keratoplasty.

Nowadays, disposable corneal trephine is used. Donor cornea is placed on the Teflon block before trephination.

PIN-HOLE (PH) (FIG. 4.49)

Identification: It is a black disc with a small central hole, attached to a small handle.

Principle of pin-hole: When it is held in front of eye, only a small pencil of rays get through, which passes through the axis of dioptric system of the eye, and is therefore, unaffected by it.

Method: Patient complaining of dimness of vision, is asked to look at the Snellen's chart. Then a pin-hole is placed in front of his eye, the other eye is being closed. He is asked whether his vision is better or worse, or unchanged.
Uses: As discussed on page 8

STENOPAEIC SLIT (FIG. 4.50)

Identification: It is black disc with a large slit-like opening at the center. It has small handle.

Method: Stenopaeic slit is placed in front of the eye by means of a spectacle frame within the slot. It can be properly positioned by rotating it within the frame.

Uses:
- Detection of the axis for prescribing cylindrical lens for astigmatic correction.

Chapter 4: Common Eye Instruments

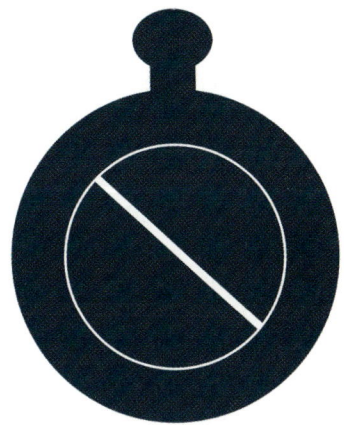

Fig. 4.50: Stenopaeic slit.

- Fincham's test to differentiate between cataract halos from glaucomatous halos.
- As a low visual aid.
- Used as a part of Maddox wing.

TRIAL FRAME AND OPHTHALMIC LENSES (FIG. 4.51)

Types of lens used in ophthalmic practice are:
- **Spherical lenses:** Convex and concave
- **Cylindrical lenses:** Convex and concave

Methods of identification of a given lens:
Close left eye. Hold the lens and look any object through the lens with the right eye for magnification or minification.

Concentrate on a distant object (some figure or a line) through the lens. Now move the lens in:
- Horizontal direction.
- Vertical direction.
- Rotatory fashion.

Note the following:
- Object is moving in the same direction with movement of the lens, or in the opposite direction.

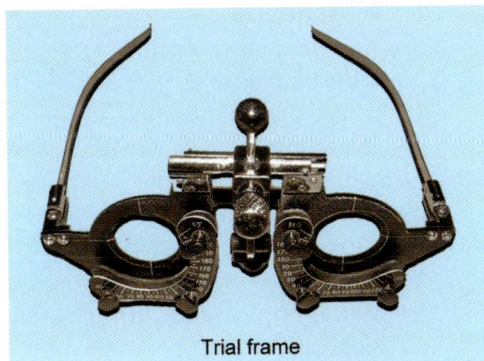
Trial frame

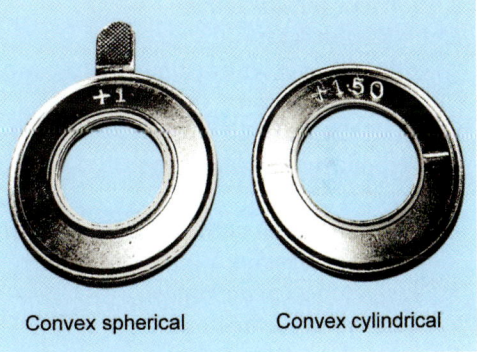
Convex spherical   Convex cylindrical

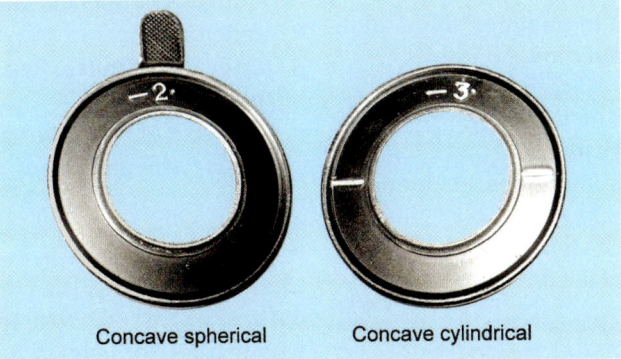
Concave spherical   Concave cylindrical

Fig. 4.51: Trial frame and trial lenses.

- Any distortion of the object while moving the lens in a rotatory fashion.

Now identification of the lens:
1. **Spherical:**
   - The object appears to move in both directions, i.e., horizontal and vertical
   - No distortion of the image of the object in rotatory movement.
2. **Cylindrical:**
   - Object appears to move in one direction only
   - Distortion of the image with rotation of the lens

Then identify whether the lens is convex or concave:
- **Convex lens (plus lens):** *Magnification of the image and the objects appears to move in the opposite direction as that of the lens.*
- **Concave lens (minus lens):** *Minification of the image and the objects appears to move in the same direction of the lens.*

So, a given lens may be either:
a. **Convex spherical:**
   - Object moves in both meridians and *opposite direction.*
   - No distortion of the image.
   - Magnification of the image.
b. **Concave spherical:**
   - Object moves in both meridians and in the *same direction.*
   - No distortion of the image.
   - Minification of the image.
c. **Convex cylindrical:**
   - Object moves in one meridian and in the *opposite direction.*
   - Distortion of the image.
   - Magnification of the image.
d. **Concave cylindrical:**
   - Object moves in one meridian and in the *same direction.*
   - Distortion of the image.
   - Minification of the image.

> **Note**
>
> **In a plane glass (Plano):** Lens with 'No' power
> - No movement of the object.
> - No distortion of the image.
> - Size remains same.

Uses:
1. **Convex spherical**
   a. *Correction of refractive status:*
      - Hypermetropia.
      - Aphakia.
      - Presbyopia.
      - As a low visual aid (magnifier).
   b. *Instrumental uses:*
      - Direct ophthalmoscope.
      - Indirect ophthalmoscope.
      - Microscope.
      - Synaptophore.
      - Corneal loupe or telescopic loupe.
   c. *Diagnostic uses:*
      - + 90D lens, or + 78D lens—to see the fundus.
      - Placido's disc (+3.0D).
      - Malingering (with high plus lens).
      - Different condensing lenses for laser therapy.
2. **Concave spherical**
   a. *In refractive error:* Myopia.
   b. *Instrumental uses:*
      - Direct ophthalmoscope.
      - Telescopic loupe (Gallelian system).
   c. *Diagnostic uses:*
      - Hruby lens (–55D).
      - Fundus contact lens (–45D).
      - Central lens of gonioscope.
      - Malingering test with high minus lens.
3. **Convex cylinder:** Regular hypermetropic astigmatism.
4. **Concave cylinder:** Regular myopic astigmatism.

   (In case of irregular astigmatism—one should use contact lens).

RETINOSCOPE (FIG. 4.52)

Identification: This is a circular plain mirror with a central aperture in a plastic frame with handle. Sometimes, a concave mirror of 2.0D may be attached with another end in a dumbbell-shaped frame.

Uses:
- It is used for determination of refraction.

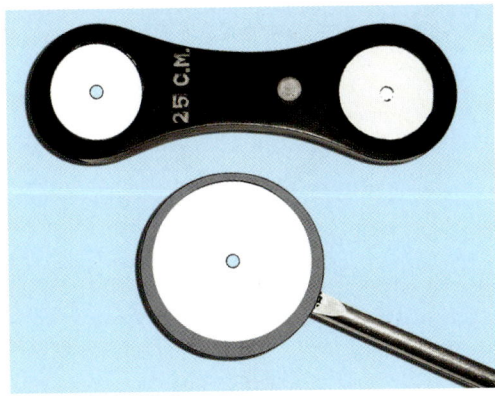

Fig. 4.52: Retinoscope.

- May be used for distant direct ophthalmoscopy (at 22 cm):
  - To know any opacity in the media.
  - To discover the edge of a subluxated or dislocated lens.
  - To recognize a retinal detachment or tumor.
  - To confirm the results found by external examination.

Optics of Retinoscopy

It entails a study of the movements of the retinal image produced by a beam of light that sweeps across the pupil.

The observer watches this illuminated retinal image through a hole in the center of a mirror (retinoscope).
- **If the eye is emmetropic:** Parallel rays of light come to a point focus on retina, so they are emerging in the same pathway.
- **If the eye is hypermetropic:** Parallel rays converge behind the retina and hence, the emerging rays are divergent.
- **If the eye is myopic:** Parallel rays converge infront of the retina and hence, the emerging rays are convergent.

The principle of retinoscopy is to make every observing eye emmetropic, so that the emerging rays should form a parallel beam.

Procedure

A. **Cycloplegia:** It is only required in children and young patients. In adults and old patients, it is usually not necessary.
   - *If the patient is less than 5 years:* Atropine eye ointment (1%) is to be applied three times daily for 3 days.
   - *If the patient is between 5 and 15 years:* 1% cyclopentolate, or 2% homatropine eye drop is instilled for 3 times, about 1 hour before examination.
   - *If the patient is between 15 and 20:* The same procedure may be undertaken.

   The refraction under cycloplegia is always pathological because the shape of the lens has been altered. **A post-cycloplegic test (PCT)** is therefore advisable after 3 days to 3 weeks depending upon the cycloplegic used.

B. **Dark-room test:** Retinoscopy should preferably be conducted in dark room.
   - Examiner sits at 1 meter from the patient (point of reversal is at 1.0D).
   - It is even more convenient to sit at arm's length, i.e., 2/3 meter away, so that the trial lenses can be held in the other hand while the light beam is passed. The point of reversal is then 1.5D.
   - The patient is normally seated and looking towards the far end of the room (relaxed eye).
   - Source of light is from behind the patient.
   - The surgeon looks through a plane mirror with central perforation, and light is reflected into the patient's eye.
   - The mirror is slowly moved from side to side in different meridians, and movement of the shadow is noted.
   - In hypermetropia, emmetropia and myopia <1.0D the reflex moves in the same direction.
   - In myopia of –1.0D = there is no movement of shadow.
   - In myopia of >ID = the shadow moves in the opposite direction.
   - Increasing convex (if the movement is on same side) or concave (if opposite side) lenses are placed before the eye until the point of reversal is reached.
   - At this point there will be no movement of the shadow, and pupil will be brightly illuminated.

➤ The procedure is done in each meridian separately.
  ♦ In simple spherical refractive error—the movement and the point of reversal will be same in both meridians.
  ♦ In astigmatism, they are different. If the axes are oblique, the shadow themselves will seem to move obliquely and the mirror is then tilted accordingly.
C. **Calculation:** Refraction of patient's eye—lens required to reach end point = –1D (myopia). [Since the doctor is sitting at 1 meter distance, and if he is at 2/3rd meter, it will be –1.5D (myopic)].
So, the refraction of the eye = –1.0D + lens.

Example:
a. *If the end point is with +4.0D Lens:*
   Refraction = –1.0D + 4.0D = +3:0D.
b. *Similarly, if, with –4.0D lens:*
   Refraction = –1.0D – 4.0D = –5.0D.
c. *If the end point is with +1.0D lens:*
   Refraction = –1.0D = 0, i.e., the patient is emmetropic.
d. In case of astigmatism, each meridian is to be calculated separately.

[**Streak retinoscopy:** Instead of circular light as obtained by a plain mirror, a self-illuminated streak of light is used. Here, the appearances of the shadow are more dramatic. Axis of the astigmatism is easily determined. Nowadays, streak retinoscopy is more common.]

It has certain other advantages:
❖ Can be done in any position of the patient.
❖ Can be done in difficult patients, e.g., in children or non-cooperative patient.
❖ Can be used peroperatively.

JACKSON'S CROSS CYLINDER (FIG. 4.53)

Identification: It is a sphero-cylindrical combination of lens in which the spherical component is half the power but of the opposite sign of the cylindrical component. *The most convenient form* is a combination of a –0.25 D spherical with +0.50 D cylinder.

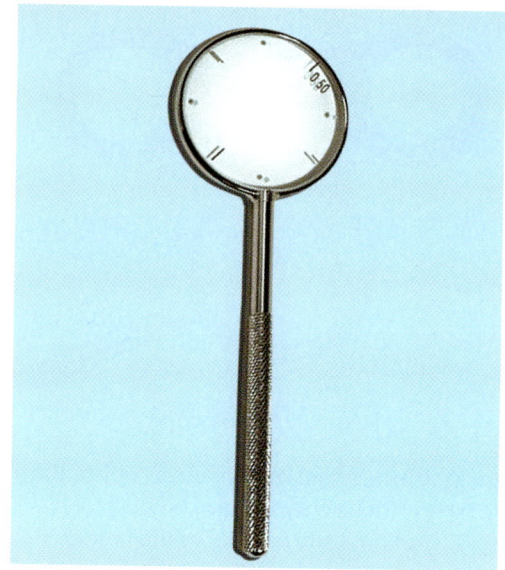

Fig. 4.53: Jackson's cross cylinder.

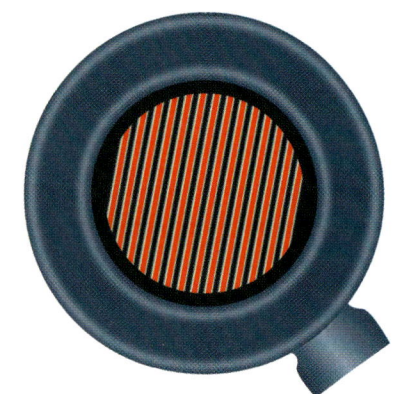

Fig. 4.54: Maddox rod.

Use: It is used for finer adjustment of the power and axis of the cylinder in refractive correction.

MADDOX ROD (FIG. 4.54)

Identification: It consists of a series of parallel high-power, plus cylinders (rods) of red glass placed side by side in a supporting disc. It can convert a point light into a red streak light at right angle to the axis of rods.

Methods: When a Maddox rod is held in a front of one eye, the image of a point source of light becomes dissimilar between the two eyes, and fusion becomes dissociated ('dissimilar image test'). This test is performed at 6 meters and at 33 cm from a bright spot light in a dark room.

Use:
- To test the latent squint for distance.
- For orthoptic exercise in cyclophoria.
- To test macular function, in presence of opaque media.

PLACIDO'S DISC (FIG. 4.55)

Identification: It is a medium size circular disc with a central hole and attached to a handle. On one surface of the disc, there are alternate black and white circle like bull's eye.

Procedure: Placido's disc is held in front of the patient's eye while examiner looks through the hole in center of the disc. The examiner then observes the corneal image of the disc as reflected from the light behind the patient.

Use: It is used to assess the corneal surface and anterior corneal curvature (astigmatism):
- A loss in sharpness of image denotes a loss of normal smoothness of the anterior corneal surface, e.g., corneal abrasion, dry eye, etc.
- Elliptical image is seen in regular astigmatism.
- Irregular image is seen in keratoconus.

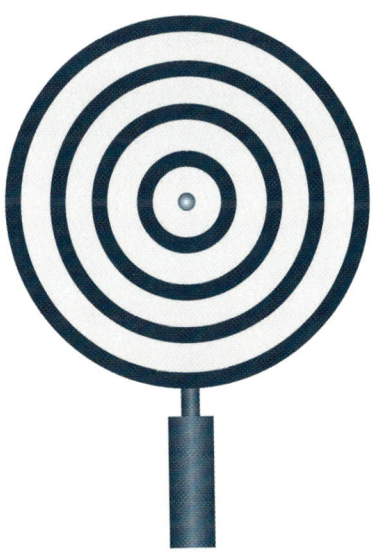

Fig. 4.55: Placido's disc.

METHODS OF STERILIZATION OF INSTRUMENTS

The methods of sterilization commonly practiced in ophthalmic surgery are: (1) Autoclave, (2) Boiling, (3) Dry heat, (4) Chemicals, (5) Gamma rays; (6) Plasma Sterilization and (7) Ultraviolet (UV) rays.

1. **Autoclave:** Steam under pressure is biocidal. A temperature of 134°C (32 lbs/sq inch pressure) for 3 minutes, or 121°C (15 lbs/sq inch pressure) for 15 minutes is used. It is used to sterilize towels, gowns, masks, sutures, dressings, irrigating solutions and blunt instruments. Sharp instruments should not be autoclaved.

2. **Boiling:** Boiling for 30 minutes usually kills most bacteria, but some spores may withstand boiling for this period. It is preferable to use distilled water to prevent salt deposition. Sharp instruments are better not to be sterilized by boiling.

3. **Dry heat:** Dry heat kills bacteria by oxidative destruction of their protoplasm. In dry heat, a temperature of 150°C is used for 90 minutes in the hot air oven. It is better not to sterilize sharp instruments by dry heat.

4. **Chemicals:**
    - *Ethylene oxide:* Its vapor can destroy all micro-organisms, including spores. As undiluted ethylene oxide is highly explosive, it is diluted with an inert gas like carbon dioxide or freon (12% ethylene oxide and 88% freon). Sharp instruments, IOLs, indirect ophthalmoscopy lens, diathermy wires, etc., can be sterilized by this method.
    - *Glutaraldehyde (Cidex):* 2% glutaraldehyde kills all micro-organisms including spores. Its full potency persists for 2 weeks, then it is to be discarded. Cidex does not reduce the sharpness of the cutting instruments. In 10 minutes all micro-organisms are killed and in 3 hours all spores are destroyed. The instruments after removed from cidex, are thoroughly rinsed with sterile water and hollow instruments are to be flushed.

- *Alcohol (rectified spirit):* Sharp cutting instruments and sutures may be dipped in 90% alcohol for 30 minutes for sterilization. It is not a commonly used method.
- *Isopropyl alcohol (70%):* This may be used for sterilization of all kinds of metallic instruments. Dip the instruments for 15 minutes and then wash it with sterile water or saline before use.
- *Formalin vapor:* Instruments are kept in formalin vapor in a chamber (vapor released from formalin tablets) for overnight. Rinse thoroughly before use. It is carcinogenic and now banned in many countries.

5. **Gamma irradiation:** Gamma rays from Cobalt-60. This type of sterilization is used commercially, for disposable needles, disposable syringes, infusion sets, etc.
6. **Plasma sterilization:** A nontoxic fast procedure for thermolabile and thermostable microsurgical instruments as well as IA tubings. It inactivates micro-organisms primarily by the combined use of hydrogen peroxide gas and the generation of free radicals (hydroxyl and hydroperoxyl free radicals) during the plasma phase of the cycle.
7. **Ultraviolet germicidal irradiation (UVGI):** It is a disinfection method that uses short-wavelength ultraviolet (ultraviolet C or UV-C) light to kill micro-organisms including coronavirus by destroying nucleic acids and disrupting their DNA, leaving them unable to perform vital cellular functions. UVGI is currently used as operating room air disinfectant.

CHAPTER 5

Few Common Eye Surgeries

CATARACT SURGERY

Types, Steps, Intraoperative and Postoperative Complications of Extracapusular Cataract Extraction Surgery *(OP 7.4)*

Types of Cataract Surgery

1. **Extracapsular cataract extraction (ECCE):**
   - Conventional ECCE
   - Manual small incision cataract surgery (MSICS)
   - Phacoemulsification
   - Femto laser assisted cataract surgery (FLACS)

   Intraocular lens implantation with any of the above techniques.

2. **Intracapsular cataract extraction (ICCE):** It is very rarely done (in grossly subluxated or dislocated lens), resulting aphakia.

3. **Lensectomy (with vitrectomy):** It is in children or in grossly subluxated/dislocated lens.

   Intraocular lens implantation may or may not be possible in ICCE or lensectomy cases.

4. **Combined surgery:**
   - *With glaucoma surgery:* It is combined with any types of ECCE with IOL implantation.
   - *With vitreoretinal surgery:* It is combined with any types of ECCE with IOL implantation.
   - *With keratoplasty:* It is combined with lens extraction with or without IOL implantation.

Extraction of Cataract
Preparation of the Patient
- The face is washed with soap and water.
- Shaving in male patient.
- Eyelashes of both lids of operated eye may be trimmed.
- Antibiotic drop in both eyes frequently.
- Light breakfast in the morning.

Pupillary Dilation
- The pupil is dilated with combination drop of phenylephrine (5%) and tropicamide (0.8%)—3 times at 5 minutes interval.
- NSAID drops (e.g., flurbiprofen or nepafenac) is also given along with mydriatics for sustained pupillary dilation during operation.

Anesthesia
- **Topical anesthesia:** By 4% lignocaine or 0.5% proparacaine eye drops 3 times at an interval of 5 minutes.
- **Block (infiltration) anesthesia:** It is of following types:
  1. Facial and retrobulbar (ciliary) block by two different injections.
  2. Peribulbar block by a single injection.
  3. Sub-Tenon's block

Block anesthesia is best given by mixing:
- Half volume of 2% lignocaine with or without adrenaline
- Half volume of 0.5% bupivacaine or 0.75% ropivacaine
- Both mixed with injection hyaluronidase

Facial block:
- **O'Brien technique:** About 4–5 mL of anesthetic solution is infiltrated at the neck of the mandible just in front of tragus
- **van Lint technique:** 4 mL of solution is infiltrated along the superolateral and

inferolateral orbital margins in a V-shaped manner.

Effect: It causes paralysis of orbicularis oculi which prevents closure and squeezing of the eyelids during operation.

Retrobulbar (ciliary) block: About 2 mL of anesthetic solution is injected deep into the orbit by piercing the skin with a long needle (35 mm) at the junction of medial 2/3 and lateral 1/3 of lower orbital margin almost in the muscle cone. The aim is to block ciliary ganglion and to paralyze the extraocular muscles.

Effects:
- Mydriasis
- Anesthesia of the intraocular tissues (e.g., iris).
- Akinesia of extraocular muscles (except superior oblique).
- It lowers IOP to some extent especially with bulbar massage.
- It induces proptosis of the eyeball in deep seated eyes.
- It decreases the oculocardiac reflex.

Peribulbar block: It is a better technique in which about 5–6 mL of anesthetic solution is injected into the peripheral space of orbit with a 24-G needle. The injection-site is at the junction of medial 2/3 and lateral 1/3 of the lower orbit. A good and gentle bulbar massage for 5–10 minutes is important to achieve good anesthetic effect.

Effects: It has both the effects of surface anesthesia and facial and retrobulbar injections as mentioned earlier.

Sub-Tenon's block: Sub-Tenon's space is exposed by cutting the conjunctiva and Tenon's in the inferomedial conjunctival quadrant.

2–3 mL of anesthetic agent is injected in the sub-Tenon's space using canula.

This is a non-needle technique of achieving good anesthesia.

Preparatory steps before operation:
- Cleaning of eyelids and adjacent area with *10% povidone iodine* and rectified spirit.
- *5% povidone iodine drop* in conjunctival sac for 3–5 minutes—followed by normal saline.
- Broad-spectrum antibiotic drops.
- Application of head-towel and eye-towel.
- Surgi-drape to cover the lid margins with eyelashes and separate the operative field.

Surgical Steps of Extracapsular Cataract Extraction (ECCE) *(OP 7.4)*

Conventional ECCE

- **Separation of the eyelids:** Lid speculum or lid stitches
- **Superior rectus stitch** (Bridle suture)
- **Conjunctival flap preparation**
- **Hemostasis of bleeding points:** Wet-field cautery or thermocautery
- **Limbal-groove incision:** About 1/2 to 3/4th thickness at the limbus with a blade (No. 15 or No. 11) or razor blade fragment.
- **Anterior chamber entry:** With No. 11 blade and is filled with viscoelastic
- **A can-opener anterior capsulotomy** or a continuous curvilinear capsulorhexis (CCC) is performed with the tip of the 26-gauge needle (cystitome).
- **Limbal section is enlarged** with corneal scissors for 10–12 mm (1200–1500) at superior limbus
- **Anterior capsule is removed.**
- **Lens nucleus is delivered** by scleral depression with the help of a lens hook and lens spatula, or vectis.
- **Simultaneous irrigation and aspiration** (I/A) with a two-way cannula to clear all cortical matter. The cannula is fitted with an infusion system of balanced salt solution (BSS) or Ringer's lactate.
- **Viscoelastic is injected** into the capsular-bag and anterior chamber.
- **PC IOL implantation:** IOL is grasped by the optic with McPherson forceps. The leading loop is placed in the inferior portion of the capsular bag or ciliary sulcus. The trailing loop is flexed towards the optic and engaged slightly posterior to the capsular bag or in the ciliary sulcus.

- ❖ **The IOL is then dialed** into horizontal position and checked for correct centration.
- ❖ **Removal of viscoelastic** substance by I/A cannula.
- ❖ **Constriction of the pupil** with pilocarpine (0.125%) if required and subsequently wash.
- ❖ **Closure of the wound** with 4 to 5 interrupted 10-0 nylon sutures with buried knots.
- ❖ **Reformation of the anterior chamber** with BSS or Ringer's lactate solution.
- ❖ **Conjunctival closure**
- ❖ **Subconjunctival injection** of gentamicin and dexamethasone may be given.
- ❖ Topical antibiotic and steroid ointment.
- ❖ **Pad and bandage**.

A peripheral iridectomy is not mandatory in routine cases of ECCE with PCIOL. It is required in:
- ❖ *Complicated cataract (e.g., uveitic cataract) when combined with trabeculectomy*
- ❖ *If posterior capsular rent occurs during surgery, or in case of ACIOL*

Manual Small Incision Cataract Surgery (MSICS)

- ❖ **Separation of the eyelids:** Lid speculum
- ❖ **Superior rectus stitch** (Bridle suture)
- ❖ **Conjunctival flap preparation**
- ❖ **Hemostasis of bleeding points:** Wet-field cautery or thermocautery
- ❖ **Sclerocorneal tunnel** (5.5–6.5 mm) incision with crescent blade
- ❖ **Anterior chamber entry:** With 2.8 mm keratome and is filled with viscoelastic
- ❖ **Capsulorhexis:** 5.5 mm with forceps or needle; or may be can opener capsulotomy.
- ❖ **Hydrodissection** of the lens nucleus from its capsule.
- ❖ **Nuclear prolapse into anterior chamber** and A/C again filled with viscoelastic
- ❖ **Nucleus delivery** by irrigating vectis or phaco-sandwich or fishhook technique
- ❖ **Cortical cleaning** by Simcoe I/A cannula
- ❖ **Viscoelastic agent to fill the bag** and anterior chamber

- ❖ **Intraocular lens placement in-the-bag** or may be in ciliary sulcus
- ❖ **Anterior chamber wash** and reformation
- ❖ **Conjunctival closure**

Some surgeons use anterior chamber maintainer during manual SICS.

Irrigating vectis technique is the most popular methods for nucleus delivery in manual SICS.

Phacoemulsification (Phaco)

- ❖ Most of the surgeons preferred **under topical anesthesia.**
- ❖ A 2.2–2.8 mm **clear corneal incision on temporal side.** This is for foldable IOL. It is preferable to create stepped (bi- or tri-planar) incision.
- ❖ **Viscoelastic agent is injected** into the anterior chamber.
- ❖ **Continuous curvilinear capsulorhexis (CCC)** is performed using a bent-tipped 26-gauge needle or rhexis (Utarata) forceps.
- ❖ **Hydrodissection and hydrodelamination** to separate lens nucleus and cortex from the capsular bag.
- ❖ **Sculpting the lens nucleus** from the anterior surface.
- ❖ A phaco chopper is passed into the anterior chamber through a separate stab incision.
- ❖ **Phaco-fragmentation and aspiration:** The chopper keeps the nucleus away from the corneal endothelium, simultaneously fragments the nucleus and feeds smaller pieces of nucleus into the ultrasonic tip, until the whole nucleus is fragmented and aspirated.

The different techniques used are: "Chip and flip technique" for soft nucleus; four quadrants "divide and conquer technique"; "stop and chop technique" or "direct chop" technique for nuclear fragmentation and emulsification.

- ❖ **Epinucleus removal** by phaco handpiece.
- ❖ **Lens cortex is aspirated** completely from the peripheral part, using bimanual (or coaxial) irrigation and aspiration cannulas.
- ❖ Polishing of the posterior capsule if necessary.

- Viscoelastic is injected to inflate the capsular bag.
- A foldable PC IOL is implanted within capsular bag using IOL injector system
- Viscoelastic material is washed thoroughly.
- Hydration of the side ports and main incision port.
- No suture (sutureless surgery) is required for foldable IOL with 2.2–3.0 mm incision
- No pad and bandage if under topical anesthesia.

Femtosecond Laser Assisted Cataract Surgery (FLACS)

It is the latest development in cataract surgery. Femtosecond-assisted procedure is guided by in-built anterior segment imaging system which *gives maximum precision in cataract surgery.*

Femtosecond laser is used in some steps of ECCE:
- Creation of single and multiplane perfect incisions in the cornea
- Astigmatic limbal relaxing incisions (LRI) to correct pre-existing astigmatism
- A perfect and precisely centred capsulorhexis
- Phaco-fragmentation (by micro-photolysis of the lens nucleus in multiple small fragments)

Nevertheless, the need for ultrasound phaco is still there—further, to emulsify the nuclear fragments and to aspirate them. Other steps are similar to phaco.

Intraoperative and Postoperative Complications

Intraoperative Complications

Anesthesia-related: Retrobulbar hemorrhage (RBH), injury to the optic nerve, globe perforation, lignocaine shock, acute anaphylaxis, and convulsion following injection into the optic nerve or its sheaths. Rare complication such as—brainstem anesthesia may occur, which may cause apnea and and sudden death.

Surgery-related (intraoperative):
- Subconjunctival hemorrhage
- Poor wound construction
- Runaway rhexis
- Iridodialysis
- Hyphema
- Positive vitreous pressure (upthrust)
- Zonular dialysis
- Posterior capsular tear (rent)
- Vitreous prolapse (loss)
- Nucleus drop or lens—fragment or IOL drop in the vitreous
- Descemet's tear and detachment
- Corneal endothelial damage
- Expulsive hemorrhage

Postoperative Complications

Early postoperative (within 1 week):
- Wound leak
- Tunnel or side ports infection
- Striate keratopathy (SK)
- Shallow anterior chamber due to—wound leak, pupillary block, choroidal detachment and malignant glaucoma
- Hyphema
- Iris prolapse
- Postoperative uveitis
- Retained lens matter (cortex or nuclear fragment).
- Postoperative secondary glaucoma
- Bacterial endophthalmitis
- Toxic anterior segment syndrome (TASS)

Late Postoperative (Weeks to Months)
- Cystoid macular edema (CME) or Irvine-Gass syndrome
- Unpredictable astigmatism
- Persistent chronic uveitis
- Intraocular lens related complications
- Corneal edema and bullous keratopathy (pseudophakic or aphakic)
- Late postoperative endophthalmitis
- Retinal detachment
- Posterior capsular opacification (PCO) or after cataract

Operative Complications: Unique to Specific Type of ECCE

Conventional ECCE/PCIOL:
- Complications of peribulbar or retrobulbar block (PBB/RBB)
- Positive vitreous upthrust
- Expulsive hemorrhage
- Suture-related problems—tight or loose sutures, suture infection
- High astigmatism
- Improper cortical cleaning

Manual SICS:
- Complications of PBB/RBB
- With sclerocorneal tunnel preparation:
  - Button-holing of sclera
  - Premature entry into A/C
  - Bleeding within the tunnel
- Zonular dialysis during prolapsing the nucleus into A/C
- Inferior iridodialysis during nucleus delivery
- Hyphema

Phacoemulsification:
- Posterior capsule blow-out rupture during forcible hydrodissection in case of smaller rhexis.
- **Wound burn** with phaco-probe especially with hard cataract, with high astigmatism
- Unintentional grabbing of iris with phaco-tip and bleeding
- **Intermittent floppy iris syndrome (IFIS)** with its problem. It happens with patient taking oral alpha-1 adrenergic receptor antagonists (e.g., tamsulosin) for prostate problem.
- Zonular dialysis
- **Nuclear fragments drop into the vitreous after PC rent**

INTRAOCULAR LENS (IOL)

Intraocular (IOL) implantation is the standard surgical procedure in the management of cataract. The main idea is to replace the function of natural crystalline lens and to restore the vision to pre-cataractous stage. IOL implantation is usually performed along with extraction of cataract at the same sitting called *primary implantation*, or any time postoperatively, called *secondary implantation*.

[*IOL implantation was first done by Dr Sir Harold Ridley on 29th November 1949 at St. Thomas Hospital, London. It was a posterior chamber lens.*]

Indications

Any type of cataract unless there is contraindication.

Relative contraindications:
- Congenital bilateral cataract (age <2 years)
- Gross subluxation or dislocated lens in one-eyed individual
- Recurrent anterior or posterior uveitis of unknown etiology

Types of IOL implantation: They are mainly of two types, depending upon the site of IOL placement: (A) Anterior chamber IOL (AC IOL) and (B) Posterior chamber IOL (PC IOL).

A. **Anterior chamber IOL (Fig. 5.1):** They are placed in the anterior chamber after intracapsular cataract extraction (ICCE). Here the optic of the lens lies in front of the pupil and the haptics in the anterior chamber angle (angle-supported, e.g., Kelman multiflex) or is fixed with iris (iris-supported, e.g., Worst-Singh's iris claw lens).

AC IOL implantation is *practically discarded as a primary procedure owing to its complications.* They are corneal decompensation (edema), iris capture, UGH (vveitis, glaucoma and hyphema) syndrome, etc. It may be used as secondary

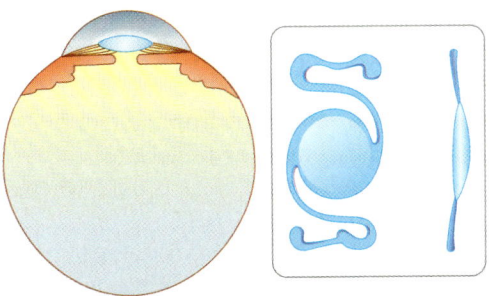

Fig. 5.1: Anterior chamber IOL (Kelman multiflex).

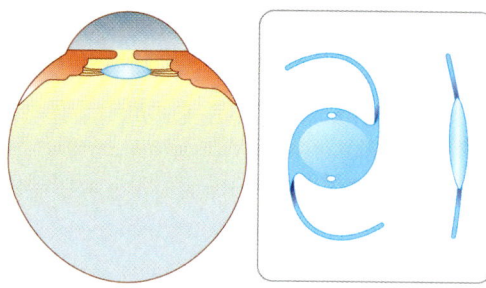

Fig. 5.2: Posterior chamber IOL (single-piece).

implantation where ICCE was done as a primary procedure long time back or during large posterior capsular rent in ECCE.
B. **Posterior chamber IOL (Fig. 5.2):** They are placed in the posterior chamber after ECCE. The lenses are intended for placement either within the "capsular bag (in-the-bag)" or in the "ciliary sulcus". It is more of anatomical to place the IOL "in-the-bag" with least complications. PCIOLs are of two types, e.g., multi-piece and single piece.

Parts of IOL

Intraocular lens has got **two parts:** (1) Optic and (2) Haptics.
1. **Optic:** Diameter—5.5, 6.0 or 6.5 mm (commonly 6.0 mm)
2. **Haptic:** J or C shaped, made of same material in single-piece; in multipiece—it is made of prolene or nylon. The main function of the haptics is to anchor the lens in position.
    Overall diameter of IOL: 12.5 mm or 13.0 mm

Types of PC IOL

PCIOLs can be classified by:
- **Optic material:** Polymethyl methacrylate (PMMA), acrylic (hydrophobic or hydrophilic), silicone or hydrogel lens.
- **Rigid or foldable:** PMMA is rigid, whereas others are foldable IOLs
- **Haptic style:** Plate haptic or loops
- **Sphericity:** Spherical, aspheric or toric (to correct astigmatism)
- **Edge-finish:** Round-edge or square-edge design
- **Focality:** Monofocal or bifocal, trifocal or multifocal
- **Wavelength feature:** UV-blocking IOLs or blue-blocking IOLs
- **Features of accommodation:** Accommodative IOLs

Trabeculectomy

It is a 'guarded' filtration operation, widely used as a surgical procedure for glaucoma.
Anesthesia: Same as cataract extraction.
Steps:
1. **Conjunctival flap** is reflected over the cornea.
2. A partial (2/3) thickness triangular, or square (5 mm × 5 mm)
3. **Scleral flap** is made and hinged at the limbus.
4. **A deep rectangular block of sclera** (1.5 mm × 3 mm), near the cornea, is excised along with trabecular tissue (using Kelly's punch).
5. A **peripheral iridectomy** is performed.
6. The **superficial scleral flap** is repositioned and **sutured**.
7. The **conjunctival flap** is closed by a running **water-tight suture**.

In trabeculectomy, the aqueous humor is drained via the lamellar scleral flap into the subconjunctival space and also through the opened canal of Schlemm. The amount of drainage can be controlled by varying the thickness of scleral flap and to some extent by the tightness of sutures.

Dacryocystectomy (DCY or DCT)

Anesthesia:
- 2 drops of 4% lignocaine into the conjunctival sac.
- **Infiltration:** Anesthetic agents are injected at the following sites:
    - In the inferior orbital margin—at the beginning of anterior lacrimal crest—0.5 mL solution is injected, and then along the line of incision to a point 3 mm above the medial palpebral ligament.

➢ *Second injection:* Needle is directed posteriorly for 8 mm and 0.5 mL solution is injected in the tissues around the lacrimal sac. The needle is then carried out further downwards to the upper half of posterior lacrimal crest and 0.5 mL solution is injected.

Steps:
1. **A slightly curved incision** with its concavity towards inner canthus. Care is taken *to avoid injury to angular vein.* Incision length is about 2.5 cm and one-third of it lies above the medial palpebral ligament.
2. **Dissection of skin, subcutaneous tissue and orbicularis oculi** along the line of incision with lacrimal dissector and retracted with Muller's retractor.
3. **Medial palpebral ligament is exposed and disinserted** from the anterior lacrimal crest by a Rougine.
4. **Lacrimal sac is separated** from the floor of the lacrimal fossa with Rougine and the rest of the parts are dissected with blunt lacrimal dissector.
5. **After sac is well dissected, it is grasped with a straight artery forceps** up to its lower part and twisted until the duct is torn off.
6. Cut end of the **nasolacrimal duct is curetted by scoop.** Thereafter, it is cauterized with 10% povidone iodine.
7. **Skin is closed** by interrupted or continuous 5-0 or 6-0 silk.
8. **Pad and pressure bandage** are applied for 24 hours. Stitches are removed after 6–7 days.

DACRYOCYSTORHINOSTOMY (DCR)

Anesthesia:
❖ In case of children—under GA
❖ **In adult:** Same as DCT (better with anesthetic mixture).

Nasal pack: In DCR, before starting the surgery, a nasal pack is given on the same side with a roller gauze soaked with 4% lignocaine and adrenaline for hemostasis.

Steps:
1. to 3. Same as dacryocystectomy
4. **Lacrimal sac is separated** from the medial wall and the floor.
Lacrimal fossa is now exposed.
5. **A 10 mm bony ostium is made** into the nose by cutting the *lacrimal bone, part of adjacent nasal bone and frontal process of maxilla.* Nasal mucous membrane of the middle meatus is thus exposed.
6. **Two horizontal 'H' shaped incisions are made on the nasal mucosa and medial wall of the lacrimal sac**, and thereby creating two anterior flaps and two posterior flaps. First posterior and then anterior flaps are sutured with a 5-0 or 6-0 Vicryl.
Sometimes, it is difficult to suture both anterior and posterior flaps. In that case, only anterior flaps are sutured while the posterior flaps are removed from both sides.
7. **Skin is sutured by** 5-0 or 6-0 silk.
8. **Pressure bandage** is applied for 24 hours.
9. **Nasal pack is removed** after 24 to 48 hours.

ENUCLEATION

Special consent: A specially informed written consent is a must prior to surgery, indicating that the patient will not get back his vision in future.

Anesthesia:
❖ As the operation is psychologically traumatic, all cases should preferably be operated under general anesthesia.
❖ In adults where GA is contraindicated, it is done under *LA:*
   ➢ Surface by 4% lignocaine eye drop
   ➢ Infiltration by 2% lignocaine (with adrenaline) in all four quadrants of the retrobulbar space.

Steps:
1. Universal **eye speculum.**
2. **360° peritomy:** Conjunctival with Tenon's capsule around the limbus are dissected and undermined peripherally with a blunt-tipped scissors.

3. Each **rectus muscle is hooked** with a squint hook and cut with scissors in the order of superior, lateral, inferior and medial rectus (SLIM).
4. Speculum is depressed and the eyeball is made to be luxated out.
5. **Enucleation scissors are introduced** with closed tip under Tenon's capsule from the lateral side and optic nerve is felt by the tip of the scissors.
6. Scissors are opened and **optic nerve** is caught between the two blades and **severed** with scissors. A sound may be heard during severing the optic nerve. Attention is always paid to get a long optic nerve stump.
7. Lastly, two oblique muscles along with some connective tissues are cut with the same scissors.
8. **Bleeding is stopped** by applying pressure for 5 minutes.
9. **Tenon's capsule and the conjunctiva are sutured separately,** in horizontal and vertical fashion respectively.
10. **Pressure bandage** is applied for 24 hours.

EVISCERATION

Anesthesia: Same as enucleation.
Special consent: As enucleation, a specially informed written consent has to be taken prior to surgery regarding nature of operation and its outcome.

Steps:
1. **Universal eye speculum** is applied.
2. **Peritomy:** Conjunctiva is dissected around the limbus.
3. Whole cornea is removed with the help of blade and corneal scissors.
4. After fixing the sclera, evisceration scoop is introduced between the sclera and uveal tissue (ciliary body) and **the whole content of the globe is removed by** 360° sweeping movement of the evisceration scoop.
5. Precaution should be taken **to remove all the uveal tissue** especially those around the vortex veins and the optic disc.
6. **Bleeding is stopped** by applying pressure with a warm saline soaked gauze.
7. Usually, conjunctiva is not sutured.

PTERYGIUM OPERATION

Indications of surgery:
- Progressive pterygium
- Recurrent pterygium
- Pterygium causing much astigmatism
- Purely cosmetic

    Before doing surgery, surgeon should give caution regarding:
- Permanent corneal opacity may remain near the limbus after operation.
- 5–10% of recurrence after operation.

Anesthesia:
- Surface anesthesia with 4% lignocaine drop.
- Infiltration with 2% lignocaine with or without adrenaline into the body of the pterygium.

Pterygium operation with conjunctival autograft:
- Universal **eye speculum**.
- **Head of the pterygium** is carefully **resected** from the cornea with a fine blade.
- When it reaches the neck (i.e., at the limbus), **two radial cuts** are given with scissors along the upper and lower border of the pterygium. The conjunctiva is undermined.
- Then, the **subconjunctival dissection of pterygium** is done with scissors and it is removed.
- Cauterize the bleeding vessels
- A rectangular piece of bulbar conjunctiva is dissected from *upper temporal area* and taken out as graft tissue. This is usually from the same eye, but rarely from the other eye.
- The tissue is placed over the bare area to cover it. Limbal side of the graft is matched carefully.
- Grafted tissue is sutured by 8-0 Vicryl or 10-0 nylon. Donor site may also be closed by same suture. *Alternately, the grafted tissue is secured in place with fibrin (tissue) glue.*
- **Pad and bandage** for few hours.
- The nylon sutures may be removed after 3 weeks.

CHALAZION OPERATION

Most chalazion require incision and curettage, for very rarely does spontaneous resolution occur.

Anesthesia:
- Surface with 4% lignocaine drop.
- Infiltration with 2% lignocaine with adrenaline into the skin around the site of chalazion.

Steps: *Incision and curettage or incision and scooping.*
- **Chalazion is fixed with a chalazion forceps** (the solid plate is towards the skin surface and the fenestrated plate is towards the conjunctival surface). The **lid is then everted**. The screw is tightened further.
- A **vertical incision** is given at the middle with a sharp knife.
- All the **contents** of the chalazion (i.e., cheesy materials) are **scooped out** with the chalazion scoop. Through curettage is done by rotatory movement of the scoop.
- Chalazion forceps is then removed, and pressure is given with a pellet inside and thumb outside for 2 minutes to secure hemostasis.
- Pad and bandage for 1–2 hours.

INDICATIONS AND METHODS OF TARSORRHAPHY (OP 4.7)

Tarsorrhaphy is the joining of part of the upper and lower eyelids so as to partially close the eye.

Types:
1. **Temporary:** It is used to help corneal healing or to protect the cornea during a short period of exposure or disease.
2. **Permanent:** It is used to permanently protect the cornea from a long-term risk of damage. It usually closes the lateral eyelids, so that the patient can still see through the central opening and the eye can be examined.

Indications
To protect the cornea:
- Lagophthalmos—due to facial nerve palsy or cicatricial damage to the eyelids caused by an injury
- Neurotrophic keratitis
- Proptosis or thyroid exophthalmos—causing a risk of corneal exposure
- After cerebellopontine angle (CPA) tumor operation
- Severe dry eye
- Comatose patients

To promote corneal healing:
- Non-healing corneal ulcer
- Progressive corneal thinning or descemetocele
- Persistent epithelial defect after keratoplasty

Other indications:
- To reduce abnormal length of the palpebral fissure (euryblepharon)
- To retain a conformer—in children after evisceration or enucleation.
- In keratoprosthesis surgery

Methods
1. **Temporary tarsorrhaphy:** Horizontal mattress sutures (at least 2) are placed through upper and lower lids and tie over bolsters on skin.
   Drawstring temporary central tarsorrhaphy: This allows repeated opening and closure of lids for examining the eye.
   Temporary glue tarsorrhaphy: Manually upper and lower eyelids are opposed with slight eversion and then apply cyanoacrylate glue to lid margin and lashes.
2. **Permanent tarsorrhaphy:** De-epithelialize lateral portion of upper and lower eyelid margins for adherence. Vertical incisions are given in upper and lower tarsus. Absorbable sutures are then placed in horizontal mattress fashion joining upper and lower lid tarsal groove.

Steps of surgery: Apart from placement of sutures both the operations almost follow the same technique.
1. Dissection of the mucous membrane from the margin of lower lid
2. **Just posterior to the gray line** in rectangular (5–6 mm long) fashion.
3. The edge of the upper lid is similarly dissected at the corresponding position.
4. A horizontal mattress suture is passed through the rubber beads and the skin, so that they come out at the posterior edge of the bare surface of both lids.
5. Suture is then tied firmly.
6. The lids will be firmly adherent within a few days (7–10 days) when the suture and rubber beads are removed.

Advanced permanent tarsorrhaphy: It needs oculoplasty clinic referral. Mobilization of tarso-conjunctival flaps and sutured.

Release of temporary tarsorrhaphy is usually done after 6–12 weeks, when the corneal lesion heals completely.
Firm pressure is given to the bridge of skin with small artery forceps for few minutes. Then cut the bridge with scissors or knife.
Apply an antibiotic ointment two-three times daily for few days.

INCISION AND DRAINAGE OF LACRIMAL ABSCESS

Principle: Rapid control of infection

Anesthesia: In adult patients under LA, but in children under GA.
2 mL 2% lignocaine with adrenaline injected to infraorbital nerve by palpating infraorbital foramen located 1 mm below the inferior orbital rim at the junction of medial 1/3rd and lateral 2/3rd.

Steps:
1. Surgical site is prepared with 10% povidone iodine
2. A vertical stab incision is made at the apex of abscess (typically below the medial canthal tendon and the direction along the anterior lacrimal crest).
3. With the help of Stevens' scissors or mosquito forceps the submuscular loculated pocket of the abscess are lysed for better drainage of pus and debris
4. Lacrimal sac curettage is done with chalazion scoop
5. Wound is irrigated with normal saline and packed with 5% povidone iodine soaked gauze
6. The wound left open to heal by secondary intention.

Microbiology: Pus is send for Gram staining and bacterial culture

Prognosis: Majority of the lacrimal abscess heal by 2 weeks and then advised for permanent solution, e.g., DCR surgery after 6 weeks.

Complications: Lacrimal fistula, skin scar, cicatricial ectropion.

INCISION AND DRAINAGE OF LID ABSCESS

Anesthesia: In adult under LA, but in children under GA.
Local infiltration anesthesia van Lint method

Steps:
1. Surgical site is prepared with 10% povidone iodine
2. Horizontal stab incision is given with No. 11 or 15 blade at the apex point of lid abscess.
3. With the help of mosquito forceps, the submuscular abscess pockets are lysed for better drainage of pus.
4. Active bleeders are cauterized and proper hemostasis is secured
5. Wound irrigated with normal saline and pressed for 5 minutes with 5% povidone iodine soaked gauze.
6. Wound left open to heal by secondary intention.

Microbiology work up: Pus send for Gram staining and KOH preparation; and for bacterial and fungal cultures.

Prognosis: Majority of the lid abscess heal by 7–10 days.

Index

Page numbers followed by *f* refer to figure and *t* refer to table.

A

Abducens nerve palsy 144, 145
Acanthamoebal keratitis 41f
Accommodation, fate of 182
Acetylcysteine 100
Achromatopsia 80
Acyclovir 75
Adherent leucoma 14, 15, 21, 45, 45f, 46
    causes of 46
    complications of 46
    mechanism of 46
Adhesion, recurrence of 101
Aflibercept 74, 76
Age-related macular degeneration 2, 22, 131, 149
Albinism 4
Alcian blue 13
Alcohol 176
    retrobulbar injection of 120
Alkali burn 104
Allergic problems 75
Allopurinol 79
Alpha-1 adrenergic blockers 23
Alpha-2 agonist 78
Amantadine 79
Amaurotic cat's eye reflex 6, 17, 93, 148
Amblyopia 79, 85
    anisometropic 86
    ex anopsia 86
    reverse 86
Amblyopic eye, characteristics of 86
Ametropia 81
    curable 81
Amikacin 74
Amiodarone 79
Amphotericin-B 74
Amsler grid test 132
Analgesics 42
Anatomical standardize uveitis nomenclature classification 57t
Anesthesia 117, 177, 180, 183-186
    topical 104, 177

Angle-closure glaucoma 3, 5, 15, 16, 96, 119, 123
    acute 57
        attack of 3, 5, 14, 16
    primary 119
    stages of 119
Angular keratome 161, 161f
Anhydrotic ectodermal dysplasia 104
Aniridia 4
Anisometropia 84
    problems of 84
Ankylosing spondylitis 114
Annular scotoma 118
Antacids 42
Anterior chamber 15, 22, 24, 27, 29, 31, 35, 37, 39, 43, 45, 47, 49, 54, 56, 64, 68, 113, 149, 142
    abnormal contents of 15
    angle of 116
    entry 178, 179
    intraocular lens 181, 181f
    paracentesis, indications of 115
    reformation of 179
    wash 179
Anterior ischemic optic neuropathy 79, 133
Anterior necrotizing scleritis
    with inflammation 112
    without inflammation 112
Anterior segment 68, 137
Anterior staphyloma 21, 46, 47
    complications of 48
    formation, probable mechanism of 48
    treatment for 48
Anterior synechia 16, 46
    causes of 16
Antibiotics, topical 42
Antidiabetic medicines 23
Antifungals 42
Antiglaucoma medications 78, 122
Antihistaminics 104
    topical 100
Antipsychotic drug 104
Antivascular endothelial growth factors 76
Aphakia 15, 17, 21, 26, 27, 27f, 28-30, 30t, 172
    causes of 27

Index

Aphakic bullous keratopathy 105
Aphakic glasses 28
   disadvantages of 28
Aqueous humour, circulation of 116
Arcuate keratotomy 84
Argyll Robertson pupil 115
Arteriosclerosis 38
Artery
   anterior ciliary 72
   forceps 152, 152f
Arthritis, juvenile idiopathic 114, 121
Artificial cornea transplantation 107
Artificial tears 76
Asthenopia 83
Astigmatism 81, 82, 84
   irregular 83
   oblique 83
   regular 83
   types of 83
Atrophic bulbi 49, 49t, 59
Atrophic pterygium 34f, 35
Atropine 17, 59, 79, 137
   eye ointment 106
   sulphate 42
Attack
   acute 3, 5, 14, 16, 119, 120
   recurrent 111
Autoclave 175
Autoimmune 57
Auto-oxidation 124
Axial ametropia 81
Axial hypermetropia 82
Axial myopia 81
Azoles 75

B

Bacterial diseases 121
Band-shaped keratopathy 59
Bard Parker handle 153
Bare sclera 35
Barraquer's wire speculum 152
Barrett universal II formula 31
Behcet's disease 114
Behcet's syndrome 122
Bell's phenomenon 135, 136
Beta-blockers 78, 104
Betamethasone 75
Bevacizumab 74, 76
Bimatoprost 78
Binocular diplopia 6
   causes of 6
Binocular loupe 11
Binocular movements 10
Binocular vision
   grade of 73
   state of 137

Bioptics 85
Bitot's spot 21, 53, 105
   bilateral 54f
   pathogenesis of 54
   treatment for 55
Bjerrum's scotoma 118
Black ball hyphema 115
Blade breaker 153, 154f
Bleeding 184
   points, hemostasis of 178, 179
Blepharitis 4, 21, 65, 66f, 86
   causal factors for 66
   complications of 66
   posterior 67
   sequalae of 66
   types of 66, 104
   ulcerative 66, 66t
Blepharospasm 5
   essential 5
Blindness 139, 149
   childhood 141
   curable 139
Blink reflex 84
Blood 15
   dyscrasias 38
   pressure 23
   sugar 23
   thinners 23
Blue sclera 15
Blue vision 79
Blunt
   injury 142
   trauma 38, 115
Board-spectrum antibiotic ointment 106
Bone
   formation 50
   gouge 166, 167f
   hypoplasia, temporal 149
   punch 166, 166f
Bony orbit 73
Borrelia burgdorferi 121
Bowman's membrane 33, 71
Bowman's needle 32
Branch retinal
   artery occlusion 128
   vein occlusion 3, 128, 130
Bridle suture 178, 179
Bromfenac 76
Bruch's membrane 94
Bulbar congestion 97
Bulbar conjunctiva 12
   examination of 12
   lower part of 12
Bull's eye maculopathy 79
Bullous keratopathy 107
Buphthalmos 4, 15, 27, 117

C

Caliper 169, 170f
Capsulorhexis 179
    continuous curvilinear 179
    forceps 158, 159f
Capsulotome 158
Carbohydrate metabolism 124
Carbonic anhydrase inhibitors 78
    topical 78
Carbon-steel blade 154f
Cat's paw retractor 166
Cataract 17, 22, 79, 115, 123, 125, 141, 145, 149
    anatomical aspect of 145
    blindness, prevalence of 22
    complications of 124, 125
    congenital 6, 126, 141
    cortical 26, 26t
    developmental 126
    etiopathogenesis of 124, 125t
    extraction of 177
    hypermature 15, 18, 18f, 21, 24, 25f
    immature 4, 6, 18, 21, 23, 26, 26t
    incipient 125
    intumescent 15
    mature 18, 18f, 21, 24, 25, 25f, 26, 26t
    nuclear 5, 26, 26t
    operation 23
    stages of maturation of 23, 124, 125
    steroid-induced 75
    surgery 24, 25, 126, 177
        informed consent for 126
        types of 30, 126, 177
Cataracta nigra 17
Cavernous sinus thrombosis 91, 92
Ceftazidime 74
Cells, malignant 15
Cellulose polymers 76
Central anterior chamber depth 68
Central corneal thickness 71
Central retinal artery
    obstruction 3, 128
    occlusion 145
        anatomical aspect of 145
Central retinal vein occlusion 128, 130
Cerebrospinal fluid 135
Chalazion 21, 50, 51, 51f, 51t, 98, 185
    forceps 163, 164f, 185
    histopathology of 51
    operation 185
    scoop 164, 164f
    treatment for 52
Chemical 175
    burns 100
    conjunctivitis 4, 98
    injury 3, 142, 143
Chemotherapy 93
Cherry red spot 129
Chiasmal field deficits 144
Chisel 166, 167f
Chlamydia
    oculogenitalis 4
    trachomatis 97
Chloroma 92
Chloroquine 79
Chlorpromazine 79
Cholinergic miotics 77
Choriocapillary 72
Choroid 142
    blood supply of 72
    structures of 72
Choroidal
    blood vessels 20
    coloboma 6
    detachment 15
    melanoma 93
    neovascular membrane 76
    tuberculoma 115
    tumors 93
Choroidoretinopathy, central serous 130
Cicatricial entropion 98
Cicatricial eyelid diseases 89
Cilia forceps 162
Ciliary body 142
    functions of 72
    nerve supply of 72
    structures of 72
    tumors 93
Ciliary congestion 13, 97, 97t
Ciliary muscles 72
Ciliary staphyloma 37, 48
Ciliary sulcus 179
Closed globe injury 142
Closed-circuit television system 150
Coat's disease 6, 76
Cold compress 100
Colibri forceps 157, 158f
Collagen vascular diseases 103, 121
Color blindness 80, 145
Color sense 80
Color vision 86, 135
    testing 9
    theories of 80
Colored halos 5, 119
    causes of 22
Computer vision syndrome 104
Concave lens 173
Concomitant squint 19, 137, 138, 138t
Confrontation method 10
Congestion 15
Conjunctiva 12, 22, 24, 27, 29, 31, 33, 35, 37, 38, 43, 45, 47, 50, 52, 53, 55, 56, 61, 64-66, 95, 98, 120, 142, 184
    anatomy of 70

limbal 12, 13
palpebral 12
Conjunctival autograft 184
Conjunctival congestion 13, 97, 97t
Conjunctival flap preparation 178, 179, 182
Conjunctival impression cytology 55
Conjunctival lepromas 115
Conjunctival xerosis 53, 105
    treatment for 55
Conjunctivitis 4, 94, 114
    acute 3, 57, 96
    allergic 94, 95, 98
    bacterial 4, 95, 98
    differential diagnosis of 95, 95t
    gonococcal 4
    hemorrhagic 37
    inclusion 4
    infective 94
    membranous 100
    phlyctenular 21, 35, 36, 36f
    vernal 99
    viral 95, 98
Contact lens
    advantages of 28
    correction 82
    disadvantages of 28
    wear 14
Contrast sense 80
Convex lens 172
Cornea 4, 13, 22, 24, 27, 29, 31, 33, 35, 37, 38, 43, 45, 47, 49, 50, 52, 54-56, 61, 64-66, 71, 98, 103, 120, 142
    abnormal curvature of refractive surfaces of 81
    anatomy of 71
    hypoxia of 103
    nerve supply of 71
    nutrition of 71
    optical power of 80
    plana 15
    structures of 71
Corneal abrasion 3-5
Corneal blindness 141
    causes of 105
Corneal ectasia 105
Corneal edema 5, 79
    causes of 103
    long-standing 14
Corneal endothelium 71
Corneal incision procedures 84
Corneal injury 105
Corneal inlay 85
Corneal loupe 10, 172
Corneal opacity 4, 44, 149
    causes of 14, 43, 44
    grade of 44, 98
    leucomatous 43f
    treatment for 44

Corneal plaque 100
Corneal reflection test 11, 137
Corneal scar 105, 107, 141
Corneal scissors 155f
Corneal sensation 14, 39, 43
    loss of 14
Corneal spring scissors 154, 155f
Corneal surface 105
Corneal surgery 14
Corneal trephine 170, 170f
Corneal ulcer 3, 5, 14, 15, 21, 38, 39, 40, 44, 46, 103, 105, 115, 116
    bacterial 41f
    fate of 40
    infective 40
    non-healing 42
    non-infective 103
    perforating 15, 16, 40, 42
    risk factors for 103
    stages of 39
    treatment for 42
    types of 39, 103
Corneal xerosis 105
Cortex 123
Corticosteroids 59
Cosmetic appearance 168
Cover test 137
COVID-19 143
Cranial nerve 14
    palsies 114
Craniosynostosis 92
Crescent knife 161, 161f
Cryosurgery 163
Cryotherapy 93
Crystalline lens 17, 123
    metabolism of 124
    surgical anatomy of 123
    transparency of 124
Curvature, radius of 71
Cyclitic membrane 59
Cyclocryotherapy 120
Cyclopentolate 79
Cyclophoria 137
Cyclophotocoagulation 120
Cycloplegia 77, 173
Cycloplegics 77
    uses of 78
Cyclotropia 137
Cylindrical lenses 171
Cysticercosis 92
Cystitome 158
Cystoid macular edema 59, 76

D

Dacryocystectomy 182

Dacryocystitis 87
  acute 61f
  chronic 21, 62
  congenital 4, 63, 89, 136
  types of 62
Dacryocystorhinostomy 62, 183
  operation, complications of 63
Dark adaptation 80
Dark-room test 173
Deep anterior
  chamber, causes of 15
  lamellar keratoplasty 45, 107
Deep vascularization 14, 44, 44t
Demodex
  folliculorum 87
  infestation 66
Depot steroid
  intra-chalazion injection of 52
  intra-lesional injection of 52
  supratarsal injection of 100
Dermoid 92
  cyst 87
Descemet's membrane 71, 117
  endothelial keratoplasty 107
Descemet's stripping endothelial keratoplasty 107
Desmarre's lid retractor 163f
Devic's disease 3
De-Wecker's iris scissors 156, 156f
Dews classification 104, 104t
Dexamethasone 74
  phosphate 75
Dextrocycloversion 10
Diabetic macular edema 76, 129, 131
Diabetic retinopathy 2, 3, 22, 129, 131, 149, 142
  types of 131
Difluprednate 75
Digital tension 22, 24, 27, 29, 31, 35, 37, 39, 43, 45, 47, 49, 56, 64
Digital tonometry 19
Dilator pupillae 72, 77
Dioptric power 11, 71
Diplopia 5, 35
  causes of 22
  charting 137
Direct light reaction 17
Direct ophthalmoscopy, method of 20
Disodium chromoglycate 100
Distance vision 7, 27, 135
  impairment 149
Distichiasis 65
Dry eye 55, 103, 114
  causes of 103, 104, 104t
  management of 103, 104
  severity of 104, 104t
  syndrome 4
Dry heat 175

Dystrophy 14
  corneal 103
  hereditary 105

E

Eales' disease 76, 115
Eccentric fixation 86
Ectasia 15
Ectopia lentis 17
Ectropion 88, 104
  uveae 56
Edinger-Westphal nucleus 146
Edridge-green lantern test 9
Egyptian ophthalmia 97
Electrical reaction 79
Electro-diathermy 163
Electrolysis 163
Electronic device 150
Electrooculography 79
Electroretinogram 135
Elschnig's pearl 32, 32f
Emmetropia 81
Emulsified silicone oil 15
Endocrine 92
Endophthalmitis 3, 74, 148
  endogenous 121
  postsurgical 121
  traumatic 121
End-organ 146
Endothelial dystrophy, congenital hereditary 103
Endothelium 71
Enophthalmos 92
Entropion 4, 88, 104
  clamp 169, 169f
  forceps 169, 169f
Enucleation 93, 94, 120, 138
  scissors 167, 167f, 184
  spoon 167, 167f
Epibulbar dermoid 87
Epidemic dropsy glaucoma 3
Epilation forceps 162
Epinucleus 123
  removal 179
Epiphora 4, 62
Epiretinal membrane 131
Episcleral manifestations 114
Episcleritis 3, 64, 64f, 96, 110, 111, 111t, 114, 115
  causes of 64
  complications of 64
  differential diagnosis of 64
  simple 110
Epithelial micro-erosions 100
Epitheliopathy 104
Epithelium 70
  posterior two layers of 72

Equatorial staphyloma 47
Erythema multiforme major 100
Esophoria 137
Esotropia 137
Ethambutol 79, 115
Ethylene oxide 175
Evisceration 184
    indications of 167
    scoop 167, 167f
Exenteration 93
Exophoria 137
Exophthalmos 92
Exotropia 137
External dacryocystorhinostomy, disadvantages of 63
Extracapsular cataract extraction
    conventional 178, 181
    surgery 126, 177
    surgical steps of 178
Extrafoveal fixation 86
Extraocular movements, examination of 135
Extraocular muscles
    actions of 73
    anatomy of 73
Exudative retinal vascular disorders 130
Eye
    anterior segment of 10
    banking 107
        functions of 109
        protocols of 109
    care 106
    donation 107, 109, 135
    drops 104
        instillation of 102
    functional anatomy of 145
    hypermetropic 82
    instruments 151
    itching of 4
    lids 12, 29, 33, 38, 43, 49, 52, 55, 56, 98
    normal dioptric power of 27
    optics of 80
    refraction of 80
    refractive errors of 81
    speculum 151, 183
    squinting of 93, 148
    surgeries 177
Eyeball 19, 48
    fixation forceps 152
    gross anatomy of 68
    layers of 145
    three concentric layers of 68
Eyelashes 12, 90
    loss of 12, 98
    lower 90
    matting of 12
    scantiness of 12
Eyelid 22, 24, 142
    anatomy of 69

    disorders 103
    functions of 70
    glands of 69
    muscles of 69
    separation of 178, 179

F

Facial
    asymmetry 19
    block 177
    cellulitis 62
    nerve palsy 89, 136
Failed graft 107
Farnsworth-Munsell 100 hue test 9
Fasanella-Servet operation 88
Fascicular ulcer 36
Femtosecond laser assisted cataract surgery 180
Festooned pupil 56
Fibrous layer 69, 70
Fincham's stenopaeic slit test 5, 119
Fixation
    behavior 137
    forceps 152, 152f
Flexner-Wintersteiner rosette 148
Flucytosine 75
Fluorescein stain 13, 55
Fluorescent treponemal antibody absorption test 121
Fluorometholone 75
Flurbiprofen 75
Flurette 148
Follicles 97
Follicular conjunctivitis 100
Forced duction test 137
Formalin vapor 176
Fornices, loss of 98
Fornix 70
Foscarnet 74
Fovea centralis 73
Foveal reflex 20
Foveolar avascular zone 73
Foveoschisis 130
Fresh small vitreous hemorrhage 6
Frontalis suspension 88
Fuchs' endothelial dystrophy 103, 107
Fuchs' heterochromic cyclitis 16
Fundal glow 20
Fundus 120, 129
    autofluorescence 132
    contact lens 172
    examination 19, 20, 130
        techniques 135
    fluorescein angiography 3, 129, 132
    general 20
    normal 20f
    peripheral 20

Fungal 41
    corneal ulcer 41f

G

Gallelian system 172
Gamma Irradiation 176
Ganciclovir 74, 75
Ganglion cell layer 72
Giant papillae 100
Giant papillary conjunctivitis 100
Glare 4
Glassy pupillary reflex 17
Glaucoma 79, 117, 121, 122, 141, 145, 149
    absolute 17, 120
    anatomical aspect of 145
    classification of 117
    congenital 4, 5, 123, 141
    inflammatory 121
    lens-induced 3, 121
    malignant 121
    neovascular 16, 76, 121
    pigmentary 121
    secondary 46, 59, 121, 148
    steroid-induced 75, 121
    traumatic 121
Glaukomflecken 119
Globe, abnormal length of 81
Glutaraldehyde 175
Goblet cell
    destruction 104
    dysfunctions 104
Goldenhar's syndrome 87
Goldmann applanation tonometer 19
Gonioscope 116
    central lens of 172
Gray eyelashes 12
Guarded eye speculum 151f, 152

H

Haab's striae 117
Hammer 166, 167f
Haptic style 182
Hard contact lens 104
Head
    injury 17
    posture 19
        abnormal 19
Headache 83
Healed infection 14
Healed ulcer 107
Heat cautery 154
Hemangioma 87, 92
Hemeralopia 5

Hemorrhage
    pontine 16
    retrobulbar 92
    subconjunctival 3, 21, 37, 37f, 38, 96
    vitreous 115
Herbert's pit 98
Herpetic keratitis 14, 41f
Hess screen 137
Heterochromia, causes of 15
Heterophoria 136
Heterotropia 137
    diagnosis of 137
High myopia 5
Hirschberg's test 11
Hoffer-Q and Holladay-2 formulas 31
Hollenhorst plaque 129
Holmgren's wools test 10
Homatropine 17
Homer-Wright rosette 148
Hordeolum
    externum 52, 52f, 53, 53f, 86
    internum 51f, 53, 53t, 86
Horner's syndrome 15, 69, 88
    anatomical basis of 144
Hospital cornea retrieval program 108
Hruby lens 172
Human immunodeficiency virus 121
Humphrey field analyser 135
Hyaloidotomy 130
Hydrocortisone acetate 75
Hydrodelamination 179
Hydrodissection 179
Hydrops, acute 103
Hydroxychloroquine 79
Hydroxycobalamine 135
Hydroxypropyl methylcellulose 76
Hypermature senile cataract, stages of 125
Hypermetropia 15, 81, 82, 84, 172
    absolute 82
    curable 82
    facultative 82
    latent 82
    types of 82
Hyperopic laser-assisted in situ keratomileusis 82
Hyperphoria 137
Hypertension 38
    ocular 119
Hypertropia 137
Hypervitaminosis A, fate of 55
Hyphema 15, 115
    grading of 115
Hypophoria 137
Hypopyon 15, 39, 115, 116
    corneal ulcer 39, 62
Hypovitaminosis A 104

Index

I

Ichthyosis 89
Immature senile cataract 21, 22f, 79
    management of 23
    stages of 125
Index ametropia 81
Index hypermetropia 82
Index myopia 81
Indirect ophthalmoscope 20, 172
Indocyanine green angiography 132
Infective keratitis 107
    differential diagnosis of 103
Inflamed pinguecula 3, 37
Inflammation, acute 19
Injury
    penetrating 16, 142, 143
    perforating 15
Inner neural layer 68
Inner nuclear layer 72
Inner plexiform layer 72
In-situ corneoscleral button 108
Instruments, methods of sterilization of 175
Intercalary staphyloma 48
Intermittent floppy iris syndrome 181
Internal limiting membrane 72
International Classification of Diseases 149
Intracapsular cataract extraction 177
Intracranial extension 149
Intracranial pressure, elevated 149
Intraocular lens 29, 181
    beyond pupillary margin, decentration of 6
    implantation 31
        advantages of 28
        disadvantages of 28
        types of 181
    normal 117
    parts of 30, 182
    placement 179
    power calculation 30
    secondary 28, 82
    types of 30
Intraocular muscles 145
Intraocular pressure 50, 103
Intraocular surgery 115
Intraocular tumors 93, 121
Intraoperative floppy iris syndrome 23
Intrastromal corneal ring segments 85
Intravitreal injections 74t, 132
Inverse hypopyon 15, 116
Iridectomy 16, 155, 156
    large peripheral 6
    method of 155
    peripheral 16, 182
    types of 155
Iridocorneal endothelial syndrome 16, 103

Iridocyclitis 16, 58, 113, 114, 114t
    acute 3, 5, 55, 56f, 57, 95, 96, 113, 113t
    causes of 57
    chronic 56, 56f, 113, 113t
    complications of 59
    pathology of 57
    recurrent 113
    treatment for 59
Iridodialysis 6
Iridodonesis 16
    causes of 16, 27
    mechanism of 27
Iridotomy 156
Iris 15, 22, 24, 27, 29, 31, 35, 37, 39, 43, 45, 47, 49, 50, 54, 56, 61, 64, 113, 120, 142
    adherence 43
    atrophy 16
    bombe 15, 16, 59
    cyst of 15, 156
    forceps 155, 155f
    neovascularization of 76, 149
    nerve supply of 72
    pearl 115
    pigmented tumor of 16
    pigments, congenital 18
    repositor 156, 157f
    shadow 18, 18f, 22, 22f, 25f
    structures of 71
    tumors 93
Iritis, acute 3, 16
Irregular anterior chamber, causes of 15
Irrigating vectis 159, 159f
Irrigation-aspiration cannula 159, 160f
Ishihara's charts 9f
Ishihara's test 9
Iso-ametropic amblyopia 86
Isopropyl alcohol 176
Itchy eyes 4

J

Jackson's cross cylinder 174, 174f
Jager's chart 8
Jet black pupillary reflex 17

K

Kelman multiflex 181, 181f
Keratectomy, photorefractive 85
Keratitis 3, 5, 14, 15, 36, 39, 104
    filamentary 114
    infectious 105
    infective 107
    interstitial 14, 115
    marginal 39, 103
    microbial 103

neuroparalytic 14
phlyctenular 36, 39, 103
sclerosing 114
Keratoconjunctivitis
   sicca 55, 104, 114
   vernal 37
Keratoconus 6, 15, 103, 107
Keratoglobus 15
Keratolysis 114
Keratomalacia 14, 105
Keratopathy 79
Keratoplasty 14, 107, 169
   conductive 85
   indications of 107
   overall indications of 107
   penetrating 14, 107
   photorefractive 82
   simple 107
   types of 107
Keratoprosthesis 107
Keratouveitis 115
Ketorolac 75
Krause glands 69, 70

L

Lacrimal abscess 61f
   drainage of 186
   incision of 186
Lacrimal apparatus 18, 142
   anatomy of 70
Lacrimal cannula 165
Lacrimal dissector 165, 165f
Lacrimal gland 70
   surgical removal of 104
Lacrimal osteomyelitis 62
Lacrimal probe 168, 168f
Lacrimal puncta 18
Lacrimal sac 18, 22, 24, 27, 29, 33, 35, 37, 39, 43, 45,
   47, 49, 50, 54, 56, 61, 64, 70, 98, 183
   regurgitation test of 91, 136
Lacrimation 4, 62
Lagophthalmos 89, 104, 115
Lamellar keratoplasty 35, 107
Lamellar separation, stages of 124
Laser photocoagulation 129, 132
Laser therapy, indications of 129
Laser-assisted in situ keratomileusis 14, 82, 84
Latanoprost 78
Left inferior rectus 10
Left lateral rectus 10
Left medial rectus 10
Left superior rectus 10
Lens 22, 24, 27, 29, 31, 35, 37, 39, 43, 45, 47, 49, 54, 56,
   61, 64, 142, 172
   abnormal position of 81

color of 17, 24
cortex 179
dislocation of 27
expressor 156, 156f
hook 156
nucleus 178
opacities classification system III 125
optical power of 80
posterior dislocation of 15, 27
subluxation of 6, 15, 27
types of 171
Lensectomy 177
Leprosy 14, 89, 115
Leptospirosis 121
Leucoma 14, 21, 42, 44
   adherent 14, 15, 21, 45, 45f, 46
Leukemia 92
Leukemic deposits 92
Leukocoria 93, 148
Levator palpebrae superioris 69
Lids 31, 35, 37, 45, 47, 50, 61, 65
   abscess 87
      drainage of 186
      incision of 186
   borders, rounding of 98
   coloboma of 104
   disorder 135
   hemangioma of 87
   lag 89
   margin 12
   notching 104
   plate 169f
   proper 12
   retractor 163
   sign 12
   spatula 168
   speculum 179
Light
   adaptation 80
   flashes of 6
   reactions 17
   reflex 145, 146
      pathology of 146
   sense 79
Lim's sclerocorneal forceps 157, 158f
Limbal dermoid 37, 87
Limbal groove incision 178
Limbal lesions 104
Limbal phlycten 36f
Limbal relaxing incision 84
Limbal section 178
Lipid abnormalities 104
Lissamine green staining 13, 55
Long posterior ciliary arteries 72
Loteprednol etabonate 75
Low vision 141
   aids 133, 172

Lower palpebral conjunctiva, examination of 12
Low-tension glaucoma 118
Low-vision devices 150
Lyme disease 121
Lymph node
    preauricular 50
    submandibular 52
Lymphadenopathy 95
Lymphangioma 92

M

Macula 14, 20, 44
Macular corneal opacity 43*f*
Macular edema 74, 76
    treatment for 129
Macular hole 131
Macular optical coherent tomography 23
Macular pathologies 6
Macular translocation 133
Madarosis 98, 115
Maddox rod 174, 174*f*
Magnetic resonance imaging 135
Manual small incision cataract surgery 179, 181
Marfan's syndrome 17
Marginal chalazion 52
Massive choroidal invasion 149
Mature cataract 18, 18*f*, 21, 24, 25, 25*f*, 26, 26*t*
    management of 25
McPherson's forceps 160, 160*f*
Measles
    immunization 141
    vaccination 141
Media, abnormal refractive indices of 81
Medial palpebral ligament 183
Meibomian gland 50, 69
    congenital absence of 104
    numbers of 50
Meibomianitis 66*f*, 67, 104
Meibomitis 87
Menace reflex 10, 84
Meningioma 92
Mesopic vision 79
Metastasis 149
Metastatic lesions, histology of 148
Methyl alcohol poisoning 3
Microagglutination test 121
Micropulse laser 130
Microscope 172
Microscopic appearance 70
Migraine 5, 6
Minimally invasive glaucoma surgery 117
Minus lens 172
Miosis, causes of 16
Miotics 77
    local 77
    uses of 77

Moll glands 69
Monocular visual field deficits 144
Mooren's ulcer 39, 103
Morphine intoxication 16
Mucin deficiency 104
Mucoid discharge 4
Mucopurulent 4
    conjunctivitis 5, 94
Muddy iris 16
Muller's muscle 69
Muller's retractor 166, 166*f*
Multifocal intraocular lens eyes 4
Multiple limbal phlycten 100
Multiple phlyctens 115
Musca sorbens 97
Muscae volitantes 6
Muscular layer 69
Mydriasis, causes of 16
Mydriatics 77
    local 77
    parasympatholytic 77
    sympathomimetic 77
    uses of 77
Myopathy 79
Myopia 15, 81, 84
    curvature 81
    degenerative 2, 3
    developmental 81
    pathological 81
    simple 81
Myopic eyes 81

N

Nagel's anamaloscope 10
Nanopulse laser 130
Nasal pack 183
Nasolacrimal duct 70
    obstruction, congenital 136
National Program for Control of Blindness 139
Near reflex 146
Near vision 8, 27, 135
    impairment 149
Nebula 14
Needle holder 157, 157*f*
Neodymium yttrium aluminum garnet laser
    capsulotomy 32
Neoplasms, secondary 149
Neovascularization 16
    treatment for 129
Nepafenac 76
Nerve damage 14
Netarsudil 78
Neuroblastoma 92
Neuron
    first-order 133, 146

second-order 133, 146
third-order 133, 146
Neuroparalytic hyposecretion 104
Neutral density filter test 86
Night blindness 5, 105
causes of 54
Nocturnal lagophthalmos 89
Nodal point 6
Nodular anterior scleritis 112
Nodular degeneration 98
Nodular episcleritis 37, 110
Nodule 15, 36
Non-optical devices 150
Non-proliferative diabetic retinopathy 131
Nonsteroidal anti-inflammatory drugs 59, 75
topical 100
Nuclear
fragments drop 181
sclerosis 125
Nucleus 124
delivery 179
Nyctalopia 5
Nystagmus 19

O

O'Brien technique 177
Occlusio pupillae 59
Occlusion therapy 86
Ocular adnexa, examination of 10
Ocular cicatricial pemphigoid 100
Ocular disorders, drugs used in 149
Ocular examination 2, 6, 24, 27, 29, 31, 33, 35, 37, 38, 43, 45, 47, 48, 52, 55, 64, 65, 135
Ocular injury 3, 142
types of 142
Ocular manifestations 114, 143
Ocular motility 52, 137
Ocular movement 10, 22, 24, , 29, 33, 38, 43, 47, 55, 56, 61, 65
Ocular muscle
balance 11
imbalance 138
Ocular pharmacology 74
Ocular surface
foreign body on 3, 4
squamous neoplasia 37
Ocular symptoms 2
Oculodigital stimulation 6
Oculomotor 144
nerve palsy 144
Oguchi's disease 5
Onchocerciasis 141
Opacity 14
grade of 14
shape of 43
site of 43

size of 43
types of 43
Open globe injury 142
Open-angle glaucoma 5, 122
primary 2, 118
Ophthalmia
neonatorum 4, 98
sympathetic 122
Ophthalmic lenses 171
Ophthalmic viscosurgical device 76
Ophthalmology 1
antibiotics used in 74
antifungals used in 75
antivirals used in 75
steroid in 75
Ophthalmoscope 19
Opponent color theory 80
Optic
atrophy 16, 17, 115, 133, 134, 144
disc 20, 120
pit 130
material 182
nerve 128, 142, 133, 184
diseases of 133
fiber layer 72
glioma of 92
invasion 149
neuritis 3, 115, 133, 134, 134t
bilateral 3
pathways 147f
tract 144
Optical biometry 30
Optical coherence tomography 132
angiography 132
Optical defects 27
Optical device 150
Optical iridectomy 155
Ora serrata 73
Oral administration 106
Oral antihistaminics 100
Oral valgancyclovir 75
Orbicularis oculi 69, 183
Orbit 142
contents of 74
surgical spaces of 74
Orbital apex syndrome 3, 114
Orbital cellulitis 62, 90, 92
Orbital dermoid 87
Orbital injury, penetrating 90
Orbital invasion 149
Orbital mucormycosis 92
Orbital pseudotumor 92
Orbital septum 69
Orbital tumors 92
Orthophoria 11
Outer nuclear layer 72
Outer plexiform layer 72

P

Pad and bandage 179, 184
Pain, acute 3
Palpebral aperture 12
Palpebral conjunctival layer 69
Palpebral oculogyric reflex 135
Pannus 97
Panophthalmitis 3, 92, 168
Papilledema 2, 3, 133, 134, 134*t*
Paranasal sinuses 91
Parasitic diseases 121
Parenchymatous xerosis 98
Pars plana 72
Pars plicata 72
Pegaptanib 76
Perfluorocarbon liquids injection 133
Perforation, relative advantages of 40, 46
Peribulbar block 178
Peripheral anterior synechiae 59
Peripheral retinal ischemic retinopathies 130
Peripheral space 74
Peritomy 183, 184
Phaco chopper 162, 162*f*
Phaco handpiece 162, 162*f*
Phacoemulsification 169, 179, 181
Phaco-fragmentation 179
Phakia 27
Phakic intraocular lens 85
Phenylephrine 17, 79
Phenytoin 79
Phlycten 36
    complications of 36
    recurrent 115
Phlyctenular keratoconjunctivitis 36
Phlyctenular pannus 36
Phlyctenulosis 100
Phoria 136
Photochemical reaction 79
Photocoagulation 93
Photodynamic therapy 130
Photokeratitis 3
Photophobia 5, 79
Photopic vision 79
Phthisis bulbi 21, 48-49, 49*f*, 49*t*, 50, 59
    causes of 49
    long-standing 50
    mechanism of 49
    treatment for 50
Pigmentation 98
    over anterior lens surface 18
Pilocarpine 16, 79
Pinguecula 21
Pin-hole 8, 8*f*, 135, 170, 170*f*
    principle of 8, 170
    test 84
Placido's disc 172, 175, 175*f*
Plasma sterilization 176
Plus lens 172
Pneumatic retinopexy 132
Polyarteritis nodosa 122
Polyarthritis 114
Polychondritis 122
Polycoria 6
Polyenes 75
Polyopia 6
    causes of 22
Post-cycloplegic test 173
Posterior capsular opacification 31
    treatment for 32
    types of 32
Posterior chamber 68
    intraocular lens 182, 182*f*
Posterior epibulbar dermoid 87
Posterior lamellar keratoplasty 107
Posterior polymorphous dystrophy 103
Post-laser-assisted in situ keratomileusis eyes 4
Post-surgical wound leak 16
Post-trabeculectomy cystic bleb 37
Pre-Descemet's layer 71
Prednisolone acetate 75
Prematurity, retinopathy of 6, 131, 141
Presbyopia 2, 3, 83, 84, 172
Pre-septal cellulitis 87, 90
Pressure
    bandage 183, 184
    over lacrimal sac 18
Primary eye-health care 140
Prism bar-cover test 137
Prism reflex test 137
Progressive pannus 97
Proliferative diabetic retinopathy 129, 131
Proptosis 92
    bilateral 92
    severe 89
    unilateral 92
Prostaglandin analogues 78
Protein
    water-insoluble 124
    water-soluble 124
Pseudocornea 48
Pseudoexfoliation glaucoma 121
Pseudohypopyon 15, 116
Pseudoisochromatic test 9
Pseudophakia 15, 17, 18, 21, 27-30, 30*f*, 30*t*
    over aphakia, advantage of 30
Pseudophakic bullous keratopathy 105
Pseudophakic corneal edema 107
Pseudophakic eye 27
Pseudo-pterygium 34, 34*t*, 98
Pseudorosette 148
Pseudo-strabismus 136
Psychosensory reflex 146
Pterygium 21, 33, 35, 100
    cystic changes of 37
    grade of 34, 34*t*

head of 184
operation 184
parts of 34, 35f
progressive 34f, 35
recurrent 33, 35
subconjunctival dissection of 184
surgery 35, 100
types of 33
Ptosis 88, 98, 136
congenital 88, 89
severe 86
surgery 170
overcorrection of 89
Punctate epithelial keratitis 100
Punctum dilator 164, 164f
Pupil 16, 22, 24, 27, 29, 31, 35, 37, 39, 43, 45, 47, 49, 50, 54, 56, 61, 64, 120, 142
constriction of 179
pharmacological dilation of 5
physiology of 145
Pupillary area, color of 17
Pupillary block 15
glaucoma 121
Pupillary dilation 177
Pupillary reflexes 145
Purkinje's images 18, 22, 24
Purkinje-Sanson images 81
Pus 5
Pyogenic granuloma after pterygium excision 37

Q

Quinine 79

R

Radial keratotomy 82, 84
Radiation neuropathy 149
Radiotherapy 92, 93
Ranibizumab 74, 76
Rapid assessment of avoidable blindness study 139
Rectus muscle 184
origin of 73
Red eye 3, 94, 95, 135
differential diagnosis of 95, 96t
Reflex blepharospasm 5
Refraction 80, 137
final visit for 126
Refractive errors 22, 81, 141, 145
full correction of 86
Refractive index 71
Refractive lens exchange 85
Refractive lenticule extraction 85
Refractive procedures 85
lens based 85
Refractive status, correction of 172

Refractive surgery
indications of 84
principles of 84
types of 84
Regurgitation on pressure over lacrimal sac test 136
Rehabilitation 150
Reiters syndrome 114
Retina 128, 142
central 73
layers of 72
peripheral 73
regions of 72, 73
Retinal artery, occlusion of 128
Retinal blood vessels 20
Retinal break 6, 130
Retinal detachment 3, 6, 130, 149
surgery 170
Retinal diseases 129, 130
Retinal dysplasia 6
Retinal lasers, indications for 129
Retinal necrosis 149
Retinal nerve fiber layer 135
Retinal photocoagulation 130
Retinal pigment epithelium 72, 79
Retinal prosthesis 133
Retinal tear 130
Retinal vascular occlusions 128, 130, 131
Retinal vasculitis 115
Retinal venous occlusion 128, 129
treatment for 129
Retinitis pigmentosa 2, 3, 5, 131
Retinoblastoma 6, 92, 93, 149
complications of 148
etiology of 148
genetics of 148
pathogenesis of 148
pathology of 148
presentation of 148
sequelae of 148
Retinochoroidal
neovascular diseases 130
vasculitis 122
Retino-cryopexy 132
Retinopathy 74, 79
central serous 3
venous stasis 114
Retinoscope 172, 173f
Retinoscopy, optics of 173
Retrobulbar block 178
Retrobulbar neuritis 3
Rhabdomyosarcoma 92
Rheumatoid arthritis 39, 104, 114, 121
Rhodopsin cycle 79
Rho-kinase inhibitors 78
Rhomboidal tip 162
Right inferior rectus 10
Right lateral rectus 10

Right medial rectus 10
Right superior rectus 10
Ripasudil 78
Rods 79
    and cones, layer of 72
    dystrophies 5
Roenne's nasal step 118
Ropy discharge 4
Rose Bengal staining 13, 55
Rougine 165, 165f
Rubeosis iridis 16

S

Sac massage 89f
Sarcoidosis 115, 121
Scalpel handle and blades 153, 153f
Schiotz tonometer 19
Schirmer's test 55
Schlemm's canal 117
Sclera 15, 29, 35, 39, 43, 45, 49, 50, 54, 56, 64, 66, 110, 142
    deep rectangular block of 182
Scleral buckling 132
Scleral flap 182
Scleral lepromas 115
Scleral procedures 85
Scleritis 3, 37, 64, 111, 111t, 112, 115
    anterior 112, 114
    posterior 112, 114
Sclerocornea 14
Sclerocorneal splitter 161
Sclerocorneal tunnel 179
Scleromalacia perforans 112, 114
Scotopic vision 79
Sculpting lens nucleus 179
Seclusio pupillae 59
Seidel's scotoma 118
Senile cortical cataract 2, 124, 125
Sensation, loss of 98
Sensitivity, contrast 80
Sensory 72
Sequalae 89
Serology testing 109
Shield ulcer 100
Short posterior ciliary arteries 72
Shrunken sclerotic hypermature cataract 27
Side-port blade 161, 161f
Siderosis bulbi 16
Sildenafil 79
Silicon oil removal 133
Simcoe cannula 160f
Sinsky's hook 160, 160f
Sinus infections 90
Sjogren's syndrome 55, 104, 114
Skin 183
    disorder 89
    dissection of 183
Sleepy eyes 98

Slightly curved incision 183
Slit-lamp
    biomicroscope 11, 11f
    examination 55
    microscope 10
Small incision
    cataract surgery 23
    lenticule extraction 82, 85
Smooth muscles 71
Snellen's distant vision chart 7, 7f, 8
Sodium hyaluronate 76
Soemmerring's ring 32
Spasmus nutans 19
Specular microscopy 23
Spherical lenses 171
Sphericity 182
Sphincter pupillae 72, 77
Squamous blepharitis 66, 66t
Squint 136, 136, 137
    hook 163
    latent 136
    measurement of angle of 137
    operation 169
    paralytic 19, 137, 138, 138t
St. Martin's forceps 157, 158f
Staphyloma 47
    anterior 21, 46, 47
    partial anterior 47f, 48
    posterior 47
    total anterior 47f, 48
Stellate-shaped scar 98
Stenopaeic slit 170, 171f
Sterile inflammations 75
Steroids 79
    topical 100
Stevens-Johnson syndrome 79, 100
Stimulus deprivation amblyopia 86
Strabismic amblyopia 86
    mechanism of 86
Strabismic anisometropia amblyopia 86
Strabismus 136, 138, 144
    classification of 136, 136
    congenital 86
    hook 163, 163f
Straight artery forceps 183
Stratified epithelium 71
Streak retinoscopy 174
Stroma 71
Sturge-Weber syndrome 87
Stye 51t, 52, 52f, 53
Subconjunctival haemorrhage
    causes of 37
    fate of 38
Subconjunctival injection 179
Subepithelial layer 70
Subepithelial surface procedures 85
Subperiosteal space 74
Sub-retinal neovascular membranes 3

Substantia propria 71
Subtarsal sulcus 101
Sub-Tenon's block 178
Sub-Tenon's injections, posterior 132
Sulphonamides 79
Superficial anterior lamellar keratoplasty 107
Superficial scleral flap 182
Superficial vascularization 14, 44, 44*t*
Superior oblique, origin of 73
Superior rectus
    holding forceps 157, 158*f*
    stitch 178, 179
Surgery 82, 91
    indications of 184
    steps of 186
    timing of 23, 25
Surgical correction 86, 138
Suture tying forceps 158, 158*f*
Swelling 19
Swinging flash light test 17, 134
Symblepharon 21, 98, 100
    anterior 101
    posterior 101
    total 101
Sympathetic miotics 77
Synaptophore 172
Synechiae 16
    anterior 16, 46
    posterior 16, 59
    total posterior 59
Synechiotomy 46
Synichiolysis 46
Syphilis 115, 121
Systemic lupus erythematosus 122

T

Tafluprost 78
Tarsal conjunctiva 4
Tarsorrhaphy 89
    advanced permanent 186
    indications of 107, 185
    methods of 107, 185
    permanent 185
    temporary 185, 186
Tear substitute 76
    eye drop 106
Tear-film break-up time 55, 104
Telescopic intraocular lens implantation 133
Tenon's capsule 184
Tenon's space 74
Tension 120, 142
    glaucoma, normal 118
Thermal burn 3
Thermocautery 154, 154*f*
Thrombophlebitis 90
Thyroid
    exophthalmos 89
    eye diseases 89
    ophthalmopathy 92
Timolol 79
    maleate 117
Tissue
    processing 109
    subcutaneous 69, 183
Tooth paste sign 66*f*
Toxic amblyopia 134
Toxic conjunctivitis 98
Toxic optic neuropathy 79, 134
Toxocara endophthalmitis 6
Toxocariasis 121
Toxoplasmosis 121
Trabecular edema 59
Trabeculectomy 169, 182
Trabeculitis 59
Trachoma 14, 97, 100, 104, 105, 141, 142, 149
    acute 97
    safe strategy for 99
    sequelae of 98
    WHO classifications of 98, 98*t*
Trachomatous nodular keratopathy 98
Transpupillary thermotherapy 130
Trauma 14
Travoprost 78
Triamcinolone 74
Trichiasis 4, 65, 65*f*, 98
    causes of 65
Trichiatic cilia 90
Trichromatic theory 80
Trochlear 144
    nerve palsy 145
True pterygium 34, 34*t*
Tubercular dacryoadenitis 115
Tubercular scleral abscess 115
Tuberculosis 115, 121
Tumor 130
    invasion 149
    malignant 168
    pituitary 143
    recurrence of 149
Tylosis 98

U

Ulcer 36, 103
Ulcerative keratitis, peripheral 114
Ultrasound B scan 132
Ultraviolet irradiation 34
Ultra-wide field fundus photography 132
Uncorrected vision 24
Uniocular diplopia, causes of 6
Universal eye speculum 151, 151*f*, 184
Upper eyelashes 90
Upper fornix, examination of 12
Upper Muller's muscle 69
Upper palpebral conjunctiva, examination of 12

Urethritis 114
Utarata forceps 158
Uvea
　anatomy of 71
　venous blood of 72
Uveal effusion syndrome 112
Uveitis 114, 121
　anterior 21, 56, 114, 115, 122
　chronic 74, 113
　classification of 57
　glaucoma-hyphema syndrome 115
　granulomatous 57, 58, 58t, 113, 115
　infectious 121
　nomenclature, standardization of 113
　non-granulomatous 57, 58, 58t, 113
　non-infectious 121
　posterior 6, 115
　types of 57
Uveoscleral outflow 116
Uyemura's fundus 106

V

Valacyclovir 75
Valsalva maneuver 38
Van Lint technique 177
Vancomycin 74
Vannas' scissors 160, 160f
Vascularization 14, 43
Vectis 159
Velvety papillary hypertrophy 97
Viral diseases 121
Viral retinal necrosis 74
Vision 22, 24, 29, 31, 38, 43, 45, 47, 48, 52, 53, 61, 65, 120
　2020: right to sight 139, 141
　dimness of 35
　distortion of 6
　field of 147
　loss 134, 149
　　permanent 79
　painless progressive loss of 2, 22
　physiology of 79, 145
　sudden loss of 3
Visual acuity 7, 33, 35, 37, 55, 56, 95, 147
　assessment 84
　normal 6
　testing 6, 137
Visual axes 4, 11
Visual cortex 86
Visual cortical circuits 86
Visual evoked potential 79, 135, 147
Visual field
　loss 134
　testing 10
Visual impairment 139
　causes of 139
Visual loss 149

Visual pathway 143, 146
　diseases of 133, 134
Visual problems 35
Visual rehabilitation 117
Vitamin A 106
　deficiency 5, 105
　　causes of 54
　prophylaxis 106
　supplementation 141
Vitrectomy 132, 177
Vitreoretinal surgeries 132
Vitreous detachment, posterior 3, 6
Vogt-Koyanagi-Harada syndrome 122
Voluntary eye donation 107
Voriconazole 74
Vortex keratopathy 79
Vossius' ring 18, 142

W

Watery discharge 4
Wavelength feature 182
Wegener's granulomatosis 122
Wet age-related macular degeneration 76
White pupillary reflex 6, 17
Wire speculum 151f
Wire vectis 159, 159f
Wolfring glands 69, 70
Worst-Singh's iris claw lens 181
Worth's four-dot test 137
Wound
　burn 181
　closure of 179
　healing, delayed 75
　leak after intraocular surgery 15

X

Xerophthalmia 105t, 106
　classification of 105
　treatment for 106
Xerophthalmic fundus 105, 106
Xerophthalmic scar 105
Xerosis 54
　types of 54

Y

YAG laser peripheral iridotomy 115, 156

Z

Zeigler's knife 32
Zeis, glands 69
Zinn annular tendon 73
Zonular attachments 124
Zonules 124